AIDS Vaccine Research

AIDS Vaccine Research

edited by

Flossie Wong-Staal
University of California, San Diego
La Jolla, California

Robert C. Gallo
Institute of Human Virology
Baltimore, Maryland

MARCEL DEKKER, INC. NEW YORK • BASEL

ISBN: 0-8247-0645-5

This book is printed on acid-free paper.

Headquarters
Marcel Dekker, Inc.
270 Madison Avenue, New York, NY 10016
tel: 212-696-9000; fax: 212-685-4540

Eastern Hemisphere Distribution
Marcel Dekker AG
Hutgasse 4, Postfach 812, CH-4001 Basel, Switzerland
tel: 41-61-261-8482; fax: 41-61-261-8896

World Wide Web
http://www.dekker.com

The publisher offers discounts on this book when ordered in bulk quantities. For more information, write to Special Sales/Professional Marketing at the headquarters address above.

Current printing (last digit):
10 9 8 7 6 5 4 3 2 1

PRINTED IN THE UNITED STATES OF AMERICA

Preface

There is perhaps no greater need in medical science at the inception of the 21st century than the development of a preventive vaccine against HIV (see Chapter 1, by Gary Nabel). It seems paradoxical that a human pathogen that medical science knows more about than virtually any other causative agent remains without a solution (Chapter 2, by Oren Cohen and Anthony Fauci, provides insight into this statement). Yet, we can draw from many analogies. We may understand everything about a mountain but not be able to reach its summit until there is a new technological advance. Is that the current situation with AIDS? Do we have the essential information and multiple tempting pathways but no sure compass to reach the top? Or is a major piece of information missing? There is no way for us to give an honest answer. It is possible that a partially—or even completely—successful preventive vaccine against HIV will be developed within the next five years, but it is also possible that this will never be achieved. However, reality is likely to lie somewhere between these two extreme predictions. Our best estimate is that we will have a partially effective vaccine before this decade ends.

There has been some debate about what a vaccine must accomplish. Some have argued that a vaccine must be able to completely prevent HIV infection (''sterilizing immunity''). Others, however, have argued that we can strive for a more limited and realistic goal: a vaccine that prevents disease but not infection. Indeed, this is the view of several of the authors of this book. Since sterilizing immunity seems out of reach, infection without disease would appear to be an acceptable alternative. However, this concession may be premature. We do not think there has been sufficient time or enough studies to justify giving up on the greater challenge of full prevention. Furthermore, one can never be sure that any infection will not ultimately lead to disease, and it would require decades of follow-up to obtain that information. Meanwhile, the premature belief that a vaccine has been effective may lead to increased risky behavior, and consequently greater incidence of infection. Of course, the opposite is also true: a vaccine that is not completely protective but reduces the amount of virus should help reduce transmissibility and ameliorate disease progression. The problem is in knowing which of the two scenarios will prevail.

What, then, are the major obstacles to the development of a preventive vaccine? They include at least the following:

1. The fact that HIV is a retrovirus, which upon infection rapidly integrates its DNA form into the host cell's chromosomal DNA, leading to persistent infection for the life of that cell and all its progeny. Thus, controlling the infection requires not only prevention of further virus spread but also destruction of the infected cells.
2. The lack of a small, readily available animal model. The only useful animal models currently involve primates infected with a simian virus (SIV) or chimeric virus (SHIV), rather than HIV-1. These primate model systems are not readily accessible to all investigators, and the results take a long time to generate.
3. The genetic variability of HIV means that an effective vaccine must be broadly active to prevent the emergence of resistant viruses (see Chapter 3, by Vladimir Lukashov, Jaap Goudsmit, and William Paxton).
4. The virus can destroy the immune system and render it ineffective.
5. HIV can co-opt the very same immune activation pathways required for successful vaccination for its own replication once infection is established.
6. There is a dearth of large companies dedicated to this pursuit, owing to the difficulty of the problem, the need for a prolonged research programs, and potential financial risk.

If we were able to achieve an early vigorous immune response that leads to virtual sterilizing immunity, obstacles 1, 4, and 5 would be irrelevant. Similarly, viral resistance would not be an issue, especially if appropriate epitope enhancement is possible (see Chapter 6, by Jay Berzofsky, Jeffrey Ahlers, and Igor Belyakov). Therefore, the only significant scientific problem left is the availability of a good animal model. We do not subscribe to the argument that because SIV is not HIV the monkey model is irrelevant. Rather, SIV—and better yet, SHIV—infection of rhesus macaques seems to be quite applicable (Chapter 11, by David Pauza and Marianne Wallace). Indeed, greater availability of this model system to scientists could be the single most important factor facilitating vaccine development. If applications of successful basic science at academic centers would not be hampered by logistical difficulties such as the need for scale-up in vaccine production, FDA approval, available target populations, and funding for population trials, then interest from the pharmaceutical industry would certainly follow. Some of these latter issues are being tackled by the International AIDS Vaccine Initiative (IAVI) (see Chapter 12, by Seth Berkley). There is no doubt that IAVI will make a great impact on HIV vaccine research and development, complementing other strategic programs at the academic centers and the National Institutes of Health.

We come to the real crux of the issue: how to develop a sufficiently early and vigorous response to HIV infection to achieve marked, if not complete, HIV suppression. This concept is the focus of most HIV vaccine research today. Mucosal immunity mediated by cytotoxic T cells is considered a key component of an effective vaccine and is generally achieved by using DNA vaccines encoding several HIV proteins. This may be done by direct inoculation of naked DNA or by using other recombinant viruses or vectors (Chapter 7, by Harriet Robinson). Alternatively, ''crippled'' forms of HIV itself may be used when pseudotyped with genes encoding envelope-like proteins from other viruses (Chapter 8, by June Kan-Mitchell and Flossie Wong-Staal). The current (and readily mutable) strategy at the Institute of Human Virology (IHV) is the combination of: 1) a carrier of HIV genes that facilitates mucosal immunity against HIV using modified *Salmonella* or *Shigella* (Chapter 9, by George Lewis, Tarek Shata, and David Hone); 2) tat toxoid, i.e., a modified, biologically inactive Tat delivered as a protein or as a gene in a bacterial carrier—tat is an important extracellular toxin that facilitates HIV spread and suppresses the immune response to HIV (Chapter 11, by David Pauza and Marianne Wallace); and 3) a gp120-CD4 chimeric protein for eliciting high serum levels of broadly neutralizing antibodies as evidenced by studies by Anthony DeVico of the Institute of Human Virology in primate, rodent, and ungulate studies.

What we are missing is a sure way to produce an almost immediate anti-HIV response. One way to achieve this would be to markedly enhance production of the anti-HIV β-chemokines because they are made within a few hours of lymphocyte activation until neutralizing antibodies (weeks) and killer T cells (days) are available to finish the task. Alternatively, we may learn how to make a vaccine that maintains a sufficiently high level of potent antibodies and CTLs so that exposure to HIV at any time will not lead to infection. We do not yet know how to achieve either of these goals. Regarding innate immunity, however, work by Thomas Lehner and his colleagues (Chapter 10) has led to the revelation that certain heat-shock proteins stimulate β-chemokine production, and that this correlates with protection in the SIV/monkey model. Although this is not practical for an HIV preventive vaccine, it is an interesting beginning.

No preface to a book on HIV vaccine development is complete without mentioning the remarkable progress made over the last five years or so in our understanding and appreciation of the cellular immune response to HIV and its important role in any HIV vaccine. This book includes two chapters by leaders in the field (Chapter 4, by Tomáš Hanke and Andrew McMichael, and Chapter 5, by Guislaine Carcelain, Lucile Mollet, and Brigitte Autran).

None of us can predict when a truly successful HIV preventive vaccine will be developed. What we can predict is that this book is a timely telling of where the field stands and should provide the reader with a clear perspective on the challenges to the biomedical research community.

Flossie Wong-Staal
Robert C. Gallo

Contents

Contributors

Jeffrey D. Ahlers, Ph.D. Staff Scientist, Molecular Immunogenetics and Vaccine Research Section, Metabolism Branch, National Cancer Institute, National Institutes of Health, Bethesda, Maryland

Brigitte Autran, M.D., Ph.D. Laboratoire d'Immunologie Cellulaire et Tissulaire, CNRS UMR 7627, Hôpital Pitié-Salpétrière, Paris, France

Igor M. Belyakov, M.D., Ph.D. Molecular Immunogenetics and Vaccine Research Section, Metabolism Branch, National Cancer Institute, National Institutes of Health, Bethesda, Maryland

Seth Berkley, M.D. President and Chief Executive Officer, The International AIDS Vaccine Initiative, New York, New York

Jay A. Berzofsky, M.D., Ph.D. Chief, Molecular Immunogenetics and Vaccine Research Section, Metabolism Branch, National Cancer Institute, National Institutes of Health, Bethesda, Maryland

Guislaine Carcelain, M.D., Ph.D. Laboratoire d'Immunologie Cellulaire et Tissulaire, CNRS UMR 7627, Hôpital Pitié-Salpétrière, Paris, France

Oren J. Cohen, M.D. Assistant Director for Medical Affairs, National Institute of Allergy and Infectious Diseases, National Institutes of Health, Bethesda, Maryland

Anthony S. Fauci, M.D. Director, National Institute of Allergy and Infectious Diseases, National Institutes of Health, Bethesda, Maryland

Jaap Goudsmit, M.D., Ph.D. Department of Human Retrovirology, Academic Medical Center, University of Amsterdam, Amsterdam, The Netherlands

Tomáš Hanke, Ph.D. MRC Human Immunology Unit, The Weatherall Institute of Molecular Medicine, The John Radcliffe, Oxford, England

David M. Hone, Ph.D. Associate Professor, Division of Vaccine Research, Institute of Human Virology, University of Maryland Biotechnology Institute, Baltimore, Maryland

June Kan-Mitchell, Ph.D. Karmanos Cancer Institute, Departments of Pathology, Immunology, and Microbiology, Wayne State University School of Medicine, Detroit, Michigan

Thomas Lehner, M.D., F.R.C.Path. Professor of Basic and Applied Immunology, Peter Gorer Department of Immunobiology, Guy's, King's & St Thomas' School of Medicine, London, England

George K. Lewis, Ph.D. Professor and Director, Division of Vaccine Research, Institute of Human Virology, University of Maryland Biotechnology Institute, Baltimore, Maryland

Vladimir V. Lukashov, M.D., Ph.D. Department of Human Retrovirology, Academic Medical Center, University of Amsterdam, Amsterdam, The Netherlands

Andrew J. McMichael, M.B., Ph.D. MRC Human Immunology Unit, The Weatherall Institute of Molecular Medicine, The John Radcliffe, Oxford, England

Lucile Mollet, Ph.D. Laboratoire d'Immunologie Cellulaire et Tissulaire, CNRS UMR 7627, Hôpital Pitié-Salpétrière, Paris, France

Gary J. Nabel, M.D., Ph.D. Director, Vaccine Research Center, National Institute of Allergy and Infectious Diseases, National Institutes of Health, Bethesda, Maryland

C. David Pauza, Ph.D. Professor, Institute of Human Virology, University of Maryland Biotechnology Institute, Baltimore, Maryland

William A. Paxton, Ph.D. Department of Human Retrovirology, Academic Medical Center, University of Amsterdam, Amsterdam, The Netherlands

Harriet L. Robinson, Ph.D. Asa Griggs Candler Professor, Emory Vaccine Center and Yerkes Primate Research Center, Emory University, Atlanta, Georgia

M. Tarek Shata, M.D., Ph.D. Postdoctoral Fellow, Division of Vaccine Research, Institute of Human Virology, University of Maryland Biotechnology Institute, Baltimore, Maryland

Marianne Wallace, Ph.D. Department of Medical Microbiology and Immunology, University of Wisconsin, Madison, Wisconsin

Flossie Wong-Staal, Ph.D. Florence Riford Professor in AIDS Research, Departments of Biology and Medicine, and Center for AIDS Research/AIDS Research Institute, University of California, San Diego, La Jolla, California

AIDS Vaccine Research

1

AIDS Vaccines

Challenges and Opportunities

Gary J. Nabel
National Institute of Allergy and Infectious Diseases
National Institutes of Health
Bethesda, Maryland

The limitations of current antiretroviral drug therapy have underscored the need to develop effective vaccines against human immunodeficiency virus (HIV) infection in an effort to limit the spread of acquired immunodeficiency syndrome (AIDS) worldwide. Typically, naturally occurring, protective immune responses provide the paradigm for such vaccine development; however, evidence that the immune system can provide protection against HIV infection is limited. Selected individuals exposed to HIV develop an immune response against the virus and apparently clear the infection, and some long-term nonprogressors display antiviral immune responses that presumably delay disease. Animal models have also shown limited efficacy in vaccine studies. Live-attenuated virus vaccines in the simian immunodeficiency virus (SIV) model have proven successful, but safety concerns presently limit their utility. A number of problems must therefore be solved to develop a highly effective AIDS vaccine. The identification of immunogens that elicit broadly neutralizing antibodies, an understanding of the molecular and cellular basis for immune responses to HIV components, the appropriate forms of viral proteins for antigen presentation, stimulation of relevant T-cell types, and enhancement of antigen-presenting, dendritic cell function require further study. A high priority for vaccine development will be the establishment of methods for the systematic quantitation of immune responses in animals and in humans, as well as expanded evaluation of candidate vaccines for testing in clinical trials.

A number of discoveries changed lifestyles and the quality of life in the last century. For example, seminal inventions—the light bulb, automobile, airplane, computer—transformed our patterns of daily living and the landscape of the world. No less remarkable has been the extent to which emerging infectious agents have affected the human race. Several global epidemic infections marked this era; pathogens such as influenza, polio, tuberculosis, malaria, and HIV/AIDS have extracted a high toll on the world's population. In the case of HIV, it is sobering to consider the impact of a simple virus, only 10,000 base pairs in size, on human health. Its exponential spread in the 20 years since it was first recognized documents our susceptibility to infectious diseases. Its full effects on human life and suffering, as well as its social and economic consequences, are yet to be realized. The implications of HIV/AIDS infections on children exemplify the dimensions of the problem. More than 11 million children have become orphans because of HIV/AIDS (18). Despite vigorous efforts to develop antiviral drugs intended to contain the disease, their distribution has remained limited, and they do not provide a cure for AIDS. As a result, the development of an AIDS vaccine has become a leading imperative for the biomedical research community. As noted by Bill Snow of the AIDS Vaccine Advocacy Coalition, the AIDS vaccine has become the greatest scientific, humanitarian, and public health challenge of our age (1).

Nearly 20 years after the identification of HIV as the causative agent of AIDS, it is difficult to understand why an effective vaccine for this disease has not been developed. The limited success is not for lack of effort. Despite the innovation and perseverance of biomedical researchers in academia, government, and industry, an effective AIDS vaccine is not at hand, and the prospects have sometimes appeared bleak.

Vaccines have perhaps provided the most successful examples of medical interventions for human disease. The development of the smallpox vaccine stands as a model for the successful application of biomedical research in preventing the spread of devastating infectious diseases. The smallpox vaccine, developed more than 200 years ago, has served as a paradigm for development of a highly effective vaccine. In the case of smallpox, as with other successful vaccines, the guiding principles for vaccine development are based upon the observation that immunity to disease can be acquired naturally. For smallpox, Edward Jenner and others observed that some individuals became resistant to infection—specifically, milkmaids who had previously contracted cowpox. Following the lead provided by an experiment of nature, Jenner was able to recreate the conditions that conferred immunity with vaccinia virus. For nearly every successful vaccine, the existence of natural immunity has been essential to its development.

The study of the mechanisms of acquired immunity has led to the scientific basis for understanding protective immunity. The major immunological components of this protection include the development of antibodies that can bind to virus and neutralize its infectivity. From the work of Zinkernagel, Doherty, and others, the role of cytotoxic T cells in the recognition of proteins processed by antigen-presenting cells was established (20,21). This mechanism allows for the detection and elimination of virally infected cells that are synthesizing virus but have not yet produced assembled virus that might be neutralized by antibodies.

For successful vaccines, the analysis of the immune response has provided an understanding of the mechanisms of protection and the development of surrogate markers that may be useful for identifying a vaccine. In the case of AIDS, natural immunity to infection is rare. Reports from Sarah Rowland-Jones, Andrew McMichael, Francis Plummer, and their colleagues in Kenya on HIV-exposed seronegative sex workers have demonstrated a high level of immunity, though they are not completely immune to viral infection (16). Cytotoxic T lymphocytes have been detected in HIV-exposed individuals who remain healthy after exposure to HIV-contaminated fluids (14). Notwithstanding the information from these small studies, the absence of known prototypic immunity for HIV infection requires that empiric strategies be employed for the development of a successful vaccine.

Investigators in the field have exploited three strategies. These include the use of live-attenuated viruses that can generate persistent viral gene expression, which can maintain cytolytic T-cell responses and perhaps also directly interfere with virus replication. Second, the enhancement of cell-mediated immunity has been developed. Finally, efforts to develop neutralizing antibodies for long-lasting protection have been a major part of the research agenda.

Live-attenuated virus provides perhaps the most compelling example of protection against a lentiviral infection in an animal model. As demonstrated by Desrosiers and colleagues (5–7,11), a nef-deleted virus was used to infect monkeys, and subsequent challenges with either the nef-deleted virus or the pathogenic wild-type SIVmac 251 failed to yield recoverable SIV from peripheral blood mononuclear cells (PBMCs). Notwithstanding potential differences between this model and natural infection in humans, it provides our best example of protection against lentiviral infection.

Despite the promise of this model, two observations tempered enthusiasm for this approach. Several reports of patients with mutations in nef and/or the LTR have appeared who have less aggressive disease progression; however, declining CD4 counts and increases in viral load were eventually seen in these patients. Ruprecht et al. (2,3) and the Desrosiers lab (19) raised additional concerns for this vaccine strategy. Challenge with these ''attenuated SIVs'' led to significant pathogenicity and disease in both infant and adult macaques. Therefore, from a vaccine perspective, live-attenuated viruses in their present form are not suitable for human trials.

The advantages of the live-attenuated viruses are their persistent gene expression, induction of cell-mediated immunity, and other mechanisms of viral interference. The disadvantages are the unacceptably high rate of pathogenic infection, the possibility of enhanced replication during immune suppression, and consequences of persistent immune stimulation and integration that may occur as a result of ongoing viral replication.

Studies of exposed seronegative individuals in Nairobi have shown that individuals resistant to infection manifest potent cytolytic T-cell responses to the virus. The importance of cytolytic T cells in controlling viral infection has been shown convincingly recently by Letvin, Reimann and colleagues (17), and Ho and colleagues (8) in rhesus macaques chronically infected with SIV. Depletion of CD8 T cells using a monoclonal antibody resulted in a marked increase in viral load in these infected animals. From these studies, it is clear that cytolytic T cells, even when unable to prevent infection completely, contain viremia, and control the symptoms of infection.

The advantages of cytolytic T cell–based vaccines are their ability to recognize viral infected cells, to detect multiple linear epitopes and eliminate virus producer cells, possibly reducing the magnitude of the latent reservoir of infected cells. On the other hand, it is not yet known that cytotoxic T lymphocytes (CTLs) can persist for a sufficiently long period of time to provide long-lasting protection against infection. There may also be mechanisms to evade immune detection, including the inability to recognize virus in the absence of MHC or specific mechanisms that cause down-modulation of major histocompatibility complex (MHC), as Nef does in vivo.

Central to long-lasting protection against many viral infections is the ability to develop neutralizing antibodies. Although it is possible to generate antibodies against the envelope protein of HIV using a variety of methods, such antibodies have shown limited utility because they neutralized lab-adapted CXCR4-tropic strains but were minimally effective against primary, CCR-5 tropic isolates and were strain-specific (13). The inability to elicit broadly neutralizing antibodies has proven a major impediment. Despite the many desirable features of antibody-based vaccines, such as the ability to neutralize virus, prevent new infection of cells, and activate the inflammatory system, the current limitations of this approach, such as limited reactivity and restricted neutralizing activity, selection of resistant strains, and the risk of generating antibodies that may exacerbate infection, remain real. There is some hope from passive transfer studies (12) and suggestions that fusion intermediates might generate such broadly neutralizing antibodies (10), but it has not yet been possible to achieve this effect consistently.

Important to the development of an AIDS vaccine is the ability to make and analyze vaccine candidates in humans. There have been an increasing number of trials that assess vaccine efficacy. To date, more than 70 phase I studies, 5 phase II studies, and 2 phase III studies have been performed or are in progress. Recombinant virus vaccines (canarypox) followed by a protein boost have been explored in humans in phase I/II trials, though efficacy data is not yet available. The ability of DNA vaccines to safely induce immunity with strong CTL responses makes them strong candidates as a component of HIV vaccines in humans; however, these responses have not been so potent that they would be expected to be highly effective alone in clinical settings. In the absence of clear examples of natural immunity to HIV, it is important to test the efficacy of different vaccine strategies and to compare these candidates. The necessary safety studies must first be performed in conjunction with rigorous immunological analyses. Selected candidates must then be tested in relevant clinical populations. The phase III trial becomes the ultimate test of the hypothesis that a specific type of immune response elicited by a vaccine candidate can be successful in preventing infection in humans. The relatively limited number of vaccine candidates and complex nature of developing vaccines has underscored the fact that vaccine development requires multidisciplinary teams that can collaborate closely and work together.

In terms of developing effective immunogens to elicit broadly neutralizing antibody responses, the recent x-ray crystallographic studies from Sodroski, Hendrickson, et al. (9) have provided structural data on gp160/gp120 relevant to this effort. The interactions of CD4 with gp120 and the recessed nature of the CD4-binding site provide better guidance for the generation of broadly neutralizing antibodies. The molecular definition of the helical coiled-coil region from the Kim (4) and Wiley labs has defined highly conserved epitopes of the viral envelope critical to its function that are attractive targets for neutralizing antibodies.

There are unprecedented opportunities for the use of genomics and bioinformatics in both basic and clinical studies of vaccines. Genetic information is contained within individual gene products that determine alternative immune responses, for example, comparing gp160 and Nef. The same methods of immunization for these two alternative gene products induce distinct immune responses for each—predominantly CTLs for env and antibodies (abs) for Nef. The information that controls this response is determined by the primary amino acid sequences of these proteins, and it should be possible to predict such responses based on genetic sequence. By defining such relationships, vaccine technology can be advanced. There are also opportunities for the judicious use of genotyping in human trials to identify genes that determine responsiveness to antigens in given human populations. Though this must be done in a way that maintains patient confidentiality, such information may provide opportunities to make vaccines more effective on a population basis.

An important aspect of human clinical trials is the analysis of human immune responses. In this regard, progress has been made in the development of assays that allow for comparison of immune responses within and between individuals. Such evaluation will be needed to identify vaccine candidates that provide the strongest immune responses of different types and potentially the broadest protection. Although cytotoxic T-cell assays were initially used to make such assessments, it is clear that they are cumbersome, costly, and time-consuming, and such analyses cannot be readily performed in large patient populations, particularly for phase III vaccine trials. Two assays have more recently shown promise in their ability to quantify human immune responses. These include the cytokine ELISA assays, which provide broad, sensitive, and consistent assays of immune function. Another excellent analytical tool has become evident through the work of Picker, Koup, and colleagues (15). Analysis of intracellular cytokine induction by flow cytometry not only provides insight into the expression of immunologically activated genes but also into the analysis of T-cell subsets that are stimulated by different immunogens.

It will be important to anticipate the outcomes of large-scale clinical efficacy trials and to consider the implications of alternative outcomes. In some instances, sterilizing immunity, the ability to prevent infection entirely, may be observed. On the other hand, partial immunological protection may be found that might nonetheless be useful. Partial protection could manifest itself in several ways. For example, complete protection may occur in a certain percentage of vaccinees. Alternatively, reduced disease pathogenicity and/or transmission might be seen at the same frequency as in unvaccinated controls. It also remains possible that disease could be converted to latency or that the setpoint of viral load could be reduced. It will be critical to define the implications of these possible outcomes in the natural history of the disease that might be affected by vaccination. Animal models might best serve this purpose; for example, if the prevention of symptoms is not accompanied by a reduction in transmissibility, a problem may be created. Such analyses will inform decisions about the appropriateness of vaccine candidates in large patient populations. Despite the need to evaluate vaccines in humans, it is important that safety studies be rigorously conducted, and the urgency for developing the vaccine must be balanced against the need to do so carefully and to minimize adverse events.

To summarize, a number of critical hurdles remain to be addressed in HIV vaccine development, but the field has progressed significantly and is poised to make significant advances. Immunogens have been identified that induce broad and long-lasting CTL responses, whose efficacy will be tested within the next few years in human studies. Crystallographic structures have been defined that are relevant to the development of broadly neutralizing antibodies. Greater understanding of immune correlates of protection in humans and nonhuman primates has been achieved. The importance of CTL immunity has become evident and will guide vaccine development. Immune recognition of alternative clades or alternative strains has not yet been addressed, but it is evident that despite this heterogeneity, these alternative clades are available for incorporation into multivalent vaccine candidates. Human studies require expansion, including the need to prepare clinical grade vaccine and to improve methods to assess immune responses in humans. In addition to these scientific and clinical opportunities, the role of biotechnology and pharmaceutical industries in vaccine production is essential. It will be extremely difficult to develop, market, and distribute effective AIDS vaccines without their involvement. This collective effort of academia, industry and government will require time, but builds on a vaccine effort that has made substantial progress over the years. This work on AIDS vaccines has implications that extend beyond HIV/AIDS. This research will apply to other infectious diseases, including known viral pathogens, emerging viruses, parasites, and bacteria that threaten human populations. There are also important potential applications to cancer treatment and prevention, to neurological diseases, cardiovascular diseases, allergies, and autoimmunity. The AIDS vaccine effort may therefore not only curb the expanding HIV pandemic, but also set the stage for future progress in the treatment of a range of human diseases.

REFERENCES

1. Avrett S, Carroll S, Collins C, Fast P, Gold D, Snow B, Vazquez R, Wakefield S, Warne T. HIV Vaccine Handbook: Community Perspectives on Participating in Research, Advocacy, and Progress. Washington, DC: AIDS Vaccine Advocacy Coalition, 1999.
2. Baba TW, Jeong YS, Pennick D, Bronson R, Greene MF, Ruprecht RM. Pathogenicity of live, attenuated SIV after mucosal infection of neonatal macaques. Science 1995; 267:1820–1825.
3. Baba TW, Liska V, Khimani AH, Ray NB, Dailey PJ, Penninck D, Bronson R, Greene MF, McClure HM, Martin LN, Ruprecht RM. Live attenuated, multiply deleted simian immunodeficiency virus causes AIDS in infant and adult macaques. Nat Med 1999; 5:194–203.
4. Chan DC, Fass D, Berger JM, Kim PS. Core structure of gp41 from the HIV envelope glycoprotein. Cell 1997; 89:263–273.
5. Daniel MD, Kirchhoff F, Czajak SC, Sehgal PK, Desrosiers RC. Protective effects of a live attenuated SIV vaccine with a deletion in the nef gene. Science 1992; 258:1938–1941.
6. Deacon NJ, Tsykin A, Solomon A, Smith K, Ludford-Menting M, Hooker DJ, McPhee DA, Greenway AL, Ellett A, Chatfield C. Genomic structure of an attenuated quasi species of HIV-1 from a blood transfusion donor and recipients. Science 1995; 270:988–991.
7. Greenough TC, Sullivan JL, Desrosiers RC. Declining CD4 T-cell counts

in a person infected with nef-deleted HIV-1. N Engl J Med 1999; 340:236–237.

8. Jin X, Bauer DE, Tuttleton SE, Lewin S, Gettie A, Blanchard J, Irwin CE, Safrit JT, Mittler J, Weinberger L, Kostrikis LG, Zhang L, Perelson AS, Ho DD. Dramatic rise in plasma viremia after CD8+ T cell depletion in simian immunodeficiency virus-infected macaques. J Exp Med 1999; 189: 991–998.
9. Kwong PD, Wyatt R, Robinson J, Sweet RW, Sodroski J, Hendrickson WA. Structure of an HIV gp120 envelope glycoprotein in complex with the CD4 receptor and a neutralizing human antibody. Nature 1998; 393: 648–659.
10. LaCasse R, Follis K, Trahey M, Scarborough J, Littman DR, Nunberg JH. Fusion-competent vaccines: broad neutralization of primary isolates of HIV. Science 1999; 283:357–362.
11. Learmont JC, Gexzy AF, Mills J, Ashton LJ, Raynes-Greenow CH, Garsia RJ, Dyer WB, McIntyre L, Oelrichs RB, Rhodes DI, Deacon NJ, Sullivan JS. Immunologic and virologic status after 14 to 18 years of infection with an attenuated strain of HIV-1. N Engl J Med 1999; 340:1715–1722.
12. Mascola JR, Lewis MG, Stiegler G, Harris D, VanCott TC, Dayes D, Louder MK, Brown CR, Sapan CV, Frankel SS, Lu Y, Robb ML, Katinger H, Birx DL. Protection of macaques against pathogenic simian/human immunodeficiency virus 89.6PD by passive transfer of neutralizing antibodies. J Virol 1999; 73:4009–4018.
13. Mascola JR, Snyder SW, Weislow OS, Belay SM, Belshe RB, Schwartz DH, Clements ML, Dolin R, Graham BS, Gorse GJ, Keefer MC, McElrath MJ, Walker MC, Wagner KF, McNeil JG, McCutchan FE, Burke DS. Immunization with envelope subunit vaccine products elicits neutralizing antibodies against laboratory-adapted but not primary isolates of human immunodeficiency virus type 1. J Infect Dis 1996; 173:340–348.
14. Pinto LA, Sullivan J, Berzofsky JA, Clerici M, Kessler HA, Landay AL, Shearer GM. Env-specific cytotoxic T lymphocyte responses in HIV seronegative health care workers occupationally exposed to HIV-contaminated body fluids. J Clin Invest 1995; 96:867–876.
15. Pitcher CJ, Quittner C, Peterson DM, Connors M, Koup RA, Maino VC, Picker LJ. HIV-1-specific CD4+ T cells are detectable in most individuals with active HIV-1 infection, but decline with prolonged viral suppression. Nat Med 1999; 5:518–525.
16. Rowland-Jones SL, Dong T, Fowke KR, Kimani J, Krausa P, Newell H, Blanchard T, Ariyoshi K, Oyugi J, Ngugi E, Bwayo J, MacDonald KS, McMichael AM, Plummer FA. Cytotoxic T cell response to multiple conserved HIV epitopes in HIV-resistant prostitutes in Nairobi. J Clin Invest 1998; 102:1758–1765.

17. Schmitz JE, Kuroda MJ, Santra S, Sasseville VG, Simon MA, Lifton MA, Racz P, Tenner-Racz K, Dalesandro M, Scallon BJ, Ghrayeb J, Forman MA, Montefiori DC, Rieber EP, Letvin NL, Reimann K. Control of viremia in simian immunodeficiency virus. Science 1999; 283:857–860.
18. UNAIDS. AIDS epidemic update: December 1999. Geneva: Joint United Nations Programme on HIV/AIDS, 1999.
19. Wyand MS, Manson KH, Montefiori D, Lifson JD, Johnson RP, Desrosiers R. Protection by live, attenuated simian immunodeficiency virus against heterologous challenge. J Virol 1999; 73:8356–8363.
20. Zinkernagel R, Doherty P. Major transplantation antigens, viruses, and specificity of surveillance T cells. Contemp Topics Immunobiol 1977; 7: 179–220.
21. Zinkernagel R, Doherty P. MHC-restricted cytotoxic T cells: studies on the biological role of polymorphic major transplantation antigens determining T-cell restriction-specificity, function, and responsiveness. Adv Immunol 1979; 27:51–177.

2

Immunopathogenesis of HIV Infection

Oren J. Cohen and Anthony S. Fauci
National Institute of Allergy and Infectious Diseases
National Institutes of Health
Bethesda, Maryland

INTRODUCTION

The human immunodeficiency virus (HIV) has a unique capacity to infect cells of the human immune system, leading eventually to frank immunodeficiency. The virus has usurped a variety of molecules of the immune system, such as CD4 and chemokine receptors, to gain entry into cells. HIV can utilize the millieu of an activated immune system to its own replicative advantage; thus, activation and mobilization of the immune response, which are intended to thwart the virus, instead fuel its replication and spread.

Understanding the pathogenesis of HIV infection is an important guide to the development of preventive and therapeutic strategies. In this regard, therapeutic strategies targeted to the viral entry and fusion process and to the viral enzymes reverse transcriptase, protease, and integrase have been developed and informed by HIV pathogenesis research. Development of a safe and effective vaccine against HIV is hampered by the lack of clear correlates of protective immunity; further delineation of the intimate interactions between the virus and the immune system will be critical in this effort.

IMMUNE SYSTEM MOLECULES NECESSARY FOR HIV ENTRY

HIV enters cells through interactions with the CD4 molecule and one of a number of seven-transmembrane G-protein–coupled chemokine coreceptors. CD4 was identified as the major receptor for HIV fusion and entry in 1984 (1–3). Although transfection of CD4 into CD4-negative human cells renders them infectable with HIV (4), murine cells remain resistant to HIV infection despite expression of human CD4. This result suggested that other factor(s) were necessary for HIV fusion and entry (5,6), although the identity of these additional factors remained elusive for several years.

In late 1995 and early 1996, several lines of investigation into diverse areas of HIV pathogenesis converged, revealing the identity of several cofactors necessary for HIV entry (Fig. 1). Investigators studying HIV suppressor factors secreted by CD8+ T cells reported in 1995 that the CC-chemokines macrophage inflammatory protein (MIP)-1α, MIP-1β, and RANTES (regulated on activation, normal T cell expressed and secreted) were major components of CD8+ T-cell–derived HIV suppressor activity (7). These chemokines inhibited the infection

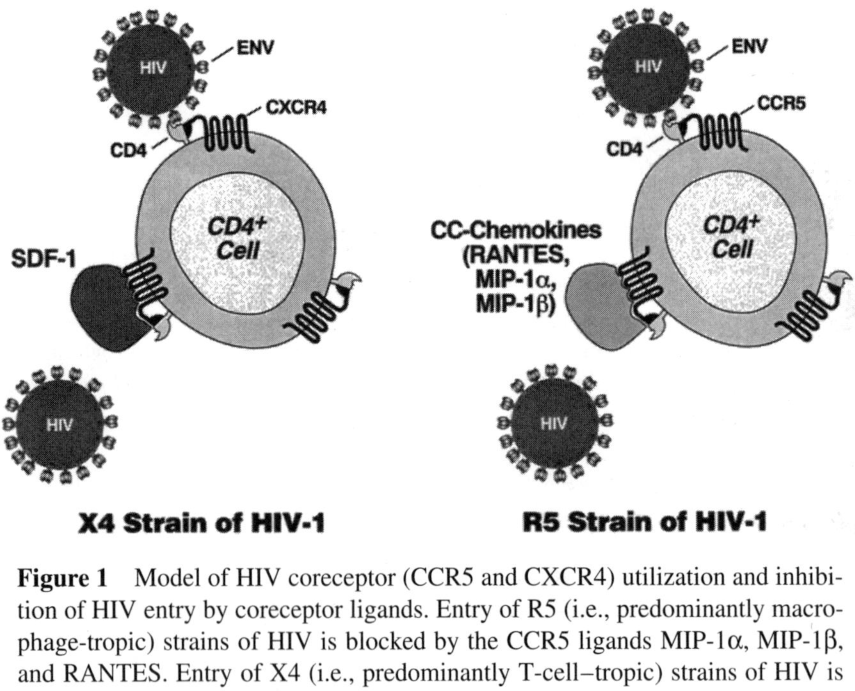

Figure 1 Model of HIV coreceptor (CCR5 and CXCR4) utilization and inhibition of HIV entry by coreceptor ligands. Entry of R5 (i.e., predominantly macrophage-tropic) strains of HIV is blocked by the CCR5 ligands MIP-1α, MIP-1β, and RANTES. Entry of X4 (i.e., predominantly T-cell–tropic) strains of HIV is blocked by the CXCR4 ligand SDF-1.

of activated CD4+ T cells by certain strains of HIV-1, HIV-2, and simian immunodeficiency virus (SIV). Of note, these CC-chemokines selectively inhibited infection of cells by different strains of HIV-1. They potently inhibited infection by viral strains that infect macrophages and peripheral blood mononuclear cells (i.e., macrophage (M)–tropic strains) but not strains that infect T-cell lines and peripheral blood mononuclear cells (i.e., T-cell (T)–tropic strains). In a somewhat unrelated line of investigation, a gene was identified that allowed HIV envelope–mediated cell fusion in the presence of CD4 (8,9). The encoded protein, called fusin (later renamed CXC chemokine receptor 4, or CXCR4), is a seven transmembrane G-protein–coupled chemokine receptor. This receptor, together with CD4, was required for cell fusion with envelopes from T-tropic strains of HIV but was not used by M-tropic envelopes. The natural ligand for CXCR4 was later determined to be stromal cell derived factor (SDF)-1 (10,11).

In a separate line of research, Paxton and coworkers were studying a population of individuals who had been exposed to HIV-infected partners but remained uninfected (i.e., ''exposed-uninfected,'' or E-U) (12). They identified two subjects whose CD4+ T cells were refractory to infection with M-tropic strains of HIV in vitro, but were easily infectable with T-tropic strains. In addition, cells from these individuals produced high levels of CC-chemokines, which had been identified as suppressors of infection with M-tropic strains of HIV. Subsequently, a new CC-chemokine receptor, CC-chemokine receptor (CCR)-5, was identified; interestingly, the natural ligands that bind to this receptor were identified as MIP-1α, MIP-1β, and RANTES (13–15). In light of the previous work showing that the CCR5 ligands inhibit cellular entry of M-tropic strains of HIV, the obvious question that arose was whether CCR5 might function as a co-receptor for such strains. A series of five papers simultaneously showed this to be the case (16–20). Other chemokine receptors, including CCR1, CCR2b, and CCR3, were also identified in these reports as potential coreceptors for certain HIV strains. Recently, other chemokine receptors have been shown to be potential HIV coreceptors (21–26); however, CCR5 and CXCR4 appear to be the most physiologically relevant coreceptors for HIV entry. Strains of HIV are now classified according to their coreceptor utilization preferences; strains that use CCR5 for entry (i.e., most M-tropic strains) are referred to as R5 strains, and those that use CXCR4 (i.e., most T-tropic strains) are referred to as X4 strains (27).

The interactions between the HIV envelope, CD4, and the relevant coreceptor molecule that is necessary for HIV entry are complex (Fig. 2). M-tropic HIV envelope molecules bind first to CD4; this interaction creates a high-affinity binding site for CCR5 as a consequence of a conformational change in the envelope (28–34). Although the chemokine ligands of CCR5 appear to interact only with the receptor's second extracellular loop, HIV envelope can interact with multiple CCR5 domains; in fact, the HIV coreceptor activity of CCR5 maps to all of the receptor's extracellular domains including the N-terminal domain and all three

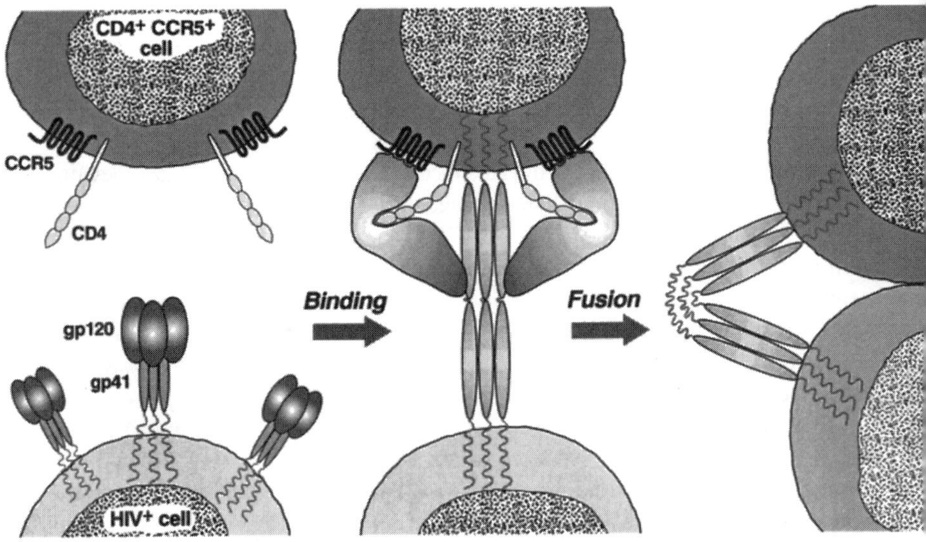

Figure 2 Binding of the HIV envelope glycoprotein gp120 to the CD4 molecule on the cell surface enables a subsequent interaction with a coreceptor molecule. A conformational change occurs in the HIV envelope, and the fusion process is initiated. Envelope epitopes that are exposed during this conformational change may be so transient that they are not recognized by the imune system.

extracellular loops (35–46). Multiple points of contact may be made between the coreceptor and HIV envelope molecules; however, clearly, the V3 loop of the HIV envelope is critical in mediating this interaction (28,29,31–33,47–50). Although signal transduction through the chemokine receptor is not necessary for coreceptor activity (36,39,47,51,52), it may have important effects on viral replication after viral entry (53–55). Many of the characteristics of the interactions between HIV envelope, CD4, and CCR5 appear to be operative in the case of CXCR4 as well. T-tropic HIV envelope molecules interact with CD4 and CXCR4 (56), with multiple domains of CXCR4 playing a role in binding (57). Of note, T-tropic HIV envelope molecules have a higher affinity for CD4 compared with M-tropic envelope molecules (58).

Transmission of HIV is almost always associated with replication of M-tropic strains of HIV in the newly infected individual (59,60). The reasons for this ''bottleneck'' in transmission are unclear, but it may be due to the expression of CCR5 and lack of expression of CXCR4 on cells that may serve as initial targets of HIV infection (i.e., Langerhans cells in genital mucosa) (61). The critical role of CCR5 in the ability of HIV to be transmitted hinted at a possible explanation for cases of individuals who were exposed to HIV but remained uninfected (see above). Indeed, two exposed, uninfected individuals were shown to be homozygous for identical 32 base-pair (bp) deletions in the *CCR5* gene (*CCR5-Δ32*), resulting in a truncated version of the receptor that is not expressed at the cell surface, and therefore does not serve as a functional coreceptor for HIV infection (62). Molecular epidemiological studies in HIV-uninfected populations have found that approximately 20% of Caucasians of northern and western European background are heterozygous for this mutation and 1% are homozygous; the frequency of the *CCR5-Δ32* allele appears to be exceedingly rare in Asian and African populations (63–66). Among HIV-infected Caucasians, no subjects homozygous for *CCR5-Δ32* were initially identified, suggesting complete protection from infection (63–66); however, rare cases of infection of homozygous individuals subsequently have been reported, likely reflecting rare transmission of T-tropic strains of HIV (67–70). Although *CCR5-Δ32* heterozygotes are not protected against HIV infection, they are afforded a modest degree of protection against disease progression and are overrepresented among cohorts of HIV-infected long-term nonprogressors (64–66,71–73). The mechanism of delayed disease progression in *CCR5-Δ32* heterozygotes may involve a lower viral load "setpoint" following acute HIV infection and a slower rate of CD4+ T-cell depletion (65). These effects may be due to a decrease in expression of CCR5 on CD4+ cells from *CCR5-Δ32* heterozygotes (74,75), allowing less efficient spread of HIV infection to new target cells (76); however, it is clear that *CCR5-Δ32* is not the sole determinant of delayed progression of HIV disease (72).

Mutations in chemokine receptor and chemokine genes other than *CCR5-Δ32* can confer protection against HIV infection or partial protection against disease progression. A rare point mutation in the *CCR5* gene (m303) results in a premature stop codon, preventing expression of a functional coreceptor; the *CCR5-Δ32/m303* genotype confers a high degree of resistance to HIV infection, similar to that afforded by homozygosity for *CCR5-Δ32* (77). Polymorphisms in the CCR5 promoter also influence rates of disease progression (78–81). A mutation in the *CCR2* gene involving a conservative amino acid change in a transmembrane domain of the receptor results in a significant delay in disease progression among HIV-infected individuals (82–84); this effect may be related to the ability of the mutant form of the CCR2 protein to form heterodimers with CXCR4 and CCR5, thus limiting the functional availability of these important HIV coreceptors (85).

A polymorphism in the RANTES promoter is associated with enhanced transcription of the RANTES gene; not surprisingly, this polymorphism is also associated with a slower rate of HIV disease progression (86). A mutation in the 3′ untranslated region of the *SDF-1* gene, *SDF1–3′A*, also plays a role in protecting against disease progression in HIV-infected individuals (87). Homozygosity for the *SDF1–3′A* allele may be associated with high levels of expression of SDF-

1, which may occupy CXCR4 and thereby inhibit replication of X4 strains of HIV. Consistent with this hypothesis, the protective effect of the *SDF-1* mutation is observed late in the course of HIV disease, when T-tropic strains may predominate. Downregulation of coreceptor expression and/or upregulation of chemokines may also recapitulate phenotypes similar to those created by the genetic polymorphisms described above (12,75,88–92).

Delineation of the role of chemokine receptors as HIV entry cofactors and of the role of the chemokine ligands of these receptors as potential inhibitors of HIV cellular entry has led to the development of new therapeutic strategies (93). Chemokine analogs that bind to HIV coreceptors and prevent entry of virus without transducing an intracellular signal represent an attractive class of compounds, since they are unlikely to elicit inappropriate inflammatory signals. Such a strategy is highlighted by molecules that bind to CCR5 and block infection of cells with R5 strains of HIV without delivering intracellular signals (94–96). Several small molecules (AMD3100, a bicyclam; T22, a peptide derivative of polyphemusin II; and ALX40–4C, a highly cationic oligopeptide) that compete with SDF-1 for binding to CXCR4 have also been developed. These compounds bind specifically to CXCR4 and inhibit cellular entry of X4 strains of HIV; they also inhibit SDF-1–mediated intracellular calcium mobilization (97–100). Finally, molecular genetic approaches have been taken to prevent cell surface expression of HIV coreceptors, thus recapitulating the *CCR5-Δ32* phenotype (101–103).

Another therapeutic strategy that inhibits HIV fusion and entry is targeted at the requisite conformational changes within the HIV envelope glycoproteins (104). After interaction with CD4, dramatic conformational changes occur in both the gp120 and gp41 envelope components. Within gp41, a central trimeric coiled coil structure is formed; this structure is essential to the process of fusion with the cell memebrane, and represents an excellent therapeutic target (105,106). In fact, a peptide, T20, which prevents the assembly of the coiled coil structure, has shown promise as a clinically useful antiretroviral agent (107).

ACUTE INFECTION

HIV is transmitted either by exposure of the oral, rectal, or vaginal mucosa during sex or breast feeding or by intravascular inoculation (i.e., through transfusion of contaminated blood products, use of contaminated equipment during injection drug use, or maternal-fetal circulation). In a macaque model of SIV sexual transmission, bone marrow–derived dendritic cells (DC) in the vaginal mucosa were the first cells to contain SIV DNA, which became detectable 2 days after vaginal exposure. In subsequent examinations of lymphoid organs, the pattern of appearance and spread of SIV mirrored the course taken by DC upon migrating from peripheral tissues to lymphoid organs (108). In addition to serving as direct targets of HIV infection, DC are also capable of retaining infectious virions on their surface for extended periods of time (109). This property is mediated by DC-SIGN (dendritic cell–specific ICAM-3 grabbing nonintegrin), a dendritic cell surface molecule that normally interacts with ICAM-3 on the surface of T cells (110). DC-SIGN also binds with high affinity to the HIV-1 gp120; however, the protein does not serve as an entry coreceptor, but rather enhances the viability of surface-bound virions (111). Thus, the role of DC in the initiation of HIV infection includes capturing virions at sites of entry, carrying HIV to the paracortical regions of lymphoid organs, and delivering virus to CD4+ T cells that become activated through their interaction with DCs (Fig. 3). In fact, active viral replication occurs in DC-CD4+ T-cell conjugates that are formed in vitro (112); similar conjugates of DC and CD4+ T-cells containing HIV antigen have been identified in vivo in tonsil biopsy specimens from individuals infected with HIV (113), in the peripheral blood in low quantities (109), and in the submucosal tissue after vaginal exposure to SIV (108).

CD4+ T cells and macrophages are key targets of HIV infection. The viral determinant of cellular tropism maps to the gp120 envelope protein of HIV-1,

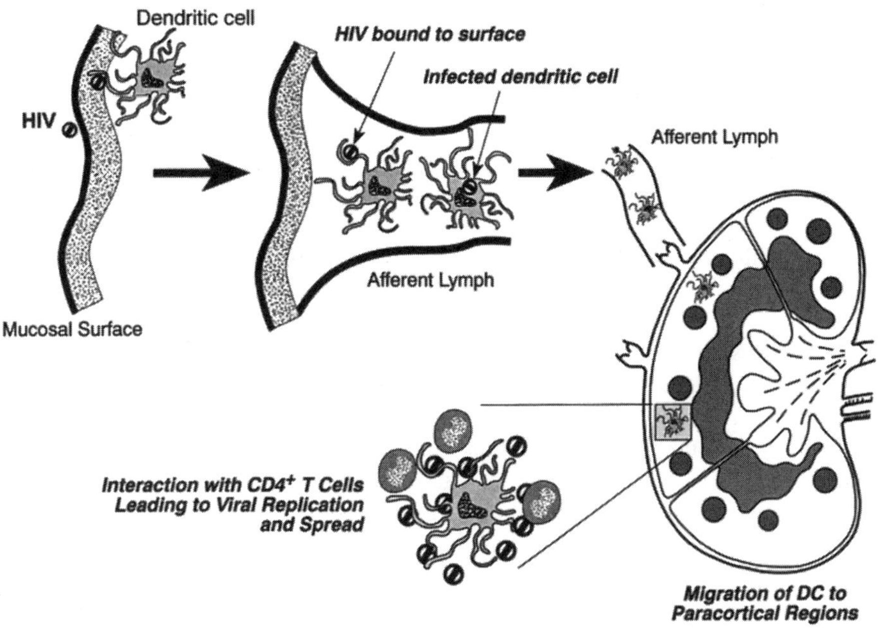

Figure 3 Role of dendritic cells (DC) in the initial stages of HIV infection. DC at the site of HIV exposure transport the virus to paracortical regions of draining lymph nodes, where CD4+ T cells become infected.

mostly to the third variable region (V3 loop) (114–117) that is also the major determinant for coreceptor usage (48). Changes in viral phenotype have been observed at different stages of HIV infection. CCR5-utilizing viruses are preferentially transmitted during primary infection and predominate at most stages of infection (59,60). In approximately 50% of HIV-infected individuals, the appearance of CXCR4-utilizing isolates late in the course of disease heralds accelerated CD4+ T-cell decline and clinical disease progression (118–121). This transition may occur by mutation of only a few amino acid residues predominantly in the envelope V3 loop (116,117,122,123). Given the high error rate of RT and the rapid kinetics of HIV replication, the surprising failure of such mutants to emerge until late in the course of the disease process indicates a change in the selective advantage of such a mutation during the course of disease progression. The nature of such a selective advantage is currently unknown; however, it may relate to the ability of X4 viruses to gain cellular entry through an expanded repertoire of coreceptor molecules.

The mechanisms responsible for the restriction of R5 viruses during primary infection is the subject of intense investigation. Freshly isolated Langerhans cells (resembling mucosal DC) express CCR5, but not CXCR4, on their surfaces (61); this finding suggests that infection of DC may be a necessary first step in acute infection and that this step is restricted by the expression pattern of HIV coreceptors on DC. However, HIV-pulsed DC from individuals lacking a functional CCR5 gene are capable of transmitting infection to CD4+ T cells in vitro (124). Thus, although infection of DC may be dependent on specific HIV coreceptor expression, the ability of DC to trap virions on their surface and infect CD4+ T cells that they encounter is at least in part a coreceptor-independent phenomenon.

In animal models of SIV infection, virus can be detected in peripheral lymph nodes within 1 week of infection (108,125,126). Most of the SIV RNA at this time is associated with individual productively infected cells in lymph nodes. This production of virus by individually infected cells in lymphoid tissue precedes and likely is responsible for the peak of viremia. Coincident with the appearance of SIV-specific immune responses, a decrease in the frequency of productively infected cells is seen during the second week after infection. By 4 weeks after infection, viremia decreases as a result of further elimination of productively infected cells by SIV-specific cell-mediated immune responses and clearance of circulating virions by the formation of immune complexes consisting of virus, antibody, and complement that are trapped within lymphoid tissue germinal centers (125,126).

Cross-sectional studies in patients evaluated soon after acute HIV infection are similar to the findings in the SIV model (Fig. 4). The kinetics of HIV viremia and HIV-specific immune responses in peripheral blood parallel those in the SIV model (127–131). Preliminary data from a limited number of lymph node biopsies obtained from acutely infected individuals suggest that the SIV model is

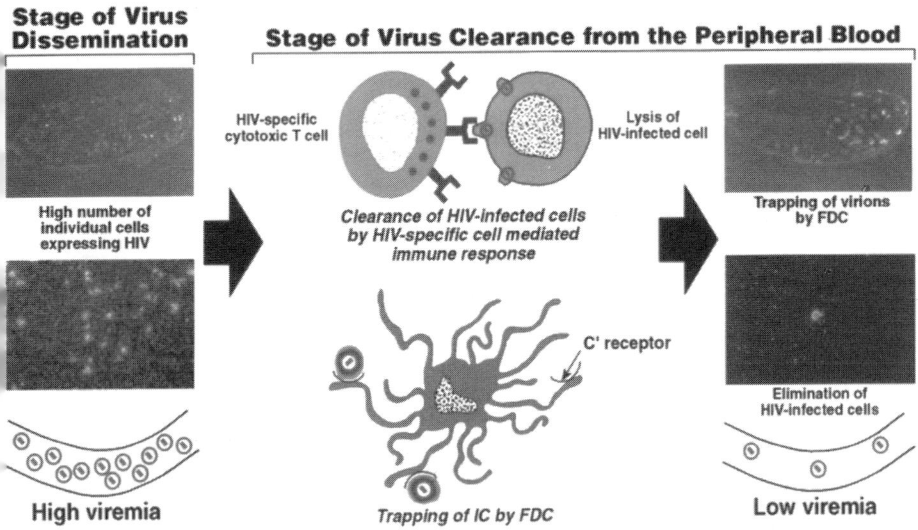

Figure 4 Cell-mediated and humoral immune mechanisms involved in the down-regulation of viremia following primary HIV infection. Prior to the emergence of HIV-specific immune responses, large numbers of individual productively infected cells are found in lymph nodes (left; low and high power photomicrographs of an in situ hybridization assay for HIV RNA in a lymph node), resulting in high levels of plasma viremia. Emergence of cytotoxic T-cell responses against HIV leads to elimination of a large number of productively infected cells (photomicrograph, lower right). In addition, HIV-specific antibodies combine with virions to form immune complexes (IC); complement (C′) binds to the immune complexes, which are then trapped in the follicular dendritic cell (FDC) network of expanding germinal centers by complement receptors (photomicrograph, upper right). (Adapted from Ref. 174.)

valid in depicting the early events associated with HIV infection in lymphoid tissue as well (132,133). In the weeks to months following acute HIV infection, a sharp decline in the frequency of productively infected cells is evident in lymphoid tissue. Germinal center formation within lymphoid follicles becomes pronounced and viral RNA corresponding to extracellular virions complexed with antibody and complement is detected in the network of follicular dendritic cell (FDC) processes (134–137). Although the immune system is capable of efficient elimination of a substantial number of productively infected cells in lymphoid tissue, the very earliest interactions between virus and host virtually ensure viral persistence. In this regard, massive numbers of virions trapped within the germinal center FDC network as well as latently infected cells, which harbor proviral DNA but do not express viral proteins (and thus elude the immune response), represent potentially continuous sources of virus for de novo infection of CD4+ T lymphocytes that are resident in or migrating through lymphoid tissue (138–142).

VIRAL DISSEMINATION

Like many other invading microorganisms, HIV is transported by antigen-presenting cells to lymphoid tissue. However, in the case of HIV, the host immune system is never able to completely control and eradicate the infection. In fact, in an impressive example of subversion of the immune system, HIV utilizes the activated milieu of lymphoid tissue toward its own replicative advantage. Close contact between immune effector cells as well as high levels of pro-inflammatory cytokines are characteristic of the lymphoid tissue microenvironment; these conditions favor viral replication in several ways. Activated CD4+ T lymphocytes migrating through lymphoid tissue serve as ideal targets for de novo infection with HIV (142–146). Activation signals such as those delivered by pro-inflammatory cytokines, found in abundance within activated lymph nodes, are potent inducers of HIV replication in latently infected cells (147–151) and also are able to increase the pool of activated cells that are susceptible to HIV infection (146,152–154). Another example of the ability of HIV to subvert the immune system for its own replicative advantage is the immune hyperactivation induced by the virus itself (155,156). Sequestration of HIV-infected cells within lymphoid tissue due to histopathological abnormalities and cytokine imbalances (157,158) may further contribute to the high levels of viral replication that occur in lymphoid tissue. Viral replication that occurs in lymphoid tissue prior to the development of a host immune response is responsible for wide dissemination of virus by lymphatic and hematogenous routes.

Viral dissemination throughout lymphoid tissue is a fundamental pathogenic event during the early phase of HIV infection. Lymphoid tissue remains the most important reservoir of infection throughout the entire course of the disease. The early chronic stage of HIV disease is characterized by heavy concentration of viral load in lymphoid tissue. In this regard, the frequency of infected cells in lymph nodes exceeds that in peripheral blood by 5- to 10-fold; differences in levels of viral replication are generally 10- to 100-fold (137,159,160). Up to 25% of CD4+ T lymphocytes present in lymph node germinal centers harbor HIV DNA, further emphasizing the role of lymphoid tissue as a critical reservoir for HIV in vivo (138). The continuous state of rapid high-level turnover of plasma viremia derives in large measure from viral replication in lymphoid tissue (161–164).

The concentration of viral load in lymphoid tissue is due in part to the normal process of follicular hyperplasia within lymphoid germinal centers following antigenic challenge (134,165–168). Expansion of the FDC network within hyperplastic lymphoid follicles is an efficient mechanism for viral trapping via interactions between antibody and complement-coated virions with complement receptors and/or adhesion molecules on the surface of FDC (136,169).

During the course of HIV disease progression, there is a shift in the lymphoid histopathological pattern from follicular hyperplasia to follicular involution (137,165–168,170–173). This shift in histopathology is associated with important changes in viral distribution. Disruption of the FDC network is characteristic during this period, leading to a decrease in the efficiency of viral trapping in germinal centers and a consequent increase in plasma viremia (137,174). Sequestration of infected cells within lymphoid tissue also becomes less efficient during follicular involution, leading to an increase in the frequency of infected cells in the peripheral blood. As the CD4+ T lymphocyte count falls below 200 cells/μl, there is a tendency for viral load to increase more rapidly in the peripheral blood compartment leading to equilibration between lymph node and peripheral blood.

Destruction of lymphoid tissue certainly is a major mechanism responsible for the severe immune dysfunction and loss of the ability to inhibit viral replication observed in advanced-stage HIV disease. The ability to maintain an effective immune response to HIV is severely impaired in the absence of intact lymphoid tissue architecture. As a consequence, increased cell-associated viral RNA becomes evident in the paracortical regions of lymph nodes, reflecting increased viral replication. Thus, during progression of HIV disease there is a reversal in the predominant forms of virus in lymph nodes, with progressive diminution of the extracellular form (i.e., trapped virus) and an increase in cell-associated virus (i.e., cells expressing HIV) (137,174). In the advanced stage of disease there is almost total dissolution of lymphoid architecture. Follicular involution, fibrosis, frank lymphocyte depletion, and fatty infiltration herald complete loss of functional lymphoid tissue, contributing to the state of immunodeficiency and the dramatically enhanced susceptibility to opportunistic infections. Disruption of the lymphoid microenvironment during the course of HIV infection remains an enigmatic process with considerable implications for future therapeutic interventions. Productive infection of FDC by HIV may occur, particularly in the late stages of HIV infection (175); however, the majority of data suggest that productive infection of FDC is rare during the period of intermediate-stage disease when dissolution of the FDC network begins (169,176). Of note, some of the HIV-related pathological changes that occur in lymphoid tissue may be at least partly reversible during potent antiretroviral therapy (177,178).

IMMUNE RESPONSES

Similar to most pathogens, HIV induces a broad array of host immune responses in an infected individual (Fig. 5). A central question of pathogenesis is how HIV

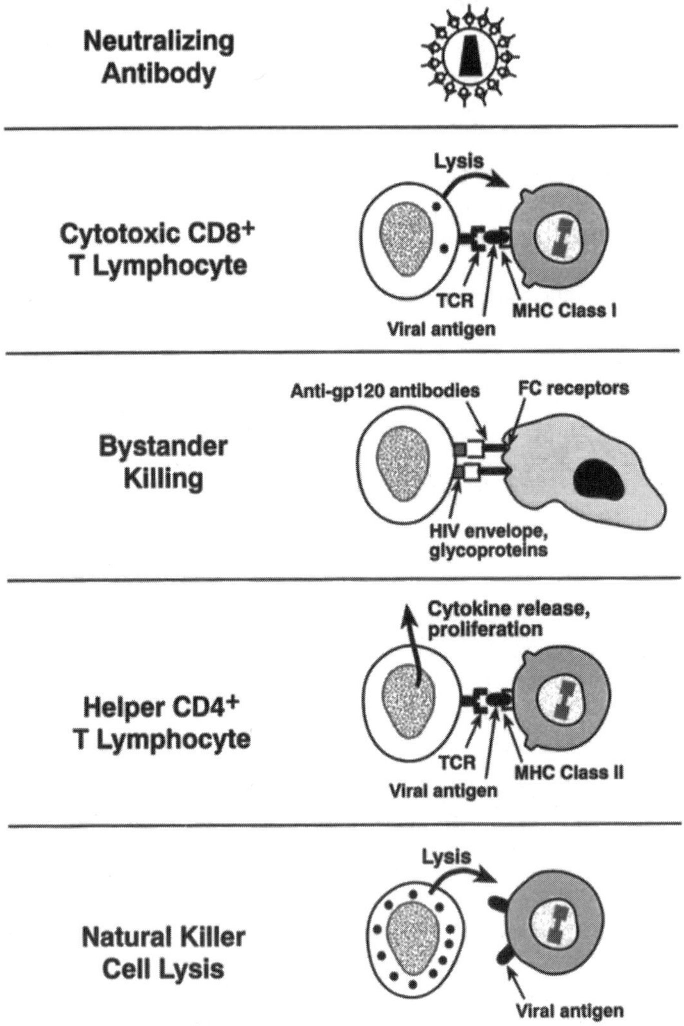

Figure 5 Immune responses against HIV. Neutralizing antibodies bind to virion components and prevent attachment to target cells. CD8+ cytotoxic T lymphocytes recognize viral antigens on the surface of infected cells in the context of MHC class I presentation and are able to directly lyse these cells. ADCC results in Fc receptor–mediated elimination of infected cells as well as uninfected cells that are coated HIV with antigen-antibody complexes. CD4+ T cells may recognize viral antigens in the context of MHC class II presentation, resulting in the release of cytokines and cellular proliferation. NK cells may also directly lyse HIV-infected cells. (Adapted from Fauci, A.S., H.C. Lane. 1998. Human immunodeficiency virus (HIV) disease: AIDS and related disorders. In: Harrison's Principles and Practice of Internal Medicine. 14th ed. New York: McGraw-Hill, p 1791.)

is able to continuously replicate and cause the inexorable decline in immune system function in the presence of these immune responses.

Humoral Immune Responses

Antibodies against the viral core protein p24 develop within weeks of acute HIV infection and may play a role in the decline of plasma viremia associated with primary infection (127,179–181). Loss of anti-p24 antibodies is associated with progression of HIV disease (127,179–183).

Antibodies that neutralize HIV infectivity may be responsible for at least partial control of viral replication in vivo (179,182). Neutralizing antibodies may be type-specific (i.e., specific for one viral isolate) or group-specific (i.e., specific for a broad range of viral isolates). Most type-specific neutralizing antibodies recognize the V3 region of the HIV envelope gp120 protein (184). Neutralizing anti-V3 loop antibodies may prevent conformational changes within gp120 necessary for HIV entry or for cell-cell fusion (185). Group-specific neutralizing antibodies recognize epitopes within the HIV envelope gp41 protein (186), discontinuous conformational epitopes around the CD4 binding site of gp120 (187), or carbohydrate determinants (188). Both type- and group-specific neutralizing antibodies are more efficient in neutralizing laboratory strains of HIV grown in T-cell lines compared to primary isolates grown in peripheral blood mononuclear cells (PBMC); this is likely due to differential exposure of the V3 loop and CD4 binding domain epitopes among these isolates (189,190). Some neutralizing antibodies interfere with the interaction between the HIV envelope and CCR5, thereby inhibiting cellular entry of R5 strains of HIV (28,29).

Neutralizing antibodies appear to be prognostically relevant to the course of HIV infection (191–193). The regularity with which viral variants that resist neutralization emerge suggests that such antibodies are potent impediments to viral replication (194). In nonhuman primate models, neutralizing antibodies are associated with slow rates of disease progression (195) and accelerate clearance of both infectious and noninfectious virions (196); furthermore, passive transfer of SHIV-neutralizing antibodies can protect macaques against a subsequent viral challenge (197–200).

Some anti-HIV antibodies bind to IgG Fc receptor-positive cells and sensitize them to mediate antibody-dependent cellular cytotoxicity (ADCC) against HIV-infected or HIV-coated cells (201,202). Most of these antibodies are directed against HIV envelope gp120 or gp41 proteins. CD16+ natural killer (NK) cells are important mediators of ADCC (203), and monocytes may also mediate this activity (204). Anti-HIV ADCC antibodies develop soon after primary infection and are detectable throughout the course of HIV disease, with some decrease in titers with the onset of AIDS (205). ADCC may also represent an immunopathogenic immune response that may be responsible for CD4+ T-cell depletion during the course of HIV infection. In this regard, a combination of high levels of plasma viremia with high HIV envelope–specific ADCC activity is correlated with rapid CD4+ T-cell depletion; this correlation may reflect ADCC-mediated "innocent bystander" killing of gp120-coated, but uninfected, CD4+ T-cells (206).

Cellular Immune Responses

Cytotoxic T Lymphocytes

Classical MHC class I–restricted, HIV-specific, CD8+ cytotoxic T lymphocyte (CTL) responses against a variety of HIV target proteins have been demonstrated in HIV-infected individuals (207,208). Using standard cell culture methods, a high frequency of HIV-specific CTLs and CTL precursors (up to 1% of peripheral blood T-cells) has been observed in asymptomatic HIV-infected patients (209,210); using HLA-peptide tetramers, the true frequency of HIV-specific CTL may be up to an order of magnitude greater than that detected by standard methods (211,212).

A critical role for CTL in the suppression of viral replication in HIV-infected individuals is suggested by the close correlation between emergence of an HIV-specific CTL response and downregulation of viremia following acute infection (130,131, 213), the association of vigorous HIV-specific CTL responses with slow progression of HIV disease (214–216), and the decline in HIV-specific CTL activity with disease progression (207,209). Quantitative studies have revealed an inverse correlation between the frequency of HIV-specific CTL and levels of plasma viral load (212,213) and between the CTL frequency and the rate of CD4+ T cell decline (213). A beneficial role for HIV-specific CTL is also suggested by their presence in the peripheral blood of individuals who are frequently exposed to HIV yet remain uninfected (217,218) and the depletion of HIV-specific CTL from lymph nodes of patients with advanced HIV disease (219). Studies in nonhuman primates have demonstrated that monkeys subjected to CD8+ T-cell depletion manifest diminished control of plasma viremia during primary SIV infection (220); in addition, CD8+ T-cell depletion during the chronic phase of SIV infection leads to a prompt and profound increase in levels of viral replication (220–222).

The quality of the HIV-specific CTL response is also an important determinant of the efficacy of these responses in controlling viral replication. The specificity of CTL responses may in part determine their salutary role; in this regard, CTL responses against viral core proteins in particular have been associated with a decreased risk of disease progression (215,223). CTL recognition of immunodominant HIV epitopes presented by certain MHC class I alleles may result in potent anti-HIV activity (224) and may in part explain the association of certain

MHC class I alleles with slower progression of HIV disease (225–230). Furthermore, the ability to recruit an HIV-specific CTL response comprised of a diverse group of T-cell receptor Vβ families that recognize multiple epitopes is associated with better control of viral replication and an improved prognosis compared with a narrow CTL response (231,232).

The loss of HIV-specific CTL activity in patients with progressive disease is likely a result of several factors. Viral proteins such as Tat, Nef, and Vpu can downregulate cellular expression of MHC class I molecules that are necessary for CTL recognition of infected cells (233–235). Increased expression of killer inhibitory receptors may also inhibit CTL activity (236). Another mechanism responsible for the loss of CTL activity is the selective accumulation of CD8+DR+ HIV-specific CTL that lack the interleukin (IL)–2 receptor and are defective in clonogenic potential (237). Finally, the ability of HIV to escape CTL responses by viral mutation or by exhaustion of CTL clones due to high concentration of antigen helps explain the loss of CTL-mediated control over viral replication (238,239).

The host CTL response against HIV is constrained by the ability of the MHC class I alleles to bind to various viral epitopes, while the virus is constrained by the degree to which an escape mutation impairs viral fitness (240–245). These host-virus dynamics are extraordinarily complex given the large number of permutations of viral epitopes and MHC class I alleles. Viral mutations within CTL recognition cpitopes (i.e., ''escape mutants'') are associated with increased levels of viral replication and progression of HIV disease (246–249); similar observations have been made in a well-controlled SIV model (250). Viral escape mutants may thrive due to the release of CTL control over their replication and also may inhibit CTL responses against the preescape viral epitope (251–253). A mathematical model of CTL-virus dynamics was provided by Nowak and coworkers, who described disease progression as a result of viral sequence variation that escapes an immunodominant CTL response and shifts the host response towards a weaker epitope (254). In this scenario, disease progression may be the result of fitness of viral escape mutants outpacing the plasticity of the host CTL response, with slow progression resulting from CTL plasticity overpowering viral escape mutants with limited fitness.

A further mechanism for loss of CTL control over viral replication may be clonal exhaustion. This appears to be a strategy for viral persistence employed by other viruses, such as certain strains of lymphocytic choriomeningitis virus that rapidly and completely mobilize the host CTL response resulting in CTL exhaustion (i.e., high zone tolerance) (255). CTL exhaustion may also occur to some degree in HIV infection: the disappearance of some CTL clonotypes can be demonstrated in the absence of viral escape mutations that might otherwise explain the phenomenon (238,239).

CD8+ T-Cell–Derived Soluble Suppressor Factors

A variety of soluble antiviral factors are elaborated by CD8+ T-cells. CD8 antiviral factor (CAF) (256–258) is noncytolytic, inhibits viral replication at the level of HIV LTR transcription (259–261), and lacks identity to known cytokines (262). Although CAF activity is non–MHC restricted, its activity is maximal in a syngeneic system (263). CAF activity decreases with disease progression, but remains potent in long term nonprogressors (89,264–266).

The combination of RANTES, MIP-1α, and MIP-1β (the natural ligands for CCR5) are also important soluble antiviral factors and are secreted by CD8+ T cells as well as other cell types (7,267). These CC-chemokines inhibit viral replication primarily at the level of cell entry. Emerging data support a role for CC-chemokines in protecting against HIV infection and disease progression (88,90–92); interestingly, the source of these chemokines does not appear to be exclusively CD8+ T cells (7,268,269) and likely includes CD4+ T cells (88,92,267) and NK cells (270). Macrophage-derived chemokine (MDC) can potently suppress replication of R5 as well as X4 strains of HIV in vitro (271); the role of MDC in controlling HIV replication in vivo is uncertain. Finally, IL-16 has been reported to be a soluble antiviral factor (272). IL-16 inhibits HIV transcription and can potently suppress HIV replication when it is expressed in HIV-infected T-cells (273,274); furthermore, IL-16 production has been correlated with protection against disease progression in HIV-infected individuals (89,275).

CD4+ T-Cell Responses

HIV proteins contain helper T-cell epitopes that may be presented by MHC class II alleles (276,277). Recognition of these epitopes by CD4+ T-cells results in secretion of cytokines and cellular proliferation. These responses may be associated with abortive infection in individuals who are exposed to HIV but who remain uninfected (278), and they decrease with HIV disease progression (276,277). An inverse correlation has been found between the magnitude of HIV-specific CD4+ T-cell response and levels of plasma viremia (279); these data are consistent with the observed inverse correlation between CTL activity and plasma viremia as well (212). The fate of HIV-specific CD4+ T cells during the course of HIV infection is controversial. Some evidence suggests that these cells are usually depleted in the early stages of disease and that initiation of potent antiretroviral therapy during acute HIV infection may prevent this loss and lead to more effective immunological control of viral replication (279). Other data suggest that HIV-specific CD4+ T cells are present throughout the course of HIV disease and that their frequency actually declines during HAART-induced viral suppression (280).

CYTOKINES AND HIV DISEASE: DYSREGULATION OF CYTOKINE PRODUCTION

Cytokines that are generated during the host immune response to an infection play an important role in determining the outcome of the infectious process. Dysregulation of the host cytokine network is characteristic of all phases of HIV infection. Many of the observed alterations in cytokine production contribute to HIV pathogenesis by further stimulating viral replication, suppressing the ability of the immune system to mount an efficient antiviral response, and inducing cytokine-mediated cytopathic effects (281–283).

HIV infection is associated with increased expression of proinflammatory cytokines; high levels of TNF-α, IL-1β, and IL-6 are secreted by PBMC and macrophages from HIV-infected subjects and are found at elevated levels in serum, cerebrospinal fluid, and tissues (reviewed in Refs. 283,284). High levels of expression of these cytokines, as well as interferon (IFN)–γ (285–287) and IL-10 (287), are particularly evident in lymphoid tissue, a major site of HIV replication throughout the course of disease (134,137,138,159). Chronically activated CD8+ T cells (288) and macrophages (289,290) are thought to be major contributors to the elevated cytokine levels observed in HIV-infected subjects.

Another major disruption in the cytokine pattern observed in HIV disease is a progressive loss in the ability to produce immunoregulatory cytokines such as IL-2 and IL-12 (291–293). IL-2 and IL-12 are critical for effective cell-mediated immune responses, as they stimulate proliferation and lytic activity of CTL and NK cells. In addition, IL-12 is essential for stimulating the production of T helper (TH)–1 type cytokines, including IL-2 and IFN-γ, which favor the development of cell-mediated immune responses (294,295). The TH1 limb of cellular immune responses is impaired during the course of HIV infection; this is especially true with regard to defects in IL-2 production and IL-2 receptor expression (293,296–301). Although the cause of this TH1 defect in HIV infection is multifactorial, it may derive in part from the ability of the HIV envelope to induce IL-10 production in monocytes, and thereby inhibit IL-2 secretion (302). Some investigators have proposed that a dominance of TH2-like responses (i.e., secretion of IL-4, IL-5, and IL-10) characterizes progression of HIV disease (293,296,297,303, 304). Most studies, however, suggest that cytokine dysregulation during the course of HIV infection is complex and cannot easily be classified in terms of TH1 and TH2 polarity (287,298,299,305).

Effects of Cytokines on HIV Replication

Soluble factors produced by activated PBMC (147), macrophages (306), and B cells (307) can dramatically upregulate HIV expression in acutely and chronically infected cells of the lymphocytic and macrophage lineage (Fig. 6). Cytokines

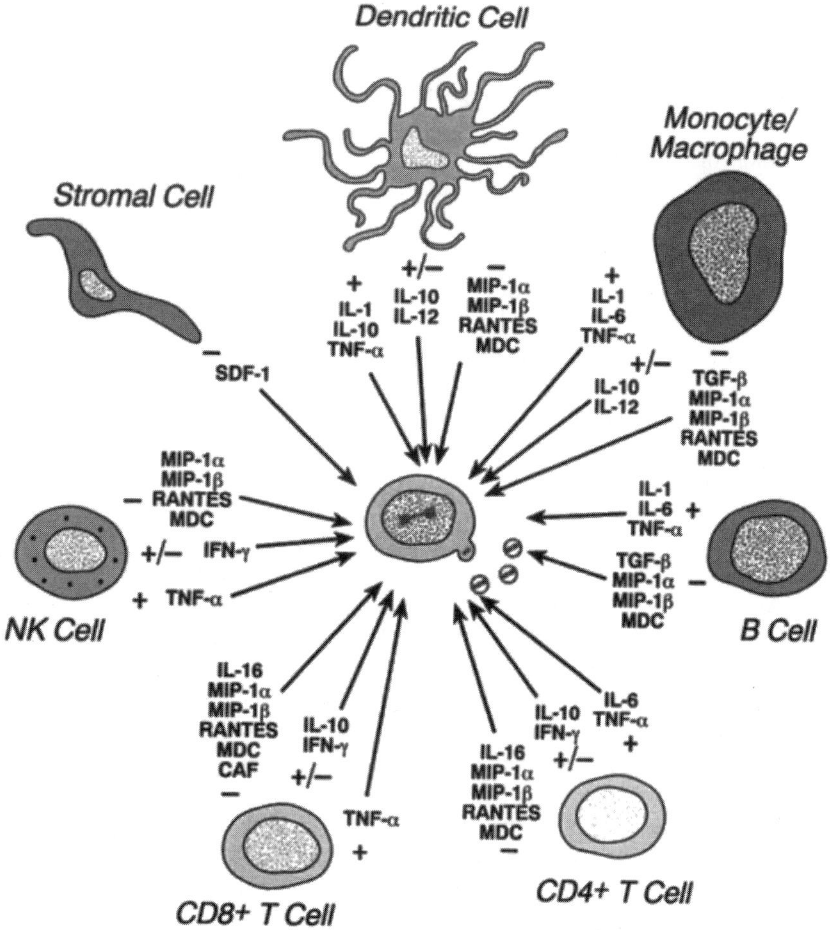

Figure 6 Cytokine networks that regulate HIV replication. Cytokines that enhance viral replication (+), inhibit viral replication (−), and enhance or inhibit viral replication depending upon the conditions (+/−) are shown.

that have been reported to upregulate HIV replication in vitro include IL-1β, IL-2, IL-3, IL-6, IL-7, IL-12, IL-15, IL-18, TNF-α, TNF-β, and the colony-stimulating factors (CSF) macrophage (M)–CSF and granulocyte-macrophage (GM)–CSF (reviewed in Ref. 283; see also Refs. 308–313). IFN-α, IFN-β, and IL-16 (275,314,315) are primarily suppressors of HIV production, whereas other cytokines, such as IL-4 (316,317), IL-10 (318–321), IL-13 (316), IFN-γ (322,323), and TGF-β (324,325), reduce or enhance viral replication depending on the infected cell type and the culture conditions. The effects of a particular cytokine are often greatly influenced by the activity of other cytokines present in the lymphoid tissue microenvironment (321,326,327).

Proinflammatory cytokines, particularly TNF-α, are considered the most potent HIV-inducing cytokines, and their mechanism of action is relatively well understood. Both TNF-α and IL-1β activate the cellular transcription factor nuclear factor (NF)κB (328,329), a strong inducer of HIV LTR-mediated transcription. IL-6 increases HIV expression primarily by a posttranscriptional mechanism; however, IL-6 can synergize with NFκB-inducing cytokines to enhance HIV transcription (326). The production of HIV by macrophages or PBMC stimulated with physiological inducers of proinflammatory cytokine production such as bacterial endotoxin or IL-2 can be partially or nearly completely abrogated by the addition of anti-proinflammatory cytokines (319,330), neutralizing antibodies to the cytokines (308), or receptor antagonists (ra), such as IL-1ra (308). In cultures of HIV-infected macrophages, the viral-suppressive activity of several cytokines, such as IL-10 and TGF-β, is attributable largely to their ability to inhibit the secretion or activity of HIV-inducing proinflammatory cytokines (319,324,330,331). HIV production by infected T cells is sensitive to both the antiproinflammatory and the antiproliferative activity of such cytokines (332).

Chemokines, or chemoattractant cytokines, are produced by numerous cell types and may influence HIV replication by binding to chemokine receptors that also serve as HIV coreceptors (333). Chemokine production, induced during inflammation, is enhanced by CD40 ligand stimulation (334,335) and by several cytokines including TNF-α, IL-1β, IL-2, and IL-15 (336–338). Chemokines that bind to CCR5 suppress HIV replication in vitro in PBMC from asymptomatic HIV-infected individuals harboring predominantly R5 strains of HIV (267), but not in PBMC from individuals with more advanced disease harboring predominantly X4 strains of HIV (267,339). Similarly, HIV isolates obtained longitudinally from individuals with rapid disease progression exhibit reduced sensitivity to inhibition by CCR5 ligands in vitro over time (339,340). Ligation of chemokine receptors in different cell types may have different effects on HIV replication; CC-chemokines inhibit replication of R5 strains of HIV in CD4+ T cells but may actually enhance replication of these strains in monocyte/macrophages (341,342). Unanticipated effects of manipulating the chemokine–chemokine receptor axis have also been observed, including CC-chemokine–mediated upregulation of CXCR4 expression and enhancement of replication of X4 strains of HIV in vitro that is dependent on intracellular signal transduction (53,54).

Immunological signals, cytokines, and chemokines influence chemokine receptor expression, which may also exert variable strain-dependent effects on HIV replication and spread (54,74). In this regard, differential regulatory patterns clearly distinguish the major HIV coreceptors, CCR5 and CXCR4 (74,343).

CCR5 expression is predominantly seen in previously activated, memory T cells (i.e., CD26^{high}CD45RO+ cells), whereas CXCR4 expression is seen in naive, unactivated cells (i.e., CD26^{low}CD45RA+ cells). Cytokines that are characteristic of TH1-type responses, such as IL-2, IL-12, TNF-α, and IFN-γ, upregulate CCR5 expression (74,344–346), whereas TH2-associated cytokines, such as IL-4 and IL-10, tend to upregulate CXCR4 expression and downregulate CCR5 expression (317,344,346–349). Stimulation of CD4+ T cells through CD3 and CD28 protects cells from HIV infection and potently downregulates HIV replication in infected cells (350–352); this effect appears to be due in part to downregulation of CCR5 (353). Finally, various components of pathogens, including HIV-1 itself, can induce expression of CXCR4 and favor replication of X4 strains of virus that use this coreceptor (354–357).

ROLE OF CELLULAR ACTIVATION IN HIV PATHOGENESIS

The end result of HIV infection is profound immunodeficiency; however, paradoxically, HIV infection is associated with hyperactivation of the immune system throughout most of the course of disease. HIV subverts the immune system by inducing immune activation and utilizing this milieu toward its own replicative advantage (282,283,358).

The replicative cycle of HIV infection is most efficiently achieved in activated cells (149–151). Cytokines that induce T-cell activation can further contribute to viral replication by inducing a state of productive infection in latently infected resting T cells (359). Several lines of evidence suggest that HIV replication in vivo is dependent upon antigen-driven activation of CD4+ T cells. HIV-infected individuals with intercurrent infections experience transient increases in plasma viremia that correlate with the degree of induced immune activation; similar observations have been made in SIV-infected macaques and in HIV-infected individuals who received immunizations against various pathogens (152–154,360,361). The amount of viral replication observed after vaccination with influenza vaccine or tetanus toxoid, or during active infection with *Mycobacterium tuberculosis*, correlated inversely with the stage of HIV disease. Individuals with late-stage HIV disease had a moderate increase in viral replication, while individuals with early-stage disease had a much greater increase in plasma viremia over baseline, suggesting a correlation between the ability of the immune system to respond to antigen and the magnitude of induction of virus replication. Furthermore, when PBMC from tetanus toxoid-immunized, HIV-infected individuals were stimulated in vitro with tetanus antigen, or when PBMC from purified protein derivative (PPD)–positive, HIV-infected individuals were stimulated in vitro with PPD or live *M. tuberculosis*, subjects with early-stage disease manifested a much stronger proliferative response to the respective antigens with a larger increase in viral replication in vitro than did individuals with advanced-stage disease (153,154,361,362). These studies suggest that the level of viral replication correlates with the level of immune system activation in response to an antigen.

Analysis of viral quasispecies and immune responses within lymphoid tissue from HIV-infected individuals reveals that within individual splenic white pulps, a restricted number of individual antigen-specific immune responses occurs (defined by the analysis of T-cell receptor Vβ gene usage), and each of the immune responses contains a single or limited number of HIV quasispecies (363). These data support the theory that within the context of individual antigen-specific immune responses, a single quasispecies of HIV, which was present at the initiation of the reaction, spread among the newly activated T cells. Thus, it is likely that the continuous daily production of HIV occurs in newly activated CD4+ T-cells that are being driven by antigen-specific activation (363,364).

IMMUNE DYSFUNCTION DURING HIV INFECTION

The pathogenesis of HIV disease is a complex, multifactorial process (283,358). A wide array of immune system deficits are associated with HIV infection; abnormalities in the function of all limbs of the immune system, including T and B lymphocytes, antigen-presenting cells, natural killer cells, and neutrophils, have been described.

CD4+ T Cells

CD4+ T cell dysfunction and depletion are hallmarks of HIV disease. The proximate cause of the susceptibility to opportunistic infections observed with advancing disease is the defects in T-cell number and function that result directly or indirectly from HIV infection. In addition to the decrease in IL-2 production and IL-2 receptor expression, the percentage of CD4+ T cells expressing CD28 (i.e., the major costimulatory receptor that is necessary for normal activation of T cells) is reduced during HIV infection compared to cells from uninfected individuals (365). CD28− cells do not respond to activation signals and express markers of terminal activation, including HLA-DR, CD38, and CD45RO (366). In addition, CD4+ T cells from HIV-infected individuals express abnormally low levels of CD40 ligand (367).

A variety of mechanisms, both directly and indirectly related to HIV infection of CD4+ T cells, are likely responsible for the observed defects in T cell function. Interference with CD4 expression by HIV gp120 (368), Nef (369), and Vpu (370), may impair the ability of the infected CD4+ T cell to interact with appropriate MHC class II molecules. Preferential infection by HIV of CD4+ memory cells and/or the preferential susceptibility of these cells to the cytopathic effects of HIV infection may in part explain the loss of memory responses to soluble antigens and consequent increase in the risk of infection with opportunistic organisms (291,371–373).

The relatively small fraction of T-cells that is infected with HIV in seropositive subjects at any given time militates against direct infection as the sole mediator of the immunopathogenesis of HIV infection (see below) (159). In addition, CD4+ T-cell dysfunction is evident even in the early stages of HIV infection, prior to quantitative depletion of this key cellular subset (291). A role for HIV envelope in the immunopathogenesis of HIV disease has been suggested by a number of studies (reviewed in Ref. 374). The presence of measurable levels of circulating soluble gp120 in HIV-infected subjects (375,376) and accumulation of high concentrations of virions (both infectious and defective) in lymphoid tissue (134,137,377) underscore the potential for envelope to contribute to T-cell dysfunction in a process distinct from infection of CD4+ T cells.

HIV envelope glycoproteins bind with high affinity to the CD4 molecule and to a number of chemokine co-receptors. Evidence of aberrant intracellular signaling induced by HIV has been available for a number of years (378,379). Intracellular signals transduced by HIV-1 envelope have been implicated in several immunopathogenic processes, including anergy (380–383), syncytium formation (384), apoptosis (385–387), and inappropriate cell trafficking (388,389). The molecular mechanisms responsible for these abnormalities include dysregulation of the T-cell receptor phosphoinositide pathway (390), p56lck activation (381,391), phosphorylation of focal adhesion kinase (392), activation of caspase-3 (387), downregulation of the costimulatory molecules CD40 ligand and CD80 (393), and activation of the MAP kinase and ras signaling pathways (394). Most of these aberrant signals were presumed to result from interactions between HIV envelope glycoproteins and CD4; however, more recently it has become clear that HIV envelope may also transduce intracellular signals through coreceptor molecules such as CCR5 (388,392,395) and CXCR4 (389).

Direct Infection as a Cause of CD4+ T-Cell Depletion

The observations that CD4+ T-cells are the principal targets of HIV infection in vivo and that HIV infection of CD4+ T-cells in vitro causes cytopathicity (2,396–399) led to a reasonable assumption that direct infection of CD4+ T cells in vivo results in their depletion. However, quantitative studies of the frequency of HIV-infected cells in vivo suggest that single cell killing by direct infection with HIV may not be the predominant mechanism of CD4+ T cell depletion (159,400). Although it increases with disease progression, the frequency of HIV-infected peripheral blood CD4+ T cells rarely exceeds 1 in 100 even in patients with AIDS (159,400–404). Viral burden and levels of virus expression are far greater in lymphoid tissue compared with peripheral blood (137,138,159); however, these levels even in lymphoid tissue do not appear to be sufficiently high to account for CD4+ T-cell depletion solely by direct mechanisms.

Multiple mechanisms of cell death appear to be operative after infection of a CD4+ T cell with HIV. Accumulation of reverse-transcribed viral DNA in the cytoplasm (399), interference by viral RNA with normal cellular RNA processing (405,406), intracellular interactions between the viral envelope gp120 and CD4 molecules (407–409), compromise of cell membrane integrity by the budding virions (410,411), and HIV-induced increases in the concentration of intracellular monovalent cations (412) all may play roles in CD4+ T-cell killing.

HIV-infected cells also may die as a consequence of viral-specific immune responses that occur before the cell succumbs directly to viral infection. Multiple effector mechanisms may be involved in the killing of HIV-infected cells, including cytotoxic T-lymphocyte, ADCC, and NK cell responses.

Indirect Mechanisms of CD4+ T-Cell Depletion

Syncytium Formation

The molecular events associated with viral entry that lead to fusion between the viral coat and cell membrane involve the interaction of the HIV envelope glycoprotein, CD4, and a coreceptor molecule. Similar events may occur when an infected cell bearing HIV envelope glycoprotein molecules on its surface encounters an uninfected CD4+ cell with an appropriate coreceptor. Fusion between infected and uninfected cells, resulting in multinucleated giant cells, or syncytia has long been observed in vitro (413–416). Syncytia have been observed only rarely in tissues obtained from HIV-infected individuals (113,166,417–421); thus, it is unlikely that syncytium formation is a major pathogenic mechanism of CD4+ T-cell depletion in vivo.

Autoimmunity

Autoimmunity may occur during the course of HIV infection as a result of molecular mimicry by viral components. Highly homologous regions exist in the carboxy terminus of the HIV-1 envelope glycoprotein and the amino-terminal domains of different HLA-DR and DQ alleles (422). Sera from a substantial number of HIV-infected individuals react with the shared determinant of gp41 and MHC class II: these sera can inhibit normal antigen-specific proliferative responses and also eliminate class II–bearing cells by ADCC (423). Similar instances of molecular mimicry between HIV-1 envelope constituents and host proteins, which may result in pathogenic autoimmune responses, include the collagen-like region of complement component C1q-A (424), MHC class I heavy chains (425), HLA-DR4 and DR2 alleles (426), variable regions of the T-cell receptor alpha, beta, and gamma chains (426), Fas (427,428), functional domains of IgG and

IgA (426), denatured collagen (429), and a number of nuclear antigens (430,431). Finally, immune recognition of normal cellular components may be induced by their association with HIV; such phenomena may be responsible for the emergence of CTL that are specific for autologous CD4+ T cells (432).

Innocent Bystander Phenomena

Immune responses that target HIV determinants on infected cells may also contribute to elimination of uninfected cells with HIV proteins (e.g., gp120) bound on their surface. Targeting of such ''innocent bystander'' cells by antibody and cellular immune responses has been described (201,433–435).

HIV-Mediated Inhibition of Hematopoiesis

Failure of normal hematopoiesis is an obvious candidate mechanism to account for depletion of CD4+ T cells during HIV infection. A subset of CD34+ progenitor cells express CD4 and HIV coreceptors and are infectable in vitro with HIV-1 (436–441). Furthermore, a substantial minority of HIV-infected patients with severe CD4+ T-cell depletion have a reservoir of HIV-infected CD34+ progenitor cells (442).

Although the role of direct infection of CD34+ progenitor cells in CD4+ T-cell depletion remains controversial, a large body of evidence suggests that viral proteins and HIV-induced cytokines can impair the survival and clonogenic potential of these cells (443–450). The subnormal mobilization of CD34+ cells into the peripheral blood following treatment with GM-CSF in HIV-infected individuals provides further evidence of reduced hematopoietic capacity and reserve in HIV infection (451).

Disruption of the thymic microenvironment (452) and HIV-induced thymocyte depletion may also contribute to the failure of CD4+ T-cell production. Thymic epithelial cells normally secrete IL-6, which can in turn increase HIV replication in infected cells (453). Subpopulations of thymic CD3-CD4-CD8- cells (i.e., ''triple negative'' cells) are susceptible to infection with HIV in vitro (454), and thymic CD3-CD4+CD8- progenitor cells from HIV-infected patients are infected in vivo. Finally, uninfected thymocytes from HIV-infected individuals are primed for apoptotic death, suggesting that indirect mechanisms of defective thymopoiesis are operative as well (455).

Apoptosis

Aberrant intracellular signals transduced by HIV may prime CD4+ T cells for apoptosis, resulting in depletion of these cells during the course of HIV infection (456,457). Acute infection of T cells with HIV in vitro can induce apoptosis

(458,459), and T cells from HIV-infected patients undergo enhanced rates of apoptosis in vitro compared with normal T cells, particularly following activation (460,461). Cross-linking of CD4 followed by ligation of the T-cell receptor is sufficient to induce apoptosis, suggesting that uninfected CD4+ T cells can be depleted inappropriately upon encountering antigen if CD4 had been cross-linked by gp120 (385,462).

Fas-dependent and Fas-independent pathways of apoptosis may be triggered by HIV. HIV-mediated Fas-independent apoptosis of CD4+ T cells has been shown in vitro by several groups (463–465); enhanced susceptibility of CD4+ T cells to Fas-dependent apoptosis has been reported as well. Mechanisms that may contribute to this susceptibility include upregulation of Fas and Fas ligand (386,466–470); upregulation and activation of caspase-1 (471), caspase-3 (387), and caspase-8 (472); activation of cyclin-dependent kinases (473); and downregulation of the anti-apoptotic Bcl-2 protein (474). Viral gene products that have been associated with enhanced susceptibility to apoptosis include the viral envelope (383,385,386,475), Nef (469,470), Tat (386,472), and Vpu (476).

The susceptibility of uninfected "bystander" cells to apoptosis is a possible mechanism by which large numbers of cells may be eliminated during HIV infection. In fact, studies in lymphoid tissue from HIV-infected individuals suggest that the majority of apoptosis occurs in uninfected bystander cells (477–479). Macrophages are efficient mediators of CD4+ T-cell bystander apoptosis. HIV-induced upregulation of Fas ligand expression on macrophages and enhanced secretion of TNF-α from these cells appear to be responsible in part for this phenomenon (466,468,480,481). Another mechanism of bystander apoptosis may involve upregulation of CD62L on lymphocytes by HIV (482). These HIV-exposed lymphocytes home to lymph nodes and undergo apoptosis upon signaling through homing receptors such as CD62L, CD44, and CD11a (483).

It remains uncertain whether HIV-induced apoptosis plays an important role in vivo in CD4+ T-cell depletion. The frequency of apoptotic CD4+ and CD8+ T cells as well as B cells is significantly higher in lymphoid tissue from HIV-infected individuals compared with uninfected controls (477,479). The relationship between the frequency of apoptotic cells and the stage of HIV infection remains controversial. Some data indicate a positive correlation between the stage of HIV disease and susceptibility of peripheral blood T cells to apoptosis (484), and another study demonstrated very low frequencies of apoptotic cells in HIV-infected long-term nonprogressors (485). However, other studies found no correlation between apoptosis and stage of disease (475,477). Compelling evidence that apoptosis may play a role in HIV pathogenesis comes from animal models wherein an increased frequency of apoptosis in CD4+ T-cells is seen in primates infected with pathogenic strains of SIV, but not in primates infected with nonpathogenic strains of SIV (486).

CD8+ T Cells

Dysregulation of CD8+ T-cell numbers and function is evident throughout the course of HIV disease. Following an initial decline associated with acute primary infection, CD8+ T cell counts usually rebound to supranormal levels and may remain elevated for prolonged periods. Increases in CD8+ T cells during all but the late stages of disease may, in part, reflect the expansion of HIV-specific CD8+ CTL (487,488).

During HIV disease progression, CD8+ T cells acquire an abnormal phenotype characterized by the expression of certain activation markers and the absence of expression of the CD25 IL-2 receptor. Alterations in the phenotype of CD8+ T cells in HIV-infected individuals may have prognostic significance. In this regard, individuals whose CD8+ T cells express HLA-DR but not CD38 after seroconversion experience a stabilization of their CD4+ T-cell counts and a less fulminant disease course, while individuals whose CD8+ T cells express both HLA-DR and CD38 experience a more aggressive course with rapid CD4+ T-cell depletion and a poorer prognosis (489–491). CD8+ T cells lacking CD28 expression are also increased in HIV disease (492–497), possibly reflecting the expansion of the CD8+CD28-CD57+ T cell subset containing in vivo activated CTL (498). The loss of CTL activity with disease progression is not restricted to HIV-specific CTL; a loss of cytotoxic activity to other common antigens including Epstein-Barr virus (EBV) and *M. tuberculosis* has also been observed (499,500). In addition to CTL activity, other CD8+ T cell functions are impaired during HIV disease progression, including loss of noncytolytic non-MHC restricted CD8+ T-cell–derived suppressor activity against HIV (264).

Depletion of HIV-specific CTL may occur as a consequence of clonal exhaustion (see above) (238,239). CD8+ T cells may also be depleted by apoptosis as ''innocent bystanders.'' This phenomenon may be mediated by macrophages in which CXCR4 has been triggered by HIV envelope; membrane-bound TNF-α is upregulated by HIV in these cells, as is TNF receptor II on CD8+ T cells (501).

Monocytes/Macrophages

Cells of the monocyte/macrophage lineage play key roles in the immunopathogenesis of HIV disease. These cells serve as reservoirs of viral infection and are responsible for a variety of tissue-specific pathological processes. Dysfunction of these cells contributes to CD4+ T-cell dysfunction and also to impaired host defense against intracellular pathogens (281,358,502).

Monocytic cells express CD4 and numerous HIV coreceptors including CCR5, CXCR4, and CCR3 on their surface (503–507), and serve as targets of HIV infection. Unlike infection of CD4+ T cells, HIV is relatively noncytopathic for cells of the monocyte/macrophage lineage, and HIV can replicate extensively in these cells in intracellular compartments (508). Chronically infected macrophages may be long-lived, and currently available antiretroviral agents are generally not capable of targeting chronically infected cells; these cells therefore represent a formidable challenge to eradication of HIV (509,510). Circulating monocytes are rarely found to be infected in vivo and are difficult to infect in vitro (511–513); however, infection can readily be demonstrated in tissue macrophages, including resident microglial cells in the brain, pulmonary alveolar macrophages, and mature macrophages derived from blood monocytes in vitro (208,508,514,515). Infection of monocytic precursors in bone marrow may be directly or indirectly responsible for certain of the hematological abnormalities observed in HIV-infected individuals. Lymphoid tissue macrophages can be prolific producers of HIV in the setting of opportunistic infections, during which the cytokine milieu in the tissue favors a highly productive state of HIV infection (516).

Infection of monocyte/macrophages with HIV or exposure of these cells to viral proteins, including envelope glycoproteins and Tat, leads to a number of functional abnormalities. Impaired accessory cell function (517,518) may result from decreased MHC class II expression, decreased IL-12 secretion, and increased IL-10 secretion (518,519); this HIV-induced dysregulation of antigen presentation may in turn be a significant cause of hyporesponsiveness of CD4+ T cells (502,517). Defects in ADCC function of monocyte/macrophages, possibly related to low levels of expression of Fc and complement receptors, have also been observed in HIV infection (520–522). Finally, HIV-associated abnormalities in antigen uptake, oxidative burst, and chemotaxis have been described in monocyte/macrophages (519,523–526).

Dendritic Cells

DC are among the first cells to encounter HIV after mucosal exposure. Virions bind to the DC surface by virtue of interactions between the envelope glycoprotein gp120 and the DC surface protein DC-SIGN (111). DC are thus able to efficiently transport HIV to lymphoid organs, facilitating infection of CD4+ T cells and viral dissemination. DC also express several different chemokine receptors that can be used as HIV coreceptors for entry (61,527,528). Although the frequency of HIV-infected DC in vivo may be low, these cells nevertheless may represent an important viral reservoir.

It has been reported that infectability of Langerhans cells (i.e., DC resident in the epidermis) may be dependent on viral subtype (529). This finding could in part explain the differences in the global epidemiology of HIV infection; an HIV subtype that can replicate well in Langerhans cells, likely a major cell type involved in the initiation of viral infection through mucosal contact (108), may be more efficiently transmitted heterosexually. It should be pointed out that these

these findings are controversial (530,531), although data do suggest a role for DC in selecting the strain of HIV that can be transmitted across a mucosal barrier (532).

The degree of DC dysfunction and depletion that occurs during HIV infection remains controversial (533,534). Emerging data suggest that a subset of DC expressing CD11c are depleted during the course of HIV infection; interestingly, these cells were not restored during highly active antiretroviral therapy (535). Further studies are needed to clarify the possible role of DC depletion and dysfunction in the pathogenesis of HIV disease.

B Lymphocytes

HIV infection is almost invariably associated with hypergammaglobulinemia and B-lymphocyte hyperactivation. A large component of the immunoglobulin specificity, at least in early stage disease, is directed against HIV antigens. It has been suggested that a majority of activated B cells produce antibodies directed against HIV during this stage of infection (reviewed in Ref. 536). In spite of the observed B-cell hyperactivation, the ability of B cells to respond specifically to antigens is reduced. B cells from HIV-infected individuals express abnormally low levels of HLA-DR on their surface (537) and also fail to normally upregulate CD70 after stimulation with activated T-cells (367); this latter defect is associated with impaired CD70-dependent immunoglobulin synthesis (367). In patients with advanced-stage HIV infection, B-cells fail to proliferate and differentiate in response to ligation of the B-cell antigen receptor and CD40, suggesting a defect in signal transduction (538). Further evidence of HIV-related B-cell dysfunction comes from an in vitro lymphoid tissue culture model of HIV infection. In this model, infection of lymphoid tissue with strains of HIV that utilize CCR5 as an entry coreceptor results in enhanced antibody responses to recall antigens upon challenge; in contrast, HIV strains that utilize CXCR4 result in profound suppression of these antibody responses (539). This effect appears to be dependent on signal transduction through CXCR4 and may be irreversible (539).

B cells from HIV-infected individuals secrete increased amounts of TNF-α and IL-6, cytokines known to enhance HIV replication (307,540), and express surface-bound TNF-α that can induce the production of HIV from infected CD4+ T cells (541). The secretion of proinflammatory cytokines and the expression of surface-bound TNF-α by B cells in the lymphoid microenvironment may contribute to T-cell activation and HIV replication in these tissues.

HIV gp120 has been observed to directly bind to an immunoglobulin variable chain (VH3) and activate these B-cells in much the same manner as a superantigen (542). This antigen-independent polyclonal activation leads in part to the hypergammaglobulinemia and B-lymphocyte hyperactivation of HIV infection. Other portions of HIV, including gp41, directly activate B cells in a nonsuperantigen-mediated manner (543). Correlates of B-cell dysfunction observed in HIV-infected individuals include an increase in spontaneous EBV transformation in vitro and may contribute to the observed increased frequency of EBV-induced lymphomas (544). In addition, the increased susceptibility to bacterial infections during the course of HIV infection likely results in part from B-cell dysregulation (545).

B cells may also serve as a viral reservoir during the course of HIV infection. In this regard, stimulation of B cells with CD40L and IL-4 upregulates expression of activation and costimulatory molecules, as well as CD4 and CXCR4. B cells stimulated in this manner are susceptible to infection with dual- and T-tropic strains of HIV (546).

Neutrophils

Neutrophils appear to be hyperactivated during the course of HIV infection, and many functional defects have been observed in these cells (547). Neutrophils from HIV-infected individuals produce more TNF-α and IL-6 in response to lipopolysaccharide (LPS) or *Candida* antigen compared to neutrophils from normal donors (548). These cells also undergo apoptosis at an increased rate compared to those from normal controls (549). When stimulated through Fc receptors or protein kinase C, neutrophils from HIV-infected individuals produced less superoxide compared with controls; this defect could be recapitulated by treatment of normal neutrophils with HIV envelope protein (550). A defect has also been observed in neutrophil complement receptor function resulting in subnormal release of IL-8 in response to cryptococcal challenge by these cells in patients with advanced HIV disease (551).

Natural Killer Cells

Abnormalities of NK cells are observed throughout the course of HIV disease, and these abnormalities increase with disease, progression. Most studies report that NK cells are normal in numbers and phenotype in HIV-infected individuals; however, decreases in numbers of the CD16+/CD56+ subpopulation of NK cells with an associated increase in activation markers has been reported (552). NK cells from HIV-infected individuals are defective in their ability to kill typical NK target cells as well as gp160-expressing cells. The abnormality in NK cell lysis is thought to occur after binding of the NK cell to its target (553). A possible mechanism for defective NK activity includes a lack of cytokines necessary for optimal function. Addition of either IL-2, IL-12, IL-15, or IFN-α to cultures enhances the defective in vitro NK cell function of HIV-infected individuals (554,555). Enhanced expression of cytolytic inhibitory receptors during the course of HIV infection may also be responsible for depressed NK cell function (556,557); in addition, selective HIV-mediated downregulation of HLA-A and

−B but not HLA-C and −E molecules may prevent NK cell killing of HIV-infected target cells (558).

NK cells are an important source of HIV-inhibitory CC-chemokines in HIV-infected individuals (270). NK cells isolated from HIV-infected individuals produce high constitutive levels of MIP-1α, MIP-1β, and RANTES; high levels of chemokine production are also seen when these cells are stimulated by IL-2, IL-15, or CD16 cross-linking, or during lytic killing (270). Thus, NK cells, like CD8+ T cells, may inhibit HIV replication by cell-mediated killing as well as by secretion of soluble HIV-inhibitory factors.

CONCLUSION

The pathogenesis of HIV infection is a complex, multifactorial process involving viral and host factors. The virus is able to utilize molecules of the human immune system to infect the very cells that should be responsible for orchestrating the immune counterattack. Furthermore, activation of the immune system provides the virus with a milieu that is highly conducive to viral replication. The virus is able to evade and disarm most components of the host immune response by a variety of direct and indirect mechanisms. A more complete understanding of these mechanisms should aid the rational development of more effective preventive and therapeutic strategies.

REFERENCES

1. Dalgleish, A.G., P.C. Beverly, P.R. Clapham, D.H. Crawford, M.F. Greaves, R.A. Weiss. 1984. The CD4(T4) antigen is an essential component of the receptor for the AIDS retrovirus. Nature 312:763–767.
2. Klatzmann, D., F. Barre-Sinoussi, M.T. Nugeyre, C. Danquet, E. Vilmer, C. Griscelli, F. Brun-Veziret, C. Rouzioux, J.C. Gluckman, J.C. Chermann. 1984. Selective tropism of lymphadenopathy-associated virus (LAV) for helper-inducer T-lymphocytes. Science 225:59–63.
3. Klatzmann, D., E. Champagne, S. Chamaret, J. Gruest, D. Guetard, T. Hercend, J.-C. Gluckman, L. Montagnier. 1984. T-lymphocyte T4 molecule behaves as receptor for human retrovirus LAV. Nature 312:767–768.
4. Maddon, P.J., A.G. Dalgleish, J.S. McDougal, P.R. Clapham, R.A. Weiss, R.A. Axel. 1986. The T4 gene encodes the AIDS virus receptor and is expressed in the immune system and the brain. Cell 47:333–348.
5. Broder, C.C., E.A. Berger. 1995. Fusogenic selectivity of the envelope glycoprotein is a major determinant of human immunodeficiency virus type 1 tropism for CD4+ T-cell lines vs. primary macrophages. Proc Natl Acad Sci USA 92:9004–9008.
6. Alkhatib, G., C.C. Broder, E.A. Berger. 1996. Cell type-specific fusion

cofactors determine human immunodeficiency virus type 1 tropism for T-cell lines versus primary macrophages. J Virol 70:5487–5494.

7. Cocchi, F., A. DeVico, A. Garzino-Demo, S. Arya, R. Gallo, P. Lusso. 1995. Identification of RANTES, MIP-1α, and MIP-1β as the major HIV suppressive factors produced by CD8+ T cells. Science 270:1811–1815.
8. Feng, Y., C. Broder, P. Kennedy, E. Berger. 1996. HIV-1 entry cofactor: functional cDNA cloning of a seven-transmembrane domain, G-protein coupled receptor. Science 272:872–877.
9. Berson, J., D. Long, B. Doranz, J. Rucker, F. Jirik, R. Doms. 1996. A seven-transmembrane domain receptor involved in fusion and entry of T-cell-tropic human immunodeficiency virus type 1 strains. J Virol 70:6288–6295.
10. Bleul, C.C., M. Farzan, H. Choe, C. Parolin, I. Clark-Lewis, J. Sodroski, T.A. Springer. 1996. The lymphocyte chemoattractant SDF-1 is a ligand for LESTR/fusin and blocks HIV-1 entry. Nature 382:829–833.
11. Oberlin, E., A. Amara, F. Bachelerie, C. Bessia, J.L. Virelizier, F. Arenzana-Seisdedos, O. Schwartz, J.M. Heard, I. Clark-Lewis, D.F. Legler, M. Loetscher, M. Baggiolini, B. Moser. 1996. The CXC chemokine SDF-1 is the ligand for LESTR/fusin and prevents infection by T-cell-line-adapted HIV-1. Nature 382:833–835.
12. Paxton, W.A., S.R. Martin, D. Tse, T.R. O'Brien, J. Skurnick, N.L. VanDevanter, N. Padian, J.F. Braun, D.P. Kotler, S.M. Wolinsky, R.A. Koup. 1996. Relative resistance to HIV-1 infection of CD4 lymphocytes from persons who remain uninfected despite multiple high-risk sexual exposures. Nat Med 2:412–417.
13. Samson, M., O. Labbe, C. Mollereau, G. Vassart, M. Parmentier. 1996. Molecular cloning and functional expression of a new human CC-chemokine receptor gene. Biochemistry 35:3362–3367.
14. Combadiere, C., S.K. Ahuja, H.L. Tiffany, P.M. Murphy. 1996. Cloning and functional expression of CC CKR5, a human monocyte CC chemokine receptor selective for MIP-1(alpha), MIP-1(beta), and RANTES. J Leukoc Biol 60:147–152.
15. Raport, C., J. Gosling, V. Schweickart, P. Gray, I. Charo. 1996. Molecular cloning and functional characterization of a novel human CC chemokine receptor (CCR5) for RANTES, MIP-1beta, and MIP-1alpha. J Biol Chem 271:17161–17166.
16. Deng, H., R. Liu, W. Ellmeier, S. Choe, D. Unutmaz, M. Burkhart, P. DiMarzio, S. Marmon, R. Sutton, C. Hill, C. Davis, S. Peiper, T. Schall, D. Littman, N. Landau. 1996. Identification of a major co-receptor for primary isolates of HIV-1. Nature 381:661–666.
17. Dragic, T., V. Litwin, G. Allaway, S. Martin, Y. Huang, K. Nagashima, C. Cayanan, P. Maddon, R. Koup, J. Moore, W. Paxton. 1996. HIV-1

entry into CD4+ cells is mediated by the chemokine receptor CC-CKR-5. Nature 381:667–673.

18. Alkhatib, G., C. Combadiere, C. Broder, Y. Feng, P. Kennedy, P. Murphy, E. Berger. 1996. CC CKR5: a RANTES, MIP-1α, MIP-1β receptor as a fusion cofactor for macrophage-tropic HIV-1. Science 272:1955–1958.
19. Choe, H., M. Farzan, Y. Sun, N. Sullivan, B. Rollins, P. Ponath, L. Wu, C. Mackay, G. LaRosa, W. Newman, N. Gerard, C. Gerard, J. Sodroski. 1996. The β-chemokine receptors CCR3 and CCR5 facilitate infection by primary HIV-1 isolates. Cell 85:1135–1138.
20. Doranz, B., J. Rucker, Y. Yi, R. Smyth, M. Samson, S. Peiper, M. Parmentier, R. Collman, R. Doms. 1996. A dual-tropic primary HIV-1 isolate that uses fusin and the β-chemokine receptors CKR-5, CKR-3, and CKR-2b as fusion cofactors. Cell 85:1149–1158.
21. Alkhatib, G., F. Liao, E.A. Berger, J.M. Farber, K.W. Peden. 1997. A new SIV co-receptor, STRL33. Nature 388:238.
22. Liao, F., G. Alkhatib, K.W. Peden, G. Sharma, E.A. Berger, J.M. Farber. 1997. STRL33, a novel chemokine receptor-like protein, functions as a fusion cofactor for both macrophage-tropic and T-cell line-tropic HIV-1. J Exp Med 185:2015–2023.
23. Deng, H.K., D. Unutmaz, V.N. KewalRamani, D.R. Littman. 1997. Expression cloning of new receptors used by simian and human immunodeficiency viruses. Nature 388:296–300.
24. Choe, H., M. Farzan, M. Konkel, K. Martin, Y. Sun, L. Marcon, M. Cayabyab, M. Berman, M.E. Dorf, N. Gerard, C. Gerard, J. Sodroski. 1998. The orphan seven-transmembrane receptor apj supports the entry of primary T-cell-line-tropic and dualtropic human immunodeficiency virus type 1. J Virol 72:6113–6118.
25. Rucker, J., A.L. Edinger, M. Sharron, M. Samson, B. Lee, J.F. Berson, Y. Yi, B. Margulies, R.G. Collman, B.J. Doranz, M. Parmentier, R.W. Doms. 1997. Utilization of chemokine receptors, orphan receptors, and herpesvirus-encoded receptors by diverse human and simian immunodeficiency viruses. J Virol 71:8999–9007.
26. Horuk, R., J. Hesselgesser, Y. Zhou, D. Faulds, M. Halks-Miller, S. Harvey, D. Taub, M. Samson, M. Parmentier, J. Rucker, B.J. Doranz, R.W. Doms. 1998. The CC chemokine I-309 inhibits CCR8-dependent infection by diverse HIV-1 strains. J Biol Chem 273:386–391.
27. Berger, E.A., R.W. Doms, E.M. Fenyo, B.T. Korber, D.R. Littman, J.P. Moore, Q.J. Sattentau, H. Schuitemaker, J. Sodroski, R.A. Weiss. 1998. A new classification for HIV-1 [letter]. Nature 391:240.
28. Trkola, A., T. Dragic, J. Arthos, J. Binley, W. Olson, G. Allaway, C. Cheng-Mayer, J. Robinson, P. Maddon, J. Moore. 1996. CD4-dependent,

antibody-sensitive interactions between HIV-1 and its co-receptor CCR-5. Nature 384:184–187.

29. Wu, L., N. Gerard, R. Wyatt, H. Choe, C. Parolin, N. Ruffing, A. Borsetti, A. Cardoso, E. Desjardin, W. Newman, C. Gerard, J. Sodroski. 1996. CD4-induced interaction of primary HIV-1 gp120 glycoproteins with the chemokine receptor CCR-5. Nature 384:179–183.
30. Hill, C.M., H. Deng, D. Unutmaz, V.N. Kewalramani, L. Bastiani, M.K. Gorny, S. Zolla-Pazner, D.R. Littman. 1997. Envelope glycoproteins from human immunodeficiency virus types 1 and 2 and simian immunodeficiency virus can use human CCR5 as a coreceptor for viral entry and make direct CD4-dependent interactions with this chemokine receptor. J Virol 71:6296–6304.
31. Wyatt, R., P.D. Kwong, E. Desjardins, R.W. Sweet, J. Robinson, W.A. Hendrickson, J.G. Sodroski. 1998. The antigenic structure of the HIV gp120 envelope glycoprotein. Nature 393:705–711.
32. Kwong, P.D., R. Wyatt, J. Robinson, R.W. Sweet, J. Sodroski, W.A. Hendrickson. 1998. Structure of an HIV gp120 envelope glycoprotein in complex with the CD4 receptor and a neutralizing human antibody. Nature 393:648–659.
33. Rizzuto, C.D., R. Wyatt, N. Hernandez-Ramos, Y. Sun, P.D. Kwong, W.A. Hendrickson, J. Sodroski. 1998. A conserved HIV gp120 glycoprotein structure involved in chemokine receptor binding. Science 280:1949–1953.
34. Doranz, B.J., S.S. Baik, R.W. Doms. 1999. Use of a gp120 binding assay to dissect the requirements and kinetics of human immunodeficiency virus fusion events. J Virol 73:10346–10358.
35. Wu, L., G. LaRosa, N. Kassam, C.J. Gordon, H. Heath, N. Ruffing, H. Chen, J. Humblias, M. Samson, M. Parmentier, J.P. Moore, C.R. Mackay. 1997. Interaction of chemokine receptor CCR5 with its ligands: multiple domains for HIV-1 gp120 binding and a single domain for chemokine binding. J Exp Med 186:1373–1381.
36. Atchison, R.E., J. Gosling, F.S. Monteclaro, C. Franci, L. Digilio, I.F. Charo, M.A. Goldsmith. 1996. Multiple extracellular elements of CCR5 and HIV-1 entry: dissociation from response to chemokines. Science 274: 1924–1926.
37. Kuhmann, S.E., E.J. Platt, S.L. Kozak, D. Kabat. 1997. Polymorphisms in the CCR5 genes of African green monkeys and mice implicate specific amino acids in infections by simian and human immunodeficiency viruses. J Virol 71:8642–8656.
38. Rucker, J., M. Samson, B.J. Doranz, F. Libert, J.F. Berson, Y. Yi, R.J. Smyth, R.G. Collman, C.C. Broder, G. Vassart, R.W. Doms, M. Parmen-

tier. 1996. Regions in β-chemokine receptors CCR5 and CCR2b that determine HIV-1 cofactor specificity. Cell 87:437–446.

39. Alkhatib, G., S.S. Ahuja, D. Light, S. Mummidi, E.A. Berger, S.K. Ahuja. 1997. CC chemokine receptor 5-mediated signaling and HIV-1 Co-receptor activity share common structural determinants. Critical residues in the third extracellular loop support HIV-1 fusion. J Biol Chem 272:19771–19776.
40. Edinger, A.L., A. Amedee, K. Miller, B.J. Doranz, M. Endres, M. Sharron, M. Samson, Z.H. Lu, J.E. Clements, M. Murphey-Corb, S.C. Peiper, M. Parmentier, C.C. Broder, R.W. Doms. 1997. Differential utilization of CCR5 by macrophage and T cell tropic simian immunodeficiency virus strains. Proc Natl Acad Sci USA 94:4005–4010.
41. Dragic, T., A. Trkola, S.W. Lin, K.A. Nagashima, F. Kajumo, L. Zhao, W.C. Olson, L. Wu, C.R. Mackay, G.P. Allaway, T.P. Sakmar, J.P. Moore, P.J. Maddon. 1998. Amino-terminal substitutions in the CCR5 coreceptor impair gp120 binding and human immunodeficiency virus type 1 entry. J Virol 72:279–285.
42. Farzan, M., H. Choe, L. Vaca, K. Martin, Y. Sun, E. Desjardins, N. Ruffing, L. Wu, R. Wyatt, N. Gerard, C. Gerard, J. Sodroski. 1998. A tyrosine-rich region in the N terminus of CCR5 is important for human immunodeficiency virus type 1 entry and mediates an association between gp120 and CCR5. J Virol 72:11601164.
43. Doranz, B.J., Z.H. Lu, J. Rucker, T.Y. Zhang, M. Sharron, Y.H. Cen, Z.X. Wang, H.H. Guo, J.G. Du, M.A. Accavitti, R.W. Doms, S.C. Peiper. 1997. Two distinct CCR5 domains can mediate coreceptor usage by human immunodeficiency virus type 1. J Virol 71:6305–6314.
44. Picard, L., G. Simmons, C.A. Power, A. Meyer, R.A. Weiss, P.R. Clapham. 1997. Multiple extracellular domains of CCR-5 contribute to human immunodeficiency virus type 1 entry and fusion. J Virol 71:5003–5011.
45. Siciliano, S.J., S.E. Kuhmann, Y. Weng, N. Madani, M.S. Springer, J.E. Lineberger, R. Danzeisen, M.D. Miller, M.P. Kavanaugh, J.A. DeMartino, D. Kabat. 1999. A critical site in the core of the CCR5 chemokine receptor required for binding and infectivity of human immunodeficiency virus type 1. J Biol Chem 274:1905–1913.
46. Genoud, S., F. Kajumo, Y. Guo, D. Thompson, T. Dragic. 1999. CCR5-Mediated human immunodeficiency virus entry depends on an amino-terminal gp120-binding site and on the conformational integrity of all four extracellular domains. J Virol 73:1645–1648.
47. Oravecz, T., M. Pall, M. Norcross. 1996. beta-chemokine inhibition of monocytotropic HIV-1 infection. Interference with a postbinding fusion step. J Immunol 157:1329–1332.
48. Cocchi, F., A.L. DeVico, A. Garzino-Demo, A. Cara, R.C. Gallo, P.

Lusso. 1996. The V3 domain of the HIV-1 gp120 envelope glycoprotein is critical for chemokine-mediated blockade of infection. Nat Med 2: 1244–1247.

49. Speck, R.F., K. Wehrly, E.J. Platt, R.E. Atchison, I.F. Charo, D. Kabat, B. Chesebro, M.A. Goldsmith. 1997. Selective employment of chemokine receptors as human immunodeficiency virus type 1 coreceptors determined by individual amino acids within the envelope V3 loop. J Virol 71:7136–7139.
50. Wang, W.K., T. Dudek, M. Essex, T.H. Lee. 1999. Hypervariable region 3 residues of HIV type 1 gp120 involved in CCR5 coreceptor utilization: therapeutic and prophylactic implications. Proc Natl Acad Sci USA 96: 4558–4562.
51. Gosling, J., F.S. Monteclaro, R.E. Atchison, H. Arai, C.L. Tsou, M.A. Goldsmith, I.F. Charo. 1997. Molecular uncoupling of C-C chemokine receptor 5-induced chemotaxis and signal transduction from HIV-1 coreceptor activity. Proc Natl Acad Sci USA 94:5061–506.
52. Farzan, M., H. Choe, K.A. Martin, Y. Sun, M. Sidelko, C.R. Mackay, N.P. Gerard, J. Sodroski, C. Gerard. 1997. HIV-1 entry and macrophage inflammatory protein-1beta-mediated signaling are independent functions of the chemokine receptor CCR5. J Biol Chem 272:6854–6857.
53. Dolei, A., A. Biolchini, C. Serra, S. Curreli, E. Gomes, F. Dianzani. 1998. Increased replication of T-cell-tropic HIV strains and CXC-chemokine receptor-4 induction in T-cells treated with macrophage inflammatory protein (MIP)-1alpha, MIP-1beta and RANTES beta-chemokines. AIDS 12: 183–190.
54. Kinter, A., A. Catanzaro, J. Monaco, M. Ruiz, J. Justement, S. Moir, J. Arthos, A. Oliva, L. Ehler, S. Mizell, R. Jackson, M. Ostrowski, J. Hoxie, R. Offord, A.S. Fauci. 1998. CC-chemokines enhance the replication of T-tropic strains of HIV-1 in CD4(+) T cells: role of signal transduction. Proc Natl Acad Sci USA 95:11880–11885.
55. Alfano, M., H. Schmidtmayerova, C.A. Amella, T. Pushkarsky, M. Bukrinsky. 1999. The B-oligomer of pertussis toxin deactivates CC chemokine receptor 5 and blocks entry of M-tropic HIV-1 strains. J Exp Med 190: 597–605.
56. Lapham, C., J. Ouyang, B. Chadrasekhar, N. Nguyen, D. Dimitrov, H. Golding. 1996. Evidence for cell-surface association between fusin and CD4-gp120 complex in human cell lines. Science 274:602–605.
57. Brelot, A., N. Heveker, O. Pleskoff, N. Sol, M. Alizon. 1997. Role of the first and third extracellular domains of CXCR-4 in human immunodeficiency virus coreceptor activity. J Virol 71:4744–4751.
58. Kozak, S.L., E.J. Platt, N. Madani, F.E. Ferro, Jr., K. Peden, D. Kabat. 1997. CD4, CXCR-4, and CCR-5 dependencies for infections by primary

patient and laboratory-adapted isolates of human immunodeficiency virus type 1. J Virol 71:873–882.
59. Zhu, T., H. Mo, N. Wang, S.D. Nam, Y. Cao, R.A. Koup, D.D. Ho. 1993. Genotypic and phenotypic characterization of HIV-1 in patients with primary infection. Science 261:1179–1181.
60. Zhang, L.Q., P. Mackenzie, A. Cleland, E.C. Holmes, A.J. Leigh-Brown, P. Simmonds. 1993. Selection for specific sequences in the external envelope protein of human immunodeficiency virus type 1 upon primary infection. J Virol 67:3345–3356.
61. Zaitseva, M., A. Blauvelt, S. Lee, C.K. Lapham, V. Klaus-Kovtun, H. Mostowski, J. Manischewitz, H. Golding. 1997. Expression and function of CCR5 and CXCR4 on human Langerhans cells and macrophages: implications for HIV primary infection. Nat Med 3:1369–1375.
62. Liu, R., W. Paxton, S. Choe, D. Ceradini, S. Martin, R. Horuk, M. MacDonald, H. Stuhlmann, R. Koup, N. Landau. 1996. Homozygous defect in HIV-1 coreceptor accounts for resistance of some multiply-exposed individuals to HIV-1 infection. Cell 86:367–377.
63. Samson, M., F. Libert, B. Doranz, J. Rucker, C. Liesnard, C. Farber, S. Saragosti, C. Lapoumeroulie, J. Cognaux, C. Forceille, G. Muyldermans, C. Verhofstede, G. Burtonboy, M. Georges, T. Imai, S. Rana, Y. Yi, R. Smyth, R. Collman, R. Doms, G. Vassart, M. Parmentier. 1996. Resistance to HIV-1 infection in Caucasian individuals bearing mutant alleles of the CCR-5 chemokine receptor gene. Nature 382:722–725.
64. Dean, M., M. Carrington, C. Winkler, G. Huttley, M. Smith, R. Allikmets, J. Goedert, S. Buchbinder, E. Vitinghoff, E. Gomperts, S. Donfield, D. Vlahov, R. Kaslow, A. Saah, C. Rinaldo, R. Detels, H.G.a.D. Study, M.A.C. Study, S.F.C. Cohort, A. Study, and S. O'Brien. 1996. Genetic restriction of HIV-1 infection and progression to AIDS by a deletion allele of the CKR5 structural gene. Science 273:1856–1862.
65. Huang, Y., W. Paxton, S. Wolinsky, A. Neumann, L. Zhang, T. He, S. Kang, D. Ceradini, Z. Jin, K. Yazdanbakhsh, K. Kunstman, D. Erickson, E. Dragon, N. Landau, J. Phair, D. Ho, R. Koup. 1996. The role of a mutant CCR5 allele in HIV-1 transmission and disease progression. Nat Med 2:1240–1243.
66. Zimmerman, P., A. Buckler-White, G. Alkhatib, T. Spalding, J. Kubofcik, C. Combadiere, D. Weissman, O. Cohen, A. Rubbert, G. Lam, M. Vaccarezza, P. Kennedy, V. Kumraraswami, J. Giorgi, R. Detels, J. Hunter, M. Chopek, E. Berger, A. Fauci, T. Nutman, P. Murphy. 1997. Inherited resistance to HIV-1 conferred by an inactivating mutation in CC chemokine receptor 5: studies in populations with contrasting clinical phenotypes, defined racial backgrounds and quantified risks. Mol Med 3:23–36.
67. Biti, R., R. French, J. Young, B. Bennetts, G. Stewart. 1997. HIV-1 infec-

tion in an individual homozygous for the CCR5 deletion allele. Nat Med 3:252–253.
68. Theodorou, I., L. Meyer, M. Magierowska, C. Katlama, C. Rouzioux. 1997. HIV-1 infection in an individual homozygous for CCR5Δ32. Lancet 349:1219–1220.
69. O'Brien, T., C. Winkler, M. Dean, J. Nelson, M. Carrington, N. Michael, G. White. 1997. HIV-1 infection in a man homozygous for CCR5Δ32. Lancet 349:1219.
70. Michael, N.L., J.A. Nelson, V.N. KewalRamani, G. Chang, O.B. SJ, J.R. Mascola, B. Volsky, M. Louder, G.C. White, 2nd, D.R. Littman, R. Swanstrom, O.B. TR. 1998. Exclusive and persistent use of the entry coreceptor CXCR4 by human immunodeficiency virus type 1 from a subject homozygous for CCR5 delta32. J Virol 72:6040–6047.
71. Michael, N., G. Chang, L. Louie, J. Mascola, D. Dondero, D. Birx, H. Sheppard. 1997. The role of viral phenotype and CCR-5 gene defects in HIV-1 transmission and disease progression. Nat Med 3:338–340.
72. Cohen, O., M. Vaccarezza, G. Lam, B. Baird, K. Wildt, P. Murphy, P. Zimmerman, T. Nutman, C. Fox, S. Hoover, J. Adelsberger, M. Baseler, J. Arthos, R. Davey, R. Dewar, J. Metcalf, D. Schwartzentruber, J. Orenstein, S. Buchbinder, A. Saah, R. Detels, J. Phair, C. Rinaldo, J. Margolick, G. Pantaleo, A. Fauci. 1997. Heterozygosity for a defective gene for CC chemokine receptor 5 is not the sole determinant for the immunologic and virologic phenotype of HIV-infected long term non-progressors. J Clin Invest 100:1581–1589.
73. Eugen-Olsen, J., A.K.N. Iversen, P. Garred, U. Koppelhus, C. Pedersen, T.L. Benfield, A.M. Sorensen. 1997. Heterozygosity for a deletion in the CKR-5 gene leads to prolonged AIDS free survival and slower CD4 T cell fall in a cohort of HIV seropositive individuals. AIDS 11:305–310.
74. Bleul, C., L. Wu, J. Hoxie, T. Springer, C. MacKay. 1997. The HIV coreceptors CXCR4 and CCR5 are differentially expressed and regulated on human T lymphocytes. Proc Natl Acad Sci USA 94:1925–1930.
75. Wu, L., W.A. Paxton, N. Kassam, N. Ruffing, J.B. Rottman, N. Sullivan, H. Choe, J. Sodroski, W. Newman, R.A. Koup, C.R. Mackay. 1997. CCR5 levels and expression pattern correlate wtih infectability by macrophage-tropic HIV-1, in vitro. J Exp Med 185:1681-1692.
76. Picchio, G., R. Gulizia, D. Mosier. 1997. Chemokine receptor CCR5 genotype influences the kinetics of human immunodeficiency virus type 1 infection in human PBL-SCID mice. J Virol 71:7124–7127.
77. Quillent, C., E. Oberlin, J. Braun, D. Rousset, G. Gonzalez-Canali, P. Metais, L. Montagnier, J.L. Virelizier, F. Arenzana-Seisdedos, A. Beretta. 1998. HIV-1-resistance phenotype conferred by combination of two separate inherited mutations of CCR5 gene. Lancet, 351:14–18.

78. Martin, M.P., M. Dean, M.W. Smith, C. Winkler, B. Gerrard, N.L. Michael, B. Lee, R.W. Doms, J. Margolick, S. Buchbinder, J.J. Goedert, T.R. O'Brien, M.W. Hilgartner, D. Vlahov, S.J. O'Brien, M. Carrington. 1998. Genetic acceleration of AIDS progression by a promoter variant of CCR5. Science 282:1907–1911.
79. McDermott, D.H., P.A. Zimmerman, F. Guignard, C.A. Kleeberger, S.F. Leitman, P.M. Murphy. 1998. CCR5 promoter polymorphism and HIV-1 disease progression. Multicenter AIDS Cohort Study (MACS). Lancet 352:866–870.
80. Mummidi, S., S.S. Ahuja, E. Gonzalez, S.A. Anderson, E.N. Santiago, K.T. Stephan, F.E. Craig, P. O'Connell, V. Tryon, R.A. Clark, M.J. Dolan, S.K. Ahuja. 1998. Genealogy of the CCR5 locus and chemokine system gene variants associated with altered rates of HIV-1 disease progression. Nat Med 4:786–793.
81. Gonzalez, E., M. Bamshad, N. Sato, S. Mummidi, R. Dhanda, G. Catano, S. Cabrera, M. McBride, X.H. Cao, G. Merrill, P. O'Connell, D.W. Bowden, B.I. Freedman, S.A. Anderson, E.A. Walter, J.S. Evans, K.T. Stephan, R.A. Clark, S. Tyagi, S.S. Ahuja, M.J. Dolan, S.K. Ahuja. 1999. Race-specific HIV-1 disease-modifying effects associated with CCR5 haplotypes. Proc Natl Acad Sci USA 96:12004–12009.
82. Smith, M.W., M. Dean, M. Carrington, C. Winkler, G.A. Huttley, D.A. Lomb, J.J. Goedert, T.R. O'Brien, L.P. Jacobson, R. Kaslow, S. Buchbinder, E. Vittinghoff, D. Vlahov, K. Hoots, M.W. Hilgartner, S.J. O'Brien. 1997. Contrasting genetic influence of CCR2 and CCR5 variants on HIV-1 infection and disease progression. Hemophilia Growth and Development Study (HGDS), Multicenter AIDS Cohort Study (MACS), Multicenter Hemophilia Cohort Study (MHCS), San Francisco City Cohort (SFCC), ALIVE Study. Science 277:959–965.
83. Kostrikis, L.G., Y. Huang, J.P. Moore, S.M. Wolinsky, L. Zhang, Y. Guo, L. Deutsch, J. Phair, A.U. Neumann, D.D. Ho. 1998. A chemokine receptor CCR2 allele delays HIV-1 disease progression and is associated with a CCR5 promoter mutation. Nat Med 4:350–353.
84. Rizzardi, G.P., R.A. Morawetz, E. Vicenzi, S. Ghezzi, G. Poli, A. Lazzarin, G. Pantaleo. 1998. CCR2 polymorphism and HIV disease. Swiss HIV Cohort. Nat Med 4:252–253.
85. Mellado, M., J.M. Rodriguez-Frade, A.J. Vila-Coro, A.M. de Ana, A.C. Martinez. 1999. Chemokine control of HIV-1 infection. Nature 400:723–724.
86. Liu, H., D. Chao, E.E. Nakayama, H. Taguchi, M. Goto, X. Xin, J.K. Takamatsu, H. Saito, Y. Ishikawa, T. Akaza, T. Juji, Y. Takebe, T. Ohishi, K. Fukutake, Y. Maruyama, S. Yashiki, S. Sonoda, T. Nakamura, Y. Nagai, A. Iwamoto, T. Shioda. 1999. Polymorphism in RANTES chemokine

promoter affects HIV-1 disease progression. Proc Natl Acad Sci USA 96: 4581–4585.

87. Winkler, C., W. Modi, M.W. Smith, G.W. Nelson, X. Wu, M. Carrington, M. Dean, T. Honjo, K. Tashiro, D. Yabe, S. Buchbinder, E. Vittinghoff, J.J. Goedert, O.B. TR, L.P. Jacobson, R. Detels, S. Donfield, A. Willoughby, E. Gomperts, D. Vlahov, J. Phair, O.B. SJ. 1998. Genetic restriction of AIDS pathogenesis by an SDF-1 chemokine gene variant. ALIVE Study, Hemophilia Growth and Development Study (HGDS), Multicenter AIDS Cohort Study (MACS), Multicenter Hemophilia Cohort Study (MHCS), San Francisco City Cohort (SFCC). Science 279: 389–393.
88. Furci, L., G. Scarlatti, S. Burastero, G. Tambussi, C. Colognesi, C. Quillent, R. Longhi, P. Loverro, B. Borgonovo, D. Gaffi, E. Carrow, M. Malnati, P. Lusso, A.G. Siccardi, A. Lazzarin, A. Beretta. 1997. Antigen-driven C-C chemokine-mediated HIV-1 suppression by CD4(+) T cells from exposed uninfected individuals expressing the wild-type CCR- 5 allele. J Exp Med 186:455–460.
89. Scala, E., G. D'Offizi, R. Rosso, O. Turriziani, R. Ferrara, A.M. Mazzone, G. Antonelli, F. Aiuti, R. Paganelli. 1997. C-C chemokines, IL-16, and soluble antiviral factor activity are increased in cloned T cells from subjects with long-term nonprogressive HIV infection. J Immunol 158:4485–4492.
90. Zagury, D., A. Lachgar, V. Chams, L. Fall, J. Bernard, J. Zagury, B. Bizzini, A. Gringeri, E. Santagostino, J. Rappaport, M. Feldman, S. O'Brien, A. Burny, R. Gallo. 1998. C-C chemokines, pivotal in protection against HIV type 1 infection. Proc Natl Acad Sci USA 95:3857–3861.
91. Ullum, H., A. Lepri, J. Victor, H. Aladdin, A. Phillips, J. Gerstoft, P. Skinhoj, B. Pedersen. 1998. Production of beta-chemokines in human immunodeficiency virus (HIV) infection: evidence that high levels of macrophage inflammatory protein-1 beta are associated with a decreased risk of HIV disease progression. J Infect Dis 177:331–336.
92. Saha, K., G. Bentsman, L. Chess, D.J. Volsky. 1998. Endogenous production of beta-chemokines by CD4+, but not CD8+, T-cell clones correlates with the clinical state of human immunodeficiency virus type 1 (HIV-1)-infected individuals and may be responsible for blocking infection with non-syncytium-inducing HIV-1 in vitro. J Virol 72:876–881.
93. Baggiolini, M., B. Moser. 1997. Blocking chemokine receptors. J Exp Med 186:1189–1191.
94. Arenzana-Seisdedos, F., J.-L. Virelizier, D. Rousset, I. Clark-Lewis, P. Loetscher, B. Moser, M. Baggiolini. 1996. HIV blocked by chemokine antagonist. Nature 383:400.
95. Simmons, G., P.R. Clapham, L. Picard, R.E. Offord, M.M. Rosenkilde,

T.W. Schwartz, R. Buser, T.N.C. Wells, A.E.I. Proudfoot. 1997. Potent inhibition of HIV-1 infectivity in macrophages and lymphocytes by a novel CCR5 antagonist. Science 276:276–279.

96. Baba, M., O. Nishimura, N. Kanzaki, M. Okamoto, H. Sawada, Y. Iizawa, M. Shiraishi, Y. Aramaki, K. Okonogi, Y. Ogawa, K. Meguro, M. Fujino. 1999. A small-molecule, nonpeptide CCR5 antagonist with highly potent and selective anti-HIV-1 activity. Proc Natl Acad Sci USA 96:5698–5703.
97. Schols, D., S. Struyf, J. Van Damme, J.A. Este, G. Henson, E. De Clercq. 1997. Inhibition of T-tropic HIV strains by selective antagonization of the chemokine receptor CXCR4. J Exp Med 186:1383–1388.
98. Murakami, T., T. Nakajima, Y. Koyanagi, K. Tachibana, N. Fujii, H. Tamamura, N. Yoshida, M. Waki, A. Matsumoto, O. Yoshie, T. Kishimoto, N. Yamamoto, T. Nagasawa. 1997. A small molecule CXCR4 inhibitor that blocks T-cell line-tropic HIV-1 infection. J Exp Med 186:1389–1393.
99. Doranz, B.J., K. Grovit-Ferbas, M.P. Sharron, S.H. Mao, M.B. Goetz, E.S. Daar, R.W. Doms, O.B. WA. 1997. A small-molecule inhibitor directed against the chemokine receptor CXCR4 prevents its use as an HIV-1 coreceptor. J Exp Med 186:1395–1400.
100. Donzella, G.A., D. Schols, S.W. Lin, J.A. Este, K.A. Nagashima, P.J. Maddon, G.P. Allaway, T.P. Sakmar, G. Henson, E. De Clercq, J.P. Moore. 1998. AMD3100, a small molecule inhibitor of HIV-1 entry via the CXCR4 co- receptor. Nat Med 4:72–77.
101. Yang, A.G., X. Bai, X.F. Huang, C. Yao, S. Chen. 1997. Phenotypic knockout of HIV type 1 chemokine coreceptor CCR-5 by intrakines as potential therapeutic approach for HIV-1 infection. Proc Natl Acad Sci USA 94:11567–11572.
102. Chen, J.D., X. Bai, A.G. Yang, Y. Cong, S.Y. Chen. 1997. Inactivation of HIV-1 chemokine co-receptor CXCR-4 by a novel intrakine strategy. Nat Med 3:1110–1116.
103. Steinberger, P., J. Andris-Widhopf, B. Buhler, B.E. Torbett, C.F. Barbas, 3rd. 2000. Functional deletion of the CCR5 receptor by intracellular immunization produces cells that are refractory to CCR5-dependent HIV-1 infection and cell fusion. Proc Natl Acad Sci USA 97:805–810.
104. Chan, D.C., P.S. Kim. 1998. HIV entry and its inhibition. Cell 93:681–684.
105. Wild, C., T. Oas, C. McDanal, D. Bolognesi, T. Matthews. 1992. A synthetic peptide inhibitor of human immunodeficiency virus replication: correlation between solution structure and viral inhibition. Proc Natl Acad Sci USA 89:10537–10541.
106. Eckert, D.M., V.N. Malashkevich, L.H. Hong, P.A. Carr, P.S. Kim. 1999. Inhibiting HIV-1 entry: discovery of D-peptide inhibitors that target the gp41 coiled-coil pocket. Cell 99:103–115.

107. Kilby, J.M., S. Hopkins, T.M. Venetta, B. DiMassimo, G.A. Cloud, J.Y. Lee, L. Alldredge, E. Hunter, D. Lambert, D. Bolognesi, T. Matthews, M.R. Johnson, M.A. Nowak, G.M. Shaw, M.S. Saag. 1998. Potent suppression of HIV-1 replication in humans by T-20, a peptide inhibitor of gp41-mediated virus entry. Nat Med 4:1302–1307.
108. Spira, A.I., P.A. Marx, B.K. Patterson, J. Mahoney, R.A. Koup, S.M. Wolinsky, D.D. Ho. 1996. Cellular targets of infection and route of viral dissemination after an intravaginal inoculation of simian immunodeficiency virus into rhesus macaques. J Exp Med 183:215–225.
109. Weissman, D., Y. Li, J. Ananworanich, L.J. Zhou, J. Adelsberger, T.F. Tedder, M. Baseler, A.S. Fauci. 1995. Three populations of cells with dendritic morphology exist in peripheral blood, only one of which is infectable with human immunodeficiency virus type 1. Proc Natl Acad Sci USA 92:826–830.
110. Geijtenbeek, T.B.H., R. Torensma, S.J. van Vliet, G.C.F. van Duijnhoven, G.J. Adema, Y. van Kooyk, C.G. Figdor. 2000. Identification of DC-SIGN, a novel dendritic cell-specific ICAM-3 receptor that supports primary immune responses. Cell 100:575–585.
111. Geijtenbeek, T.B.H., D.S. Kwon, R. Torensma, S.J. van Vliet, G.C.F. van Duijnhoven, J. Middel, I.L.M.H.A. Cornelissen, H.S.L.M. Nottet, V.N. KewalRamani, D.R. Littman, C.G. Figdor, Y. van Kooyk. 2000. DC-SIGN, a dendritic cell-specific HIV-1-binding protein that enhances trans-infection of T-cells. Cell 100:587–597.
112. Pope, M., M.G. Betjes, N. Romani, H. Hirmand, P.U. Cameron, L. Hoffman, S. Gezelter, G. Schuler, R.M. Steinman. 1994. Conjugates of dendritic cells and memory T lymphocytes from skin facilitate productive infection with HIV-1. Cell 78:389–398.
113. Frankel, S.S., B.M. Wenig, A.P. Burke, P. Mannan, L.D. Thompson, S.L. Abbondanzo, A.M. Nelson, M. Pope, R.M. Steinman. 1996. Replication of HIV-1 in dendritic cell-derived syncytia at the mucosal surface of the adenoid. Science 272:115–117.
114. York-Higgins, D., C. Cheng-Mayer, D. Bauer, J.A. Levy, D. Dina. 1990. Human immunodeficiency virus type 1 cellular host range, replication, cytopathicity are linked to the envelope region of the viral genome. J Virol 64:4016–4020.
115. Hwang, S.S., T.J. Boyle, H.K. Lyerly, B.R. Cullen. 1991. Identification of the envelope V3 loop as the primary determinant of cell tropism in HIV-1. Science 253:71–74.
116. Takeuchi, Y., M. Akutsu, K. Murayama, N. Shimuzu, H. Hoshino. 1991. Host range mutant of human immunodeficiency virus type 1: modification of cell tropism by a single point mutation at the neutralization epitope in the env gene. J Virol 65:1710–1718.

117. Cheng-Mayer, C., T. Shioda, J.A. Levy. 1991. Host range, replicative, and cytopathic properties of human immunodeficiency virus type 1 are determined by a very few amino acid changes in tat and gp120. J Virol 65:6931–6941.
118. Tersmette, M., J.M.A. Lange, R.E.Y. DeGoede, F. DeWolf, J.K.M. Eeftink-Schattenkerk, P.T.A. Schellekens, R.A. Coutinho, J.G. Huisman, J. Goudsmit, F. Miedema. 1989. Association between biological properties of human immunodeficiency virus variants and risk for AIDS and AIDS mortality. Lancet i:983–985.
119. Tersmette, M., R.A. Gruters, F. DeWolf, R.E.Y. DeGoede, J.M.A. Lange, P.T.A. Schellekens, J. Goudsmit, H.G. Huisman, F. Miedema. 1989. Evidence for a role of virulent human immunodeficiency virus (HIV) variants in the pathogenesis of acquired immunodeficiency syndrome: studies on sequential HIV isolates. J Virol 63:2118-2125.
120. Cheng-Mayer, C., D. Seto, M. Tateno, J.A. Levy. 1988. Biologic features of HIV-1 that correlate with virulence in the host. Science 240:80–82.
121. Koot, M., I.P.M. Keet, A.H.V. Vos, R.E.Y. deGoede, M.T.H.L. Roos, R.A. Coutinho, F. Miedema, P.T.H.A. Schellekens, M. Tersmette. 1993. Prognostic value of HIV-1 syncytium-inducing phenotype for rate of CD4+ cell depletion and progression to AIDS. Ann Intern Med 118:681–688.
122. Fouchier, R.A., M. Groenink, N.A. Koostra, M. Tersmette, H.G. Huisman, F. Miedema, H. Schuitemaker. 1992. Phenotype-associated sequence variation in the third variable domain of the human immunodeficiency virus type 1 gp120 molecule. J Virol 66:3183–3187.
123. Bhattacharyya, D., B.R. Brooks, L. Callahan. 1996. Positioning of positively charged residues in the V3 loop correlates with HIV type 1 syncytium-inducing phenotype. AIDS Res Hum Retroviruses 12:83–90.
124. Dybul, M., D. Weissman, A. Rubbert, E. Machado, M. Cohn, L. Ehler, O.C. M, S. Mizell, A.S. Fauci. 1998. The role of dendritic cells in the infection of CD4+ T cells with the human immunodeficiency virus: use of dendritic cells from individuals homozygous for the delta32CCR5 allele as a model. AIDS Res Hum Retroviruses 14:1109–1113.
125. Chakrabarti, L., P. Isola, M. Cumont, M. Claessens-Maire, M. Hurtrel, L. Montagnier. 1994. Early stages of simian immunodeficiency virus infection in lymph nodes. Evidence for high viral load and successive populations of target cells. Am J Pathol 144:1226–1237.
126. Reimann, K.A., K. Tenner-Racz, P. Racz. 1994. Immunopathogenic events in acute infection of rhesus monkeys with simian immunodeficiency virus of Macaques. J Virol 68:2362–2370.
127. Clark, S.J., M.S. Saag, W.D. Decker, S. Campbell-Hill, J.L. Roberson,

P.J. Veldkamp, J.C. Kappes, B.H. Hahn, G.M. Shaw. 1991. High titers of cytopathic virus in plasma of patients with symptomatic primary HIV-1 infection. N Engl J Med 324:954–960.

128. Daar, E.S., T. Moudgil, R.D. Meyer, D.D. Ho. 1991. Transient high levels of viremia in patients with primary human immunodeficiency virus type 1 infection. N Engl J Med 324:961–964.
129. Graziosi, C., G. Pantaleo, L. Butini, J.F. Demarest, M.S. Saag, G.M. Shaw, A.S. Fauci. 1993. Kinetics of human immunodeficiency virus type 1 (HIV-1) DNA and RNA synthesis during primary HIV-1 infection. Proc Natl Acad Sci USA 90:6405–6409.
130. Koup, R.A., J.T. Safrit, Y. Cao, C.A. Andrews, G. McLeod, W. Borkowsky, C. Farthing, D.D. Ho. 1994. Temporal association of cellular immune resposnes with the initial control of viremia in primary human immunodeficiency virus type 1 syndrome. J Virol 68:4650–4655.
131. Borrow, P., H. Lewicki, B.H. Hahn, G.M. Shaw, M.B.A. Oldstone. 1994. Virus-specific CD8+ cytotoxic T-lymphocyte activity associated with control of viremia in primary human immunodeficiency virus type 1 infection. J Virol 68:6103–6110.
132. Pantaleo, G., O.J. Cohen, T. Schacker, M. Vaccarezza, C. Graziosi, G.P. Rizzardi, J. Kahn, C.H. Fox, S.M. Schnittman, D.H. Schwartz, L. Corey, A.S. Fauci. 1998. Evolutionary pattern of human immunodeficiency virus (HIV) replication and distribution in lymph nodes following primary infection: implications for antiviral therapy. Nat Med 4:341–345.
133. Schacker, T., S. Little, E. Connick, K. Gebhard-Mitchell, Z.Q. Zhang, J. Krieger, J. Pryor, D. Havlir, J.K. Wong, D. Richman, L. Corey, A.T. Haase. 2000. Rapid accumulation of human immunodeficiency virus (HIV) in lymphatic tissue reservoirs during ccute and early HIV infection: implications for timing of antiretroviral therapy. J Infect Dis. 181:354–357.
134. Fox, C., K. Tenner-Rácz, P. Rácz, A. Firpo, P. Pizzo, A. Fauci. 1991. Lymphoid germinal centers are reservoirs of human immunodeficiency virus type 1 RNA. J Infect Dis 164:1051–1057.
135. Spiegel, H., H. Herbst, G. Niedobitek, H. Foss, H. Stein. 1992. Follicular dendritic cells are a major reservoir for human immunodeficiency virus type 1 in lymphoid tissues facilitating infection of CD4+ T-helper cells. Am J Pathol 140:15–22.
136. Joling, P., L. Bakker, J. Van Strijp, T. Meerloo, L. de Graaf, M. Dekker, J. Goudsmit, J. Verhoef, H. Schuurman. 1993. Binding of human immunodeficiency virus type-1 to follicular dendritic cells in vitro is complement dependent. J Immunol 150:1065–1073.
137. Pantaleo, G., C. Graziosi, J.F. Demarest, L. Butini, M. Montroni, C.H.

Fox, J.M. Orenstein, D.P. Kotler, A.S. Fauci. 1993. HIV infection is active and progressive in lymphoid tissue during the clinically latent stage of disease. Nature 362:355–358.
138. Embretson, J., M. Zupancic, J. Ribas, A. Burke, P. Rácz, K. Tenner-Rácz, A. Haase. 1993. Massive covert infection of helper T lymphocytes and macrophages by HIV during the incubation period of AIDS. Nature 362: 359–362.
139. Heath, S.L., J.G. Tew, J.G. Tew, A.K. Szakal, G.F. Burton. 1995. Follicular dendritic cells and human immunodeficiency virus infectivity. Nature 377:740–744.
140. Chun, T.-W., L. Carruth, D. Finzi, X. Shen, J.A. DiGiuseppe, H. Taylor, M. Hermankova, K. Chadwick, J. Margolick, T.C. Quinn, Y.-H. Kuo, R. Brookmeyer, M.A. Zeiger, P. Barditch-Crovo, R.F. Siliciano. 1997. Quantification of latent tissue reservoirs and total body viral load in HIV infection. Nature 387:183–187.
141. Chun, T.W., D. Finzi, J. Margolick, K. Chadwick, D. Schwartz, R.F. Siliciano. 1995. In vivo fate of HIV-1-infected T cells: quantitative analysis of the transition to stable latency. Nat Med 1:1284–1290.
142. Hufert, F.T., J. vanLunzen, G. Janossy, S. Bertram, J. Schmitz, O. Haller, P. Racz, D. vonLaer. 1997. Germinal center CD4+ T-cells are an important site of HIV replication in vivo. AIDS 11:849–857.
143. Lyerly, H.K., O.J. Cohen, K.J. Weinhold. 1987. Transmission of HIV by antigen presenting cells during T-cell activation: prevention by 3′-azido-3′-deoxythymidine. AIDS Res Hum Retroviruses 3:87–94.
144. Margolick, J.B., D.J. Volkman, T.M. Folks, A.S. Fauci. 1987. Amplification of HTLV-III/LAV infection by antigen-induced activation of T-cells and direct suppression by virus of lymphocyte blastogenic responses. J Immunol 138:1719–1723.
145. Ascher, M., H. Sheppard. 1988. AIDS as immune system activation: a model for pathogenesis. Clin Exp Immunol 73:165–167.
146. Weissman, D., T.D. Barker, A.S. Fauci. 1996. The efficiency of acute infection of CD4+ T cells is markedly enhanced in the setting of antigen-specific immune activation. J Exp Med 183:687–692.
147. Folks, T.M., J. Justement, A. Kinter, C.A. Dinarello, A.S. Fauci. 1987. Cytokine-induced expression of HIV-1 in a chronically infected promonocyte cell line. Science 238:800–802.
148. Nabel, G., D. Baltimore. 1987. An inducible transcription factor activates expression of human immunodeficiency virus in T-cells. Nature 326:711–713.
149. Zack, J.A., S.J. Arrigo, S.R. Weitsman, A.S. Go, A. Haislip, I.S. Chen. 1990. HIV-1 entry into quiescent primary lymphocytes: molecular analysis reveals a labile, latent viral structure. Cell 61:213–222.

150. Stevenson, M., T.L. Stanwick, M.P. Dempsey, C.A. Lamonica. 1990. HIV-1 replication is controlled at the level of T-cell activation and proviral integration. Embo J 9:1551–1560.
151. Bukrinsky, M., T. Stanwick, M. Dempsey, M. Stevenson. 1991. Quiescent T lymphocytes as an inducible virus reservoir in HIV-1 infection. Science 254:423–427.
152. O'Brien, W.A., K. Grovit-Ferbas, A. Namazi, S. Ovcak-Derzic, H.J. Wang, J. Park, C. Yeramian, S.H. Mao, J.A. Zack. 1995. Human immunodeficiency virus-type 1 replication can be increased in peripheral blood of seropositive patients after influenza vaccination. Blood 86:1082–1089.
153. Staprans, S., B. Hamilton, S. Follansbee, T. Elbeik, P. Barbosa, R. Grant, M. Feinberg. 1995. Activation of virus replication after vaccination of HIV-1-infected individuals. J Exp Med 182:1727–1737.
154. Stanley, S., M.A. Ostrowski, J.S. Justement, K. Gantt, S. Hedayati, M. Mannix, K. Roche, D.J. Schwartzentruber, C.H. Fox, A.S. Fauci. 1996. Effect of immunization with a common recall antigen on viral expression in patients infected with human immunodeficiency virus type 1. N Engl J Med 334:1222–1230.
155. Ott, M., S. Emiliani, C. VanLint, G. Herbein, J. Lovett, N. Chirmule, T. McCloskey, S. Pahwa, E. Verdin. 1997. Immune hyperactivation of HIV-1-infected T-cells mediated by tat and the CD28 pathway. Science 275: 1481–1485.
156. Schrager, J.A., J.W. Marsh. 1999. HIV-1 Nef increases T cell activation in a stimulus-dependent manner. Proc Natl Acad Sci USA 96:8167–8172.
157. Westermann, J., S. Persin, J. Matyas, P. van der Meide, R. Pabst. 1994. Migration of so-called naive and memory T lymphocytes from blood to lymph in the rat. The influence of IFN-gamma on the circulation pattern. J Immunol 152:1744–1750.
158. Rosenberg, Y.J., A. Cafaro, T. Brennan, J.G. Greenhouse, F. Villinger, A.A. Ansari, C. Brown, K. McKinnon, S. Bellah, J. Yalley-Ogunro, W.R. Elkins, S. Gartner, M.G. Lewis. 1997. Virus-induced cytokines regulate circulating lymphocyte levels during primary SIV infections. Int Immunol 9:703–712.
159. Pantaleo, G., C. Graziosi, L. Butini, P. Pizzo, S. Schnittman, D. Kotler, A. Fauci. 1991. Lymphoid organs function as major reservoirs for human immunodeficiency virus. Proc Natl Acad Sci 88:9838–9842.
160. Cohen, O., G. Pantaleo, M. Holodniy, C. Fox, J. Orenstein, S. Schnittman, M. Niu, C. Graziosi, G. Pavlakis, J. Lalezari, J. Bartlett, R. Steigbigel, J. Cohn, R. Novak, D. McMahon, J. Bilello, A. Fauci. 1996. Antiretroviral monotherapy in early stage human immunodeficiency virus disease has no detectable effect on virus load in peripheral blood and lymph nodes. J Infect Dis 173:849–856.

161. Cohen, O.J., G. Pantaleo, M. Holodniy, S. Schnittman, M. Niu, C. Graziosi, G.N. Pavlakis, J. Lalezari, J.A. Bartlett, R.T. Steigbigel, J. Cohn, R. Novak, D. McMahon, A.S. Fauci. 1995. Decreased HIV-1 plasma viremia during antiretroviral therapy reflects downregulation of viral replication in lymphoid tissue. Proc Natl Acad Sci USA 92:6017–6021.
162. Lafeuillade, A., C. Poggi, N. Profizi, C. Tamalet, O. Costes. 1996. Human immunodeficiency virus type 1 kinetics in lymph nodes compared with plasma. J Infect Dis. 174:404–407.
163. Haase, A.T., K. Henry, M. Zupancic, G. Sedgewick, R.A. Faust, H. Melroe, W. Cavert, K. Gebhard, K. Staskus, Z.-Q. Zhang, P.J. Dailey, H.H. Balfour, A. Erice, A.S. Perelson. 1996. Quantitative image analysis of HIV-1 infection in lymphoid tissue. Science 274:985–989.
164. Cavert, W., D.W. Notermans, K. Staskus, S.W. Wietgrefe, M. Zupancic, K. Gebhard, K. Henry, Z.-Q. Zhang, R. Mills, H. McDade, J. Goudsmit, S.A. Danner, A.T. Haase. 1997. Kinetics of response in lymphoid tissues to antiretroviral therapy of HIV-1 infection. Science 276:960–963.
165. Biberfeld, P., K. Chayt, L. Marselle, G. Biberfeld, R. Gallo, M. Harper. 1986. HTLV-III expression in infected lymph nodes and relevance to pathogenesis of lymphadenopathy. Am J Pathol 125:436–442.
166. Racz, P., K. Tenner-Racz, C. Kahl, A.C. Feller, P. Kern, M. Dietrich. 1986. Spectrum of morphologic changes of lymph nodes from patients with AIDS or AIDS-related complexes. Prog Allergy 37:81–181.
167. Pallesen, G., J. Gerstoft, L. Mathiesen. 1987. Stages in LAV/HTLV-III lymphadenitis: I. Histological and immunohistological classification. Scand J Immunol 25:83–91.
168. Turner, R., A. Levine, P. Gill, J. Parker, P. Meyer. 1987. Progressive histopathologic abnormalities in the persistent generalized lymphadenopathy syndrome. Am J Surg Pathol 11:625–632.
169. Fujiwara, M., R. Tsunoda, S. Shigeta, T. Yokota, M. Baba. 1999. Human follicular dendritic cells remain uninfected and capture human immunodeficiency virus type 1 through CD54-CD11a interaction. J Virol 73:3603–3607.
170. Ioachim, H.L., C.W. Lerner, M.L. Tapper. 1983. The lymphoid lesions associated with the acquired immunodeficiency syndrome. Am J Surg Pathol 7:543–553.
171. Fernandez, R., J. Mouradian, C. Metroka, J. Davies. 1983. The prognostic value of histopathology in persistent generalized lymphadenopathy in homosexual men. N Engl J Med 309:185–186.
172. Janossy, G., A.J. Pinching, M. Bofill, J. Weber, J.E. McLaughlin, M. Ornstein, K. Ivory, J.R. Harris, M. Favrot, D.C. MacDonald-Burns. 1985. An immunohistological approach to persistent lymphadenopathy and its relevance to AIDS. Clin Exp Immunol 59:257–266.

173. Tew, J.G., G.F. Burton, L.I. Kupp, A. Szakal. 1993. Follicular dendritic cells in germinal center reactions. Adv Exp Med Biol 329:461–465.

174. Pantaleo, G., C. Graziosi, J. Demarest, O. Cohen, M. Vaccarezza, K. Gantt, C. Muro-Cacho, A. Fauci. 1994. Role of lymphoid organs in the pathogenesis of human immunodeficiency virus (HIV) infection. Immunol Rev 140:105–130.

175. Sprenger, R., K.M. Toellner, C. Schmetz, W. Luke, C. Stahl-Hennig, M. Ernst, G. Hunsmann, H. Schmitz, H.D. Flad, J. Gerdes, J.P. Zimmer. 1995. Follicular dendritic cells productively infected with immunodeficiency viruses transmit infection to T-cells. Med Microbiol Immunol 184:129–134.

176. Schmitz, J., J. van Lunzen, K. Tenner-Racz, G. Groβschupff, P. Racz, H. Schmitz, M. Dietrich, F. Hufert. 1994. Follicular dendritic cells retain HIV-1 particles on their plasma membrane, but are not productively infected in asymptomatic patients with follicular hyperplasia. J Immunol 153:1352–1359.

177. Zhang, Z.Q., T. Schuler, W. Cavert, D.W. Notermans, K. Gebhard, K. Henry, D.V. Havlir, H.F. Gunthard, J.K. Wong, S. Little, M.B. Feinberg, M.A. Polis, L.K. Schrager, T.W. Schacker, D.D. Richman, L. Corey, S.A. Danner, A.T. Haase. 1999. Reversibility of the pathological changes in the follicular dendritic cell network with treatment of HIV-1 infection. Proc Natl Acad Sci USA 96:5169–5172.

178. Orcnstcin, J.M., M. Feinberg, C. Yoder, L. Schrager, J. Mican, D.J. Schwartzentruber, R.T.J. Davey, R.E. Walker, J. Falloon, J.A. Kovacs, C. Fox, J. Metcalf, H. Masur, M.A. Polis. 1999. Lymph node architecture preceding and following potent antiviral therapy: follicular hyperplasia persists in parallel with p24 antigen. Restoration after lymph node involution and CD4 cell depletion in an AIDS patient. AIDS 13:2219–2229.

179. Sei, Y., P.H. Tsang, F.N. Chu, I. Wallace, J.P. Roboz, P.S. Sarin, J.G. Bekesi. 1989. Inverse relationship between HIV-1 p24 antigenemia, anti-p24 antibody and neutralizing antibody response in all stages of HIV-1 infection. Immunol Lett 20:223–230.

180. Allain, J.P., Y. Laurian, D.A. Paul, D. Senn. 1986. Serological markers in early stages of human immunodeficiency virus infection in haemophiliacs. Lancet 2:1233–1236.

181. Paul, D.A., L.A. Falk, H.A. Kessler, R.M. Chase, B. Blaauw, D.S. Chudwin, A.L. Landay. 1987. Correlation of serum HIV antigen and antibody with clinical status in HIV-infected patients. J Med Virol 22:357–363.

182. Weber, J.N., P.R. Clapham, R.A. Weiss, D. Parker, C. Roberts, J. Duncan, I. Weller, C. Carne, R.S. Tedder, A.J. Pinching. 1987. Human immunodeficiency virus infection in two cohorts of homosexual men: neutralizing sera and association of anti-gag antibody with prognosis. Lancet 1:119–122.

183. Hogervorst, E., S. Jurriaans, F. deWolf, A. vanWijk, A. Wiersma, M. Valk, M. Roos, B. vanGemen, R. Coutinho, F. Miedema, J. Goudsmit. 1995. Predictors for non- and slow progression in human immunodeficiency virus (HIV) type 1 infection: low viral RNA copy numbers in serum and maintenance of high HIV-1 p24-specific but not V3-specific antibody levels. J Infect Dis 171:811–821.
184. Goudsmit, J., C. Debouck, R.H. Meloen, L. Smit, M. Bakker, D.M. Asher, A.V. Wolff, C.J. Gibbs, D.C. Gajdusek. 1988. Human immunodeficiency virus type 1 neutralization epitope with conserved architecture elicits early type-specific antibodies in experimentally infected chimpanzees. Proc Natl Acad Sci USA 85:4478–4482.
185. Freed, E.O., D.J. Myers, R. Risser. 1991. Identification of the principal neutralizing determinant of human immunodeficiency virus type 1 as a fusion domain. J Virol 65:190–194.
186. Muster, T., F. Steindl, M. Purtscher, A. Trkola, A. Klima, G. Himmler, F. Ruker, H. Katinger. 1993. A conserved neutralizing epitipe on gp41 of human immunodeficiency virus type 1. J Virol 67:6642–6647.
187. Steimer, K.S., C. Scandella, P.V. Skiles, N.L. Haigwood. 1991. Neutralization of divergent HIV-1 isolates by conformation-dependent human antiodies to Gp120. Science 254:105–108.
188. Hansen, J.E., H. Clausen, C. Nielsen, L.S. Teglbjaerg, L.L. Hansen, C.M. Nielsen, D. Dabelsteen, L. Mathiesen, S.I. Hakomori, J.O. Nielsen. 1990. Inhibition of human immunodeficiency virus (HIV) infection in vitro by anticarbohydrate monoclonal antibodies: peripheral glycosylation of HIV envelope glycoprotein gp120 may be a target for virus neutralization. J Virol 64:2833–2340.
189. Bou-Habib, D.C., G. Roderiquez, T. Oravecz, P.W. Berman, P. Lusso, M.A. Norcross. 1994. Cryptic nature of envelope V3 region epitopes protects primary monocytotropic human imunodeficiency virus type 1 from antibody neutralization. J Virol 68:6006–6013.
190. Sullivan, N., Y. Sun, J. Li, W. Hofmann, J. Sodroski. 1995. Replicative function and neutralization sensitivity of envelope glycoproteins from primary and T-cell line-passaged human immunodeficiency virus type 1 isolates. J Virol 69:4413–4422.
191. Sei, Y., P.H. Tsang, J.P. Roboz, P.S. Sarin, J.I. Wallace, J.G. Bekesi. 1988. Neutralizing antibodies as a prognostic indicator in the progression of acquired immune deficiency syndrome (AIDS)-related disorders: a double-blind study. J Clin Immunol 8:464–472.
192. Montefiori, D.C., G. Pantaleo, L.M. Fink, J.T. Zhou, J.Y. Zhou, M. Bilska, G.D. Miralles, A.S. Fauci. 1996. Neutralizing and infection-enhancing antibody responses to human immunodeficiency virus type 1 in long-term nonprogressors. J Infect Dis 173:60–67.

193. Pilgrim, A.K., G. Pantaleo, O.J. Cohen, L.M. Fink, J.Y. Zhou, J.T. Zhou, D.P. Bolognesi, A.S. Fauci, D.C. Montefiori. 1997. Neutralizing antibody responses to human immunodeficiency virus type 1 in primary infection and long-term-nonprogressive infection. J Infect Dis 176:924–932.
194. Albert, J., B. Abrahamsson, K. Nagy, E. Aurelius, H. Gaines, G. Nystrom, E.M. Fenyo. 1990. Rapid development of isolate-specific neutralizing antibodies after primary HIV-1 infection and consequent emergence of virus variants which resist neutralization by autologous sera. AIDS 4:107–112.
195. Fenyo, E.M., P. Putkonen. 1996. Broad cross-neutralizing activity in serum is associated with slow progression and low risk of transmission in primate lentivirus infections. Immunol Lett 51:95–99.
196. Igarashi, T., C. Brown, A. Azadegan, N. Haigwood, D. Dimitrov, M.A. Martin, R. Shibata. 1999. Human immunodeficiency virus type 1 neutralizing antibodies accelerate clearance of cell-free virions from blood plasma. Nat Med 5:211–216.
197. Shibata, R., T. Igarashi, N. Haigwood, A. Buckler-White, R. Ogert, W. Ross, R. Willey, M.W. Cho, M.A. Martin. 1999. Neutralizing antibody directed against the HIV-1 envelope glycoprotein can completely block HIV-1/SIV chimeric virus infections of macaque monkeys. Nat Med 5: 204–210.
198. Mascola, J.R., M.G. Lewis, G. Stiegler, D. Harris, T.C. VanCott, D. Hayes, M.K. Louder, C.R. Brown, C.V. Sapan, S.S. Frankcl, Y. Lu, M.L. Robb, H. Katinger, D.L. Birx. 1999. Protection of Macaques against pathogenic simian/human immunodeficiency virus 89.6PD by passive transfer of neutralizing antibodies. J Virol 73:4009–4018.
199. Mascola, J.R., G. Stiegler, T.C. VanCott, H. Katinger, C.B. Carpenter, C.E. Hanson, H. Beary, D. Hayes, S.S. Frankel, D.L. Birx, M.G. Lewis. 2000. Protection of macaques against vaginal transmission of a pathogenic HIV- 1/SIV chimeric virus by passive infusion of neutralizing antibodies. Nat Med 6:207–210.
200. Baba, T.W., V. Liska, R. Hofmann-Lehmann, J. Vlasak, W. Xu, S. Ayehunie, L.A. Cavacini, M.R. Posner, H. Katinger, G. Stiegler, B.J. Bernacky, T.A. Rizvi, R. Schmidt, L.R. Hill, M.E. Keeling, Y. Lu, J.E. Wright, T.C. Chou, R.M. Ruprecht. 2000. Human neutralizing monoclonal antibodies of the IgG1 subtype protect against mucosal simian-human immunodeficiency virus infection. Nat Med 6:200–206.
201. Lyerly, H.K., T.J. Matthews, A.J. Langlois, D.P. Bolognesi, K.J. Weinhold. 1987. Human T-cell lymphotropic virus IIIB glycoprotein (gp120) bound to CD4 determinants on normal lymphocytes and expressed by infected cells serves as target for immune attack. Proc Natl Acad Sci USA 84:4601–4605.
202. Ojo-Amaize, E.A., P. Nishanian, D.E. Keith, R.L. Houghton, D.F. Heitjan,

J.L. Fahey, J.V. Giorgi. 1987. Antibodies to human immunodeficiency virus in human sera induce cell-mediated lysis of human immunodeficiency virus-infected cells. J Immunol 139:2458–2463.

203. Tyler, D.S., C.L. Nastala, S.D. Stanley, T.J. Matthews, H.K. Lyerly, D.P. Bolognesi, D.J. Weinhold. 1989. GP120 specific cellular cytotoxicity in HIV-1 seropositive individuals. Evidence for circulating CD16+ effector cells armed in vivo and cytophilic antibody. J Immunol 142:1177–1182.

204. Jewett, A., J.V. Giorgi, B. Bonavida. 1990. Antibody-dependent cellular cytoxicity against HIV-coated target cells by peripheral blood monocytes from HIV seropositive asymptomatic patients. J Immunol 145:4065–4071.

205. Ljunggren, K., A. Karlson, E.M. Fenyo, J. Jondal. 1989. Natural and antibody-dependent cytotoxicity in different clinical stage of human immunodeficiency virus type 1 infection. Clin Exp Immunol 75:184–189.

206. Skowron, G., B. Cole, D. Zheng, G. Accetta, B. Yen-Lieberman. 1997. gp120-directed antibody-dependent cellular cytotoxicity as a major determinant of the rate of decline in CD4 percentage in HIV-1 disease. AIDS 11:1807–1814.

207. Walker, B.D., S. Chakrabarti, B. Moss, T.J. Paradis, T. Flynn, A.G. Durno, R.S. Blumberg, J.C. Kaplan, M.S. Hirsch, R.T. Schooley. 1987. HIV-specific cytotoxic T lymphocytes in seropositive individuals. Nature 328: 345–348.

208. Plata, F., B. Autran, L.P. Martins, S. Wain-Hobson, M. Raphael, C. Mayaud, M. Denis, J.M. Guillon, P. Debre. 1987. AIDS virus-specific cytotoxic T lymphocytes in lung disorders. Nature 328:348–351.

209. Hoffenbach, A., P. Langlade-Demoyen, G. Dadaglio, E. Vilmer, F. Michel, C. Mayaud, B. Autran, F. Plata. 1989. Unusually high frequencies of HIV-specific cytotoxic T lymphocytes in humans. J Immunol 142:452–462.

210. Moss, P.A., S.L. Rowland-Jones, P.M. Frodsham, S. McAdam, P. Grangrande, A.J. McMichael, J.I. Bell. 1995. Persistent high frequency of human immunodeficiency virus-specific cytotoxic T cells in peripheral blood of infected donors. Proc Natl Acad Sci USA 92:5773–5777.

211. Altman, J.D., P.A.H. Moss, P.J.R. Goulder, D.H. Barouch, M.G. McHeyzer-Williams, J.I. Bell, A.J. McMichael, M.M. Davis. 1996. Phenotypic analysis of antigen-specific T lymphocytes. Science 274:94–96.

212. Ogg, G., X. Jin, S. Bonhoeffer, P. Dunbar, M. Nowak, S. Monard, J. Segal, Y. Cao, S. Rowland-Jones, V. Cerundolo, A. Hurley, M. Markowitz, D. Ho, D. Nixon, A. McMichael. 1998. Quantitation of HIV-1 specific cytotoxic T lymphocytes and plasma load of viral RNA. Science 279:2103–2106.

213. Musey, L., J. Hughes, T. Schacker, T. Shea, L. Corey, M.J. McElrath.

1997. Cytotoxic-T-cell responses, viral load, and disease progression in early human immunodeficiency virus type 1 infection. N Engl J Med 337: 1267–1274.
214. Pantaleo, G., S. Menzo, M. Vaccarezza, C. Graziosi, O.J. Cohen, J.F. Demarest, D. Montefiori, J.M. Orenstein, C. Fox, L.K. Schrager, J.B. Margolick, S. Buchbinder, J.V. Giorgi, A.S. Fauci. 1995. Studies in subject with long-term nonprogressive human immunodeficiency virus infection. N Engl J Med 332:209–216.
215. Klein, M.R., C.A. vanBaalen, A.M. Holwerda, S.R.K. Garde, R.J. Bende, I.P.M. Keet, J.-K.M. Eeftinck-Schattenkerk, A.D.M.E. Osterhaus, H. Schuitmaker, F. Miedema. 1995. Kinetics of gag-specific cytotoxic T lymphocyte responses during the clinical course of HIV-1 infection: a longitudinal analysis of rapid progressors and long-term asymptomatics. J Exp Med 181:1365–1372.
216. Rinaldo, C., X.-L. Huang, Z. Fan, M. Ding, L. Beltz, A. Logar, D. Panicali, G. Mazzara, J. Liebmann, M. Cottrill, P. Gupta. 1995. High levels of anti-human immunodeficiency virus type 1 (HIV-1) memory cytotoxic T-lymphocyte activity and low viral load are associated with lack of disease in HIV-1-infected long-term nonprogressors. J Virol 69:5838–5842.
217. Rowland-Jones, S., J. Sutton, K. Ariyoshi, T. Dong, F. Gotch, S. McAdam, D. Whitby, S. Sabally, A. Gallimore, T. Corrah, M. Takiguchi, T. Schultz, A. McMichael, H. Whittle. 1995. HIV-specific cytotoxic T-cells in HIV exposed but uninfected Gambian women. Nat Med 1:59–64.
218. Rowland-Jones, S.L., T. Dong, K.R. Fowke, J. Kimani, P. Krausa, H. Newell, T. Blanchard, K. Ariyoshi, J. Oyugi, E. Ngugi, J. Bwayo, K.S. MacDonald, A.J. McMichael, F.A. Plummer. 1998. Cytotoxic T cell responses to multiple conserved HIV epitopes in HIV- resistant prostitutes in Nairobi. J Clin Invest 102:1758–1765.
219. Tenner-Racz, K., P. Racz, C. Thome, C.G. Meyer, P.J. Anderson, S.F. Schlossman, N.L. Letvin. 1993. Cytotoxic effector cell granules recognized by the monoclonal antibody TIA-1 are present in CD8+ lymphocytes in lymph nodes of human immunodeficiency virus-1-infected patients. Am J Pathol 142:1750–1758.
220. Schmitz, J.E., M.J. Kuroda, S. Santra, V.G. Sasseville, M.A. Simon, M.A. Lifton, P. Racz, K. Tenner-Racz, M. Dalesandro, B.J. Scallon, J. Ghrayeb, M.A. Forman, D.C. Montefiori, E.P. Rieber, N.L. Letvin, K.A. Reimann. 1999. Control of viremia in simian immunodeficiency virus infection by CD8+ lymphocytes. Science 283:857–860.
221. Matano, T., R. Shibata, C. Siemon, M. Connors, H.C. Lane, M.A. Martin. 1998. Administration of an anti-CD8 monoclonal antibody interferes with the clearance of chimeric simian/human immunodeficiency virus during primary infections of rhesus macaques. J Virol 72:164–169.

222. Jin, X., D.E. Bauer, S.E. Tuttleton, S. Lewin, A. Gettie, J. Blanchard, C.E. Irwin, J.T. Safrit, J. Mittler, L. Weinberger, L.G. Kostrikis, L. Zhang, A.S. Perelson, D.D. Ho. 1999. Dramatic rise in plasma viremia after CD8(+) T-cell depletion in simian immunodeficiency virus-infected macaques. J Exp Med 189:991–998.
223. Riviere, Y., M.B. McChesney, F. Porrot, F. Tanneau-Salvadori, P. Sansonetti, O. Lopez, G. Pialoux, V. Feuillie, M. Mollereau, S. Chamaret, F. Tekaia, L. Montagnier. 1995. Gag-specific cytotoxic responses to HIV type 1 are associated with a decreased risk of progression to AIDS-related complex or AIDS. AIDS Res Hum Retroviruses. 11:903–907.
224. Goulder, P.J., M. Bunce, P. Krausa, K. McIntyre, S. Crowley, B. Morgan, A. Edwards, P. Giangrande, R.E. Philips, A.J. McMichael. 1996. Novel, cross-restricted, conserved, and immunodominant cytotoxic T lymphocyte epitopes in slow progressors in HIV type 1 infection. AIDS Res Hum Retroviruses. 12:1691–1698.
225. Klein, M.R., I.P.M. Keet, J. D'Amaro, R.J. Bende, A. Hekman, B. Mesman, M. Koot, L.P. deWaal, R.A. Coutinho, F. Miedema. 1994. Associations between HLA frequencies and pathogenic features of human immunodeficiency virus type 1 infection in seroconverters from the Amsterdam Cohort of Homosexual Men. J Infect Dis 169:1244–1249.
226. Kaslow, R.A., M. Carrington, R. Apple, L. Park, A. Munoz, A.J. Saah, J.J. Goedert, C. Winkler, S.J. O'Brien, C. Rinaldo, R. Detels, W. Blattner, J. Phair, H. Erlich, D.L. Mann. 1996. Influence of combinations of human major histocompatibility complex genes on the course of HIV-1 infection. Nat Med 2:405–411.
227. Keet, I.P., J. Tang, M.R. Klein, S. LeBlanc, C. Enger, C. Rivers, R.J. Apple, D. Mann, J.J. Goedert, F. Miedema, R.A. Kaslow. 1999. Consistent associations of HLA class I and II and transporter gene products with progression of human immunodeficiency virus type 1 infection in homosexual men. J Infect Dis. 180:299–309.
228. Tang, J., C. Costello, I.P. Keet, C. Rivers, S. Leblanc, E. Karita, S. Allen, R.A. Kaslow. 1999. HLA class I homozygosity accelerates disease progression in human immunodeficiency virus type 1 infection. AIDS Res Hum Retroviruses 15:317–324.
229. Carrington, M., G.W. Nelson, M.P. Martin, T. Kissner, D. Vlahov, J.J. Goedert, R. Kaslow, S. Buchbinder, K. Hoots, S.J. O'Brien. 1999. HLA and HIV-1: heterozygote advantage and B*35-Cw*04 disadvantage. Science 283:1748–1752.
230. Saah, A.J., D.R. Hoover, S. Weng, M. Carrington, J. Mellors, C.R. Rinaldo, Jr., D. Mann, R. Apple, J.P. Phair, R. Detels, S. O'Brien, C. Enger, P. Johnson, R.A. Kaslow. 1998. Association of HLA profiles with early plasma viral load, CD4+ cell count and rate of progression to AIDS fol-

lowing acute HIV-1 infection. Multicenter AIDS Cohort Study. AIDS 12: 2107–2113.

231. Pantaleo, G., J.F. Demarest, T. Schacker, M. Vaccarezza, O.J. Cohen, M. Daucher, C. Graziosi, S.S. Schnittman, T.C. Quinn, G.M. Shaw, L. Perrin, G. Tambussi, A. Lazzarin, R.P. Sekaly, H. Soudeyns, L. Corey, A.S. Fauci. 1997. The qualitative nature of the primary immune response to HIV infection is a prognosticator of disease progression independent of the initial level of plasma viremia. Proc Natl Acad Sci USA 94:254–258.
232. Hay, C.M., D.J. Ruhl, N.O. Basgoz, C.C. Wilson, J.M. Billingsley, M.P. DePasquale, R.T. D'Aquila, S.M. Wolinsky, J.M. Crawford, D.C. Montefiori, B.D. Walker. 1999. Lack of viral escape and defective In vivo activation of human immunodeficiency virus type 1-specific cytotoxic T lymphocytes in rapidly progressive infection. J Virol 73:5509–5519.
233. Howcroft, T., K. Strebel, M. Martin, D. Singer. 1993. Repression of MHC class I gene promoter activity by two-exon tat of HIV. Science 260:1320–1322.
234. Schwartz, O., V. Marechal, S.L. Gall, F. Lemonnier, J.M. Heard. 1996. Endocytosis of major histocompatibiliyt complex class I molecules is induced by the HIV-1 Nef protein. Nat Med 2:338–342.
235. Kerkau, T., I. Bacik, J.R. Bennink, J.W. Yewdell, T. Huenig, A. Schimpl, U. Schubert. 1997. The human immunodeficiency virus type 1 (HIV-1) vpu protein interferes with an early step in the biosynthesis of major histocompatibility complex (MHC) class I molecules. J Exp Med 185:1295–1305.
236. De Maria, A., A. Ferraris, M. Guastella, S. Pilia, C. Cantoni, L. Polero, M.C. Mingari, D. Bassetti, A.S. Fauci, L. Moretta. 1997. Expression of HLA class I-specific inhibitory natural killer cell receptors in HIV-specific cytolytic T lymphocytes: impairment of specific cytolytic functions. Proc Natl Acad Sci USA 94:10285–10288.
237. Pantaleo, G., S. Koenig, M. Baseler, H.C. Lane, A.S. Fauci. 1990. Defective clonogenic potential of CD8+ T lymphocytes in patients with AIDS. J Immunol 144:1696–1704.
238. Pantaleo, G., H. Soudeyns, J. Demarest, M. Vaccarezza, C. Graziosi, S. Paolucci, M. Daucher, O. Cohen, F. Denis, W. Biddison, R. Sekaly, A. Fauci. 1997. Evidence for rapid disappearance of initially expanded HIV-specific CD8+ T cell clones during primary HIV infection. Proc Natl Acad Sci USA 94:9848–9853.
239. McKinney, D.M., D.A. Lewinsohn, S.R. Riddell, P.D. Greenberg, D.E. Mosier. 1999. The antiviral activity of HIV-specific CD8+ CTL clones is limited by elimination due to encounter with HIV-infected targets. J Immunol 163:861–867.
240. Itescu, S., S. Rose, E. Dwyer, R. Winchester. 1994. Certain HLA-DR5

and -DR6 major histocompatibility complex class II alleles are associated with a CD8 lymphocytic host response to human immunodeficiency virus type 1 characterized by low lymphocyte viral strain heterogeneity and slow disease progression. Proc Natl Acad Sci USA 91:11472–11476.

241. Kalams, S.A., R.P. Johnson, A.K. Trocha, M.J. Dynan, H.S. Ngo, R.T. D'Aquila, J.T. Kurnick, B.D. Walker. 1994. Longitudinal analysis of T cell receptor (TCR) gene usage by human immunodeficiency virus 1 envelope-specific cytotoxic T lymphocyte clone reveals a limited TCR repertoire. J Exp Med 179:1261–1271.

242. Kalams, S.A., R.P. Johnson, M.J. Dynan, K.E. Hartman, T. Harrer, E. Harrer, A.K. Trocha, W.A. Blattner, S.P. Buchbinder, B.D. Walker. 1996. T-cell receptor usage and fine specificity of human immunodeficiency virus 1-specific cytotoxic T lymphocyte clones: analysis of quasispecies recognition reveals a dominant response directed against a minor in vivo variant. J Exp Med 183:1669–1679.

243. Wolinsky, S.M., B.T.M. Korber, A.U. Neumann, M. Daniels, K.J. Kunstman, A.J. Whetsell, M.R. Furtado, Y. Cao, D.D. Ho, J.T. Safrit, R.A. Koup. 1996. Adaptive evolution of human immunodeficiency virus-type 1 during the natural course of infection. Science 272:537–542.

244. Haas, G., U. Plikat, P. Debre, M. Lucchiari, C. Katlama, Y. Dudoit, L. Bonduelle, M. Bauer, H.-G. Ihlenfeldt, G. Jung, B. Maier, A. Meyerhans, B. Autran. 1996. Dynamics of viral variants in HIV-1 Nef and specific cytotoxic T lymphocytes in vivo. J Immunol 157:4212–4221.

245. Wilson, C.C., S.A. Kalams, B.M. Wilkes, D.J. Ruhl, F. Gao, B.H. Hahn, I.C. Hanson, K. Luzuriaga, S. Wolinsky, R. Koup, S.P. Buchbinder, R.P. Johnson, B.D. Walker. 1997. Overlapping epitopes in human immunodeficiency virus type 1 gp120 presented by HLA A, B, and C molecules: effects of viral variation on cytotoxic T-lymphocyte recognition. J Virol 71:1256–1264.

246. Phillips, R.E., S. Rowland-Jones, D.F. Nixon, F.M. Gotch, J.P. Edwards, A.O. Ogunlesi, J.G. Elvin, J.A. Rothbard, C.R. Bangham, C.R. Rizza, A.J. McMichael. 1991. Human immunodeficiency virus genetic variation that can escape cytotoxic T-cell recognition. Nature 354:433–434.

247. Koenig, S., A.J. Conley, Y.A. Brewah, G.M. Jones, S. Leath, L.J. Boots, V. Davey, G. Pantaleo, J.F. Demarest, C. Carter, C. Wannebo, J.R. Yannelli, S.A. Rosenberg, H.C. Lane. 1995. Transfer of HIV-1-specific cytotoxic T lymphocytes to an AIDS patient leads to selection for mutant HIV variants and subsequent disease progression. Nat Med 1:330–336.

248. Borrow, P., H. Lewicki, X. Wei, M.S. Horwitz, N. Pefer, H. Meyers, J.A. Nelson, J.E. Gairin, B.H. Hahn, M.B.A. Oldstone, G.M. Shaw. 1997. Antiviral pressure exerted by HIV-1-specific cytotoxic T lymphocytes (CTL)

during primary infection demonstrated by rapid selection of CTL escape virus. Nat Med 3:205–211.

249. Goulder, P.J.R., R.E. Phillips, R.A. Colbert, S. McAdam, G. Ogg, M.A. Nowak, P. Giangrande, G. Luzzi, B. Morgan, A. Edwards, A.J. McMichael, S. Rowland-Jones. 1997. Late escape from an immunodominant cytotoxic T-lymhocyte response associated with progression to AIDS. Nat Med 3:212–217.
250. Evans, D.T., D.H. O'Connor, P. Jing, J.L. Dzuris, J. Sidney, J. da Silva, T.M. Allen, H. Horton, J.E. Venham, R.A. Rudersdorf, T. Vogel, C.D. Pauza, R.E. Bontrop, R. DeMars, A. Sette, A.L. Hughes, D.I. Watkins. 1999. Virus-specific cytotoxic T-lymphocyte responses select for amino-acid variation in simian immunodeficiency virus Env and Nef. Nat Med 5:1270–1276.
251. Klenerman, P., S. Rowland-Jones, S. McAdam, J. Edwards, S. Daenke, D. Lalloo, B. Koppe, W. Rosenberg, D. Boyd, A. Edwards, P. Giangrande, R.E. Phillips, A.J. McMichael. 1994. Cytotoxic T-cell activity antagonized by naturally occurring HIV-1 Gag variants. Nature 369:403–407.
252. Meier, U.-C., P. Klenerman, P. Griffin, W. James, B. Koppe, B. Larder, A. McMichael, R. Phillips. 1995. Cytotoxic T lymphocyte lysis inhibited by viable HIV mutants. Science 270:1360–1362.
253. Klenerman, P., R.M. Zinkernagel. 1998. Original antigenic sin impairs cytotoxic T lymphocyte responses to viruses bearing variant epitopes. Nature 394:482–485.
254. Nowak, M.A., R.M. May, R.E. Phillips, S. Rowland-Jones, D.G. Lalloo, S. McAdam, P. Klenerman, B. Koope, K. Sigmund, C.R.M. Bangham, A.J. McMichael. 1995. Antigenic oscillations and shifting immunodominance in HIV-1 infections. Nature 375:606–611.
255. Moskophidis, D., F. Lechner, H. Pircher, R.M. Zinkernagel. 1993. Virus persistence in acutely infected immunocompetent mice by exhaustion of antiviral cytotoxic effector T cells. Nature 362:758–761.
256. Walker, C.M., D.J. Moody, D.P. Stites, J.A. Levy. 1986. CD8+ Lymphocytes can control HIV infection in vitro by suppressing virus replication. Science 234:1563–1566.
257. Walker, C.M., J.A. Levy. 1989. A diffusible lymphokine produced by CD8+ T lymphocytes suppresses HIV replication. Immunology. 66:628–630.
258. Walker, C.M., A.L. Erickson, F.C. Hsueh, J.A. Levy. 1991. Inhibition of human immunodeficiency virus replication in acutely infected CD4+ cells by CD8+ cells involves a noncytotoxic mechanism. J Virol 65:5921–5927.
259. Chen, C.H., K.J. Weinhold, J.A. Bartlett, D.P. Bolognesi, M.L. Greenberg.

1993. CD8+ T lymphocyte-mediated inhibition of HIV-1 long terminal repeat transcription: a novel antiviral mechanism. AIDS Res Hum Retroviruses 9:1079–1086.

260. Copeland, K.F., P.J. McKay, K.L. Rosenthal. 1995. Suppression of activation of the human immunodeficiency virus long terminal repeat by CD8+ T-cells is not lentivirus specific. AIDS Res Hum Retroviruses 11:1321–1326.

261. Mackewicz, C., D.J. Balckbourn, J.A. Levy. 1995. CD8+ T cells suppress human immunodeficiency virus replicaton by inhibiting viral transcription. Proc Natl Acad Sci USA 92:2308–2312.

262. Mackewicz, C.E., H. Oretega, J.A. Levy. 1994. Effect of cytokines on HIV replication in CD4+ lymphocytes: lack of identity with the CD8+ cell antiviral factor. Cell Immunol 153:329–343.

263. Mackewicz, C.E., M.R. Garovoy, J.A. Levy. 1998. HLA compatibility requirements for CD8(+)-T-cell-mediated suppression of human immunodeficiency virus replication. J Virol 72:10165–10170.

264. Mackewicz, C.E., H.W. Ortega, J.A. Levy. 1991. CD8+ cell anti-HIV activity correlates with the clinical state of the infected individual. J Clin Invest 87:1462–1466.

265. Cao, Y., L. Qin, L. Zhang, J. Safrit, D.D. Ho. 1995. Virologic and immunologic characterization of long-term survivors of human immunodeficiency virus type 1 infection. N Engl J Med 332:201–208.

266. Barker, E., C.E. Mackewicz, G. Reyes-Teran, A. Sato, S.A. Stranford, S.H. Fujimura, C. Christopherson, S.Y. Chang, J.A. Levy. 1998. Virological and immunological features of long-term human immunodeficiency virus-infected individuals who have remained asymptomatic compared with those who have progressed to acquired immunodeficiency syndrome. Blood 92:3105–3114.

267. Kinter, A.L., M. Ostrowski, D. Goletti, A. Oliva, D. Weissman, K. Gantt, E. Hardy, R. Jackson, L. Ehler, A.S. Fauci. 1996. HIV replication in CD4+ T cells of HIV-infected individuals is regulated by a balance between the viral suppressive effects of endogenous beta-chemokines and the viral inductive effects of other endogenous cytokines. Proc Natl Acad Sci USA 93:14076–14081.

268. Price, D.A., A.K. Sewell, T. Dong, R. Tan, P.J. Goulder, S.L. Rowland-Jones, R.E. Phillips. 1998. Antigen-specific release of beta-chemokines by anti-HIV-1 cytotoxic T lymphocytes. Curr Biol 8:355–358.

269. Wagner, L., O.O. Yang, E.A. Garcia-Zepeda, Y. Ge, S.A. Kalams, B.D. Walker, M.S. Pasternack, A.D. Luster. 1998. Beta-chemokines are released from HIV-1-specific cytolytic T-cell granules complexed to proteoglycans. Nature 391:908–911.

270. Oliva, A., A.L. Kinter, M. Vaccarezza, A. Rubbert, A. Catanzaro, S. Moir,

J. Monaco, L. Ehler, S. Mizell, R. Jackson, Y. Li, J.W. Romano, A.S. Fauci. 1998. Natural killer cells from human immunodeficiency virus (HIV)-infected individuals are an important source of CC-chemokines and suppress HIV-1 entry and replication in vitro. J Clin Invest 102:223–231.

271. Pal, R., A. Garzino-Demo, P.D. Markham, J. Burns, M. Brown, R.C. Gallo, A.L. DeVico. 1997. Inhibition of HIV-1 infection by the beta-chemokine MDC. Science 278:695–698.

272. Baier, M., A. Werner, N. Bannert, K. Metzner, R. Kurth. 1995. HIV suppression by interleukin-16. Nature 378:563.

273. Maciaszek, J.W., N.A. Parada, W.W. Cruikshank, D.M. Center, H. Kornfeld, G.A. Viglianti. 1997. IL-16 represses HIV-1 promoter activity. J Immunol 158:5–8.

274. Viglianti, G.A., N.A. Parada, J.W. Maciaszek, H. Kornfeld, D.M. Center, W.W. Cruikshank. 1997. IL-16 anti-HIV-1 therapy. Nat Med 3:938.

275. Amiel, C., E. Darcissac, M.J. Truong, J. Dewulf, M. Loyens, Y. Mouton, A. Capron, G.M. Bahr. 1999. Interleukin-16 (IL-16) inhibits human immunodeficiency virus replication in cells from infected subjects, and serum IL-16 levels drop with disease progression. J Infect Dis 179:83–91.

276. Cease, K.B., H. Margalit, J.L. Cornette, S.D. Putney, W.G. Robey, C. Ouyang, H.Z. Streicher, P.J. Fischinger, R.C. Gallo, C. DeLisi, J.A. Berzofsky. 1987. Helper T-cell antigenic site identification in the acquired immunodeficiency syndrome virus gp120 envelope protein and induction of immunity in mice to the native protein using a 16-residue synthetic peptide. Proc Natl Acad Sci USA 84:4249–4253.

277. Clerici, M., N.I. Stocks, R.A. Zajac, R.N. Boswell, D.C. Bernstein, D.L. Mann, G.M. Shearer, J.A. Berzofsky. 1989. Interleukin-2 production used to detect antigenic peptide recognition by T-helper lymphocytes from asymptomatic HIV-seropositive individuals. Nature 339:383–385.

278. Clerici, M., J.M. Levin, H.A. Kessler, A. Harris, J.A. Berzofsky, A.L. Landay, G.M. Shearer. 1994. HIV-specific T-helper activity in seronegative health care workers exposed to contaminated blood. J Am Med Assoc 271:42–46.

279. Rosenberg, E.S., J.M. Billingsley, A.M. Caliendo, S.L. Boswell, P.E. Sax, S.A. Kalams, B.D. Walker. 1997. Vigorous HIV-1-specific CD4+ T cell responses associated with control of viremia. Science 278:1447-1450.

280. Pitcher, C.J., C. Quittner, D.M. Peterson, M. Connors, R.A. Koup, V.C. Maino, L.J. Picker. 1999. HIV-1specific CD4+ T cells are detectable in most individuals with active HIV-1 infection, but decline with prolonged viral suppression. Nat Med 5:518–525.

281. Fauci, A. 1988. The human immunodeficiency virus: infectivity and mechanisms of pathogenesis. Science 239:617–622.

282. Fauci, A. 1996. Host factors and the pathogenesis of HIV-induced disease. Nature 384:529–534.
283. Cohen, O., A. Kinter, A. Fauci. 1997. Host factors in the pathogenesis of HIV infection. Immunol Rev 159:31–48.
284. Poli, G., A. Fauci. 1995. Role of cytokines in the pathogenesis of human immunodeficiency virus infection. In: B. Aggarwal, R. Puri, eds. Human Cytokines: Their Role in Disease and Therapy. Blackwell Science, Cambridge, MA, pp. 421–449.
285. Emilie, D., M. Peuchmaur, M.C. Maillot, M.C. Crevon, N. Brousse, J.F. Delfraissy, J. Dormont, P. Galanaud. 1990. Production of interleukins in human immunodeficiency virus-1-replicating lymph nodes. J Clin Invest 86:148–159.
286. Boyle, M.J., M.F. Bergre, M. Tschuchnigg, J.E. Valentine, B.G. Kennedy, M. Divjak, D.A. Cooper, J.J. Turner, R. Penny, W.A. Sewell. 1993. Increased expressed of interferon-gamma in hyperplastic lymph nodes from HIV-infected patients. Clin Exp Immunol 92:100–105.
287. Graziosi, C., G. Pantaleo, K.R. Gantt, J.P. Fortin, J.F. Demarest, O.J. Cohen, R.P. Sekaly, A.S. Fauci. 1994. Lack of evidence for the dichotomy of TH1 and TH2 predominance in HIV-infected individuals. Science 265: 248–252.
288. Jassoy, C., T. Harrer, T. Rosenthal, B. Navia, J. Worth, R. Johnson, B. Walker. 1993. Human immunodeficiency virus type 1-specific cytotoxic T lymphocytes release gamma interferon, tumor necrosis factor alpha (TNF-alpha), and TNF-beta when they encounter their target antigens. J Virol 67:2844–2852.
289. Molina, J.M., D.T. Scadden, R. Byrn, C.A. Dinarello, J.E. Groopman. 1989. Production of tumor necrosis factor alpha and interleukin 1 beta by monocytic cells infected with human immunodeficiency virus. J Clin Invest 84:733–737.
290. Esser, R., H. vonBriesen, M. Brugger, M. Ceska, W. Glienke, S. Muller, A. Rehm, H. Rubsamen-Waigmann, R. Andressen. 1991. Secretory repertoire of HIV-infected human monocytes/macrophages. Pathobiology 59: 219–222.
291. Lane, H.C., J.M. Depper, W.C. Greene, G. Whalen, T.A. Waldmann, A.S. Fauci. 1985. Qualitative analysis of immune function in patients with the acquired immunodeficiency syndrome. Evidence for a selective defect in soluble antigen recognition. N Engl J Med 313:79–84.
292. Schulick, R.D., M. Clerici, M.J. Dolan, G.M. Shearer. 1993. Limiting dilution analysis of interleukin-2-producing T-cells responsive to recall and alloantigens in human immunodeficiency virus-infected and uninfected individuals. Eur J Immunol 23:412–417.
293. Clerici, M., D. Lucey, J. Berzofsky, L. Pinto, T. Wynn, S. Blatt, M. Dolan,

C. Hendrix, S. Wolf, G. Shearer. 1993. Restoration of HIV-specific cell-mediated immune responses by interleukin-12 in vitro. Science 262: 17211724.

294. Manetti, R., P. Parronchi, M.G. Giudizi, M.P. Piccinni, E. Maggi, G. Trinchieri, S. Romagnani. 1993. Natural killer cell stimulatory factor (interleukin 12 [IL-12]) induces T helper type 1 (Th1)-specific immune responses and inhibits the development of IL-4-producing Th cells. J Exp Med 177: 1199–1204.

295. Hsieh, C.S., S.E. Macatonia, C.S. Tripp, S.F. Wolf, A. O'Garra, K.M. Murphy. 1993. Development of TH1 CD4+ T cells through IL-12 produced by Listeria-induced macrophages. Science 260:547–549.

296. Clerici, M., F.T. Hakim, D.J. Venzon, S. Blatt, C.W. Hendrix, T.A. Wynn, G.M. Shearer. 1993. Changes in interleukin-2 and interleukin-4 production in asymptomatic, human immunodeficiency virus-seropositive individuals. J Clin Invest 91:759–765.

297. Clerici, M., T. Wynn, J. Berzofsky, S. Blatt, C. Hendrix, A. Sher, R. Coffman, G. Shearer. 1994. Role of interleukin-10 in T helper cell dysfunction in asymptomatic individuals infected with the human immunodeficiency virus. J Clin Invest 93:768–775.

298. Maggi, E., M. Mazzetti, A. Ravina, F. Annunziato, M. DeCarli, M. Piccinni, R. Manetti, M. Carbonari, A. Pesce, G. DelPrete, S. Romagnani. 1994. Ability of HIV to promote a TH1 to TH0 shift and to replicate preferentially in TH2 and TH0 cells. Science 265:244–248.

299. Meyaard, L., S. Otto, I. Keet, R. vanLier, F. Miedema. 1994. Changes in cytokine secretion patterns of CD4+ T-cell clones in human immunodeficiency virus infection. Blood 84:4262–4268.

300. David, D., L. Bani, J.L. Moreau, M.P. Treilhou, T. Nakarai, M. Joussemet, J. Ritz, B. Dupont, G. Pialoux, J. Theze. 1998. Regulatory dysfunction of the interleukin-2 receptor during HIV infection and the impact of triple combination therapy. Proc Natl Acad Sci USA 95:11348–11353.

301. Bailer, R.T., A. Holloway, J. Sun, J.B. Margolick, M. Martin, J. Kostman, L.J. Montaner. 1999. IL-13 and IFN-gamma secretion by activated T cells in HIV-1 infection associated with viral suppression and a lack of disease progression. J Immunol 162:7534–7542.

302. Barcova, M., L. Kacani, C. Speth, M.P. Dierich. 1998. gp41 envelope protein of human immunodeficiency virus induces interleukin (IL)-10 in monocytes, but not in B, T, or NK cells, leading to reduced IL-2 and interferon-gamma production. J Infect Dis. 177:905–913.

303. Clerici, M., G. Shearer. 1993. A TH1-TH2 switch is a critical step in the etiology of HIV infection. Immunol Today 14:107–111.

304. Klein, S.A., J.M. Dobmeyer, T.S. Dobmeyer, M. Pape, O.G. Ottmann, E.B. Helm, D. Hoelzer, R. Rossol 1997. Demonstration of the Th1 to

Th2 cytokine shift during the course of HIV-1 infection using cytoplasmic cytokine detection on single cell level by flow cytometry. AIDS 11:1111–1118.

305. Fakoya, A., P.M. Matear, E. Filley, G.A. Rook, J. Stanford, R.J. Gilson, N. Beecham, I.V. Weller, A. Vyakarnam. 1997. HIV infection alters the production of both type 1 and 2 cytokines but does not induce a polarized type 1 or 2 state. AIDS 11:1445–1452.
306. Clouse, K.A., D. Powell, I. Washington, G. Poli, K. Strebel, W. Farrar, P. Barstad, J. Kovacs, A.S. Fauci, T.M. Folks. 1989. Monokine regulation of human immunodeficiency virus-1 expression in a chronically infected human T cell clone. J Immunol 142:431–438.
307. Rieckmann, P., G. Poli, J.H. Kehrl, A.S. Fauci. 1991. Activated B lymphocytes from human immunodeficiency virus-infected individuals induce virus expression in infected T cells and a promonocytic cell line, U1. J Exp Med 173:1–5.
308. Kinter, A.L., G. Poli, L. Fox, E. Hardy, A.S. Fauci. 1995. HIV replication in IL-2-stimulated peripheral blood mononuclear cells is driven in an autocrine/paracrine manner by endogenous cytokines. J Immunol 154: 2448–2459.
309. Smithgall, M., J. Wong, K. Critchett, O. Haffar. 1996. IL-7 up-regulates HIV-1 replication in naturally infected peripheral blood mononuclear cells. J Immunol 156:2324–2330.
310. Bayard-McNeeley, M., H. Doo, S. He, A. Hafner, W.D. Johnson, Jr., J.L. Ho. 1996. Differential effects of interleukin-12, interleukin-15, and interleukin-2 on human immunodeficiency virus type 1 replication in vitro. Clin Diagn Lab Immunol 3:547–553.
311. Lucey, D.R., L.A. Pinto, F.R. Bethke, J. Rusnak, G.P. Melcher, F.N. Hashemi, A.L. Landay, H.A. Kessler, R.J. Paxton, K. Grabstein, G.M. Shearer. 1997. In vitro immunologic and virologic effects of interleukin 15 on peripheral blood mononuclear cells from normal donors and human immunodeficiency virus type 1-infected patients. Clin Diagn Lab Immunol 4:43–48.
312. Shapiro, L., A.J. Puren, H.A. Barton, D. Novick, R.L. Peskind, R. Shenkar, Y. Gu, M.S. Su, C.A. Dinarello. 1998. Interleukin 18 stimulates HIV type 1 in monocytic cells. Proc Natl Acad Sci USA 95:12550–12555.
313. Al-Harthi, L., K.A. Roebuck, A. Landay. 1998. Induction of HIV-1 replication by type 1-like cytokines, interleukin (IL)-12 and IL-15: effect on viral transcriptional activation, cellular proliferation, and endogenous cytokine production. J Clin Immunol 18:124–131.
314. Ho, D.D., K.L. Hartshorn, T.R. Rota, C.A. Andrews, J.C. Kaplan, R.T. Schooley, M.S. Hirsch. 1985. Recombinant human interferon alfa-A suppresses HTLV-III replication in vitro. Lancet 1:602–604.
315. Hartshorn, K.L., D. Neumeyer, M.W. Vogt, R.T. Schooley, M.S. Hirsch.

1987. Activity of interferons alpha, beta, and gamma against human immunodeficiency virus replication in vitro. AIDS Res Hum Retroviruses 3: 125–133.
316. Naif, H.M., S. Li, M. Ho-Shon, J.M. Mathijs, P. Williamson, A.L. Cunningham. 1997. The state of maturation of monocytes into macrophages determines the effects of IL-4 and IL-13 on HIV replication. J Immunol 158:501–511.
317. Valentin, A., W. Lu, M. Rosati, R. Schneider, J. Albert, A. Karlsson, G.N. Pavlakis. 1998. Dual effect of interleukin 4 on HIV-1 expression: implications for viral phenotypic switch and disease progression. Proc Natl Acad Sci USA 95:8886–8891.
318. Saville, M.W., K. Taga, A. Foli, S. Broder, G. Tosato, R. Yarchoan. 1994. Interleukin-10 suppresses human immunodeficiency virus-1 replication in vitro in cells of the monocyte/macrophage lineage. Blood 83:3591–3599.
319. Weissman, D., G. Poli, A.S. Fauci. 1994. Interleukin 10 blocks HIV replication in macrophages by inhibiting the autocrine loop of tumor necrosis factor alpha and interleukin 6 induction of virus. AIDS Res Hum Retroviruses 10:1199–1206.
320. Kootstra, N.A., A. van 't Wout, H.G. Huisman, F. Miedema, H. Schuitemaker. 1994. Interference of interleukin-10 with human immunodeficiency virus type 1 replication in primary monocyte-derived macrophages. J Virol 68:6967–6975.
321. Weissman, D., G. Poli, A.S. Fauci. 1995. IL-10 synergizes with multiple cytokines in enhancing HIV production in cells of monocytic lineage. J Acquir Immune Defic Syndr Hum Retrovirol 9:442–449.
322. Hammer, S.M., J.M. Gillis, J.E. Groopman, R.M. Rose. 1986. In vitro modification of human immunodeficiency virus infection by granulocyte-macrophage colony-stimulating factor and gamma interferon. Proc Natl Acad Sci USA 83:8734–8738.
323. Biswas, P., G. Poli, A.L. Kinter, J.S. Justement, S.K. Stanley, W.J. Maury, P. Bressler, J.M. Orenstein, A.S. Fauci. 1992. Interferon gamma induces the expression of human immunodeficiency virus in persistently infected promonocytic cells (U1) and redirects the production of virions to intracytoplasmic vacuoles in phorbol myristate acetate-differentiated U1 cells. J Exp Med 176:739–750.
324. Poli, G., A.L. Kinter, J.S. Justement, P. Bressler, J.H. Kehrl, A.S. Fauci. 1991. Transforming growth factor beta suppresses human immunodeficiency virus expression and replication in infected cells of the monocyte/macrophage lineage. J Exp Med 173:589–597.
325. Lazdins, J.K., T. Klimkait, E. Alteri, M. Walker, K. Woods-Cook, D. Cox, G. Bilbe, R. Shipman, N. Cerletti, G. McMaster. 1991. TGF-beta: upregulator of HIV replication in macrophages. Res Virol 142:239–242.
326. Poli, G., P. Bressler, A. Kinter, E. Duh, W.C. Timmer, A. Rabson, J.S.

Justement, S. Stanley, A.S. Fauci. 1990. Interleukin 6 induces human immunodeficiency virus expression in infected monocytic cells alone and in synergy with tumor necrosis factor alpha by transcriptional and post-transcriptional mechanisms. J Exp Med 172:151–158.

327. Poli, G., A.L. Kinter, A.S. Fauci. 1994. Interleukin 1 induces expression of the human immunodeficiency virus alone and in synergy with interleukin 6 in chronically infected U1 cells: inhibition of inductive effects by the interleukin 1 receptor antagonist. Proc Natl Acad Sci USA 91:108–112.

328. Osborn, L., S. Kunkel, G.J. Nabel. 1989. Tumor necrosis factor alpha and interleukin 1 stimulate the human immunodeficiency virus enhancer by activation of the nuclear factor kappa B. Proc Natl Acad Sci USA 86: 2336–2340.

329. Duh, E.J., W.J. Maury, T.M. Folks, A.S. Fauci, A.B. Rabson. 1989. Tumor necrosis factor alpha activates human immunodeficiency virus type 1 through induction of nuclear factor binding to the NF-kappa B sites in the long terminal repeat. Proc Natl Acad Sci USA 86:5974–5978.

330. Goletti, D., A.L. Kinter, E.C. Hardy, G. Poli, A.S. Fauci. 1996. Modulation of endogenous IL-1 beta and IL-1 receptor antagonist results in opposing effects on HIV expression in chronically infected monocytic cells. J Immunol 156:3501–3508.

331. Schuitemaker, H. 1994. IL4 and IL10 as potent inhibitors of HIV1 replication in macrophages in vitro: a role for cytokines in the in vivo virus host range? Res Immunol 145:588–592.

332. Goletti, D., D. Weissman, R.W. Jackson, F. Collins, A. Kinter, A.S. Fauci. 1998. The in vitro induction of human immunodeficiency virus (HIV) replication in purified protein derivative-positive HIV-infected persons by recall antigen response to Mycobacterium tuberculosis is the result of a balance of the effects of endogenous interleukin-2 and proinflammatory and antiinflammatory cytokines. J Infect Dis 177:1332–1338.

333. Locati, M., P.M. Murphy. 1999. Chemokines and chemokine receptors: biology and clinical relevance in inflammation and AIDS. Annu Rev Med 50:425–440.

334. Kornbluth, R.S., K. Kee, D.D. Richman. 1998. CD40 ligand (CD154) stimulation of macrophages to produce HIV-1-suppressive beta-chemokines. Proc Natl Acad Sci USA 95:5205–5210.

335. McDyer, J.F., M. Dybul, T.J. Goletz, A.L. Kinter, E.K. Thomas, J.A. Berzofsky, A.S. Fauci, R.A. Seder. 1999. Differential effects of CD40 ligand/trimer stimulation on the ability of dendritic cells to replicate and transmit HIV infection: evidence for CC-chemokine-dependent and -independent mechanisms. J Immunol 162:3711–3717.

336. Nelson, P., H. Kim, W. Manning, T. Goralski, A. Krensky. 1993. Genomic organization and transcriptional regulation of the RANTES chemokine gene. J Immunol 151:2601–2612.

337. Rathanaswami, P., M. Hachicha, M. Sadick, T. Schall, S. McColl. 1993. Expression of the cytokine RANTES in human rheumatoid synovial fibroblasts. Differential regulation of RANTES and interleukin-8 genes by inflammatory cytokines. J Biol Chem 268:5834–5839.
338. Schall, T., K. Bacon. 1994. Chemokines, leukocyte trafficking, and inflammation. Curr Opin Immunol 6:865–873.
339. Jansson, M., M. Popovic, A. Karlsson, F. Cocchi, P. Rossi, J. Albert, H. Wigzell. 1996. Sensitivity to inhibition by β-chemokines correlates with biological phenotypes of primary HIV-1 isolates. Proc Natl Acad Sci USA 93:15382–15387.
340. Connor, R.I., K.E. Sheridan, D. Ceradini, S. Choe, N.R. Landau. 1997. Change in coreceptor use correlates with disease progression in HIV-1-infected individuals. J Exp Med 185:621–628.
341. Schmidtmayerova, H., B. Sherry, M. Bukrinsky. 1996. Chemokines and HIV replication. Nature 382:767.
342. Kelly, M.D., H.M. Naif, S.L. Adams, A.L. Cunningham, A.R. Lloyd. 1998. Dichotomous effects of beta-chemokines on HIV replication in monocytes and monocyte-derived macrophages. J Immunol 160:3091–3095.
343. Unutmaz, D., D. Littman. 1997. Expression pattern of HIV-1 coreceptors on T cells: implications for viral transmission and lymphocyte homing. Proc Natl Acad Sci USA 94:1615–1618.
344. Patterson, B.K., M. Czerniewski, J. Andersson, Y. Sullivan, F. Su, D. Jiyamapa, Z. Burki, A. Landay. 1999. Regulation of CCR5 and CXCR4 expression by type 1 and type 2 cytokines: CCR5 expression is downregulated by IL-10 in CD4-positive lymphocytes. Clin Immunol 91:254–262.
345. Hariharan, D., S.D. Douglas, B. Lee, J.P. Lai, D.E. Campbell, W.Z. Ho. 1999. Interferon-gamma upregulates CCR5 expression in cord and adult blood mononuclear phagocytes. Blood 93:1137–1144.
346. Suzuki, Y., Y. Koyanagi, Y. Tanaka, T. Murakami, N. Misawa, N. Maeda, T. Kimura, H. Shida, J.A. Hoxie, W.A. O'Brien, N. Yamamoto. 1999. Determinant in human immunodeficiency virus type 1 for efficient replication under cytokine-induced CD4(+) T-helper 1 (Th1)- and Th2- type conditions. J Virol 73:316–324.
347. Wang, J., A. Harada, S. Matsushita, S. Matsumi, Y. Zhang, T. Shioda, Y. Nagai, K. Matsushima. 1998. IL-4 and a glucocorticoid up-regulate CXCR4 expression on human CD4+ T lymphocytes and enhance HIV-1 replication. J Leukoc Biol 64:642–649.
348. Galli, G., F. Annunziato, C. Mavilia, P. Romagnani, L. Cosmi, R. Manetti, C. Pupilli, E. Maggi, S. Romagnani. 1998. Enhanced HIV expression during Th2-oriented responses explained by the opposite regulatory effect of IL-4 and IFN-gamma of fusin/CXCR4. Eur J Immunol 28:3280–3290.
349. Zoeteweij, J.P., H. Golding, H. Mostowski, A. Blauvelt. 1998. Cytokines

regulate expression and function of the HIV coreceptor CXCR4 on human mature dendritic cells. J Immunol 161:3219–3223.

350. Levine, B.L., J.D. Mosca, J.L. Riley, R.G. Carroll, M.T. Vahey, L.L. Jagodzinski, K.F. Wagner, D.L. Mayers, D.S. Burke, O.S. Weislow, D.C. St. Louis, C.H. June. 1996. Antiviral effect and ex vivo CD4+ T-cell proliferation in HIV-positive patients as a result of CD28 costimulation. Science 272:1939–1943.

351. Riley, J.L., R.G. Carroll, B.L. Levine, W. Bernstein, D.C. St. Louis, O.S. Weislow, C.H. June. 1997. Intrinsic resistance to T cell infection with HIV type 1 induced by CD28 costimulation. J Immunol 158:5545–5553.

352. Roederer, M., P.A. Raju, D.K. Mitra, L.A. Herzenberg, L.A. Herzenberg. 1997. HIV does not replicate in naive CD4 T-cells stimulated with CD3/CD28. J Clin Invest 99:1555–1564.

353. Carroll, R.G., J.L. Riley, B.L. Levine, Y. Feng, S. Kaushal, D.W. Ritchey, W. Bernstein, O.S. Weislow, C.R. Brown, E.A. Berger, C.H. June, D.C. St. Louis. 1997. Differential regulation of HIV-1 fusion cofactor expression by CD28 costimulation of CD4+ T-cells. Science 276:273–276.

354. Moriuchi, H., M. Moriuchi, A.S. Fauci. 1998. Factors secreted by human T lymphotropic virus type I (HTLV-I)-infected cells can enhance or inhibit replication of HIV-1 in HTLV-I-uninfected cells: implications for in vivo coinfection with HTLV-I and HIV-1. J Exp Med 187:1689–1697.

355. Moriuchi, M., H. Moriuchi, W. Turner, A.S. Fauci. 1998. Exposure to bacterial products renders macrophages highly susceptible to T-tropic HIV-1. J Clin Invest 102:1540–1550.

356. Huang, L., I. Bosch, W. Hofmann, J. Sodroski, A.B. Pardee. 1998. Tat protein induces human immunodeficiency virus type 1 (HIV-1) coreceptors and promotes infection with both macrophage-tropic and T-lymphotropic HIV-1 strains. J Virol 72:8952–8960.

357. Secchiero, P., D. Zella, S. Capitani, R.C. Gallo, G. Zauli. 1999. Extracellular HIV-1 tat protein up-regulates the expression of surface CXC-chemokine receptor 4 in resting CD4+ T-cells. J Immunol 162:2427–2431.

358. Fauci, A. 1993. Multifactorial nature of human immunodeficiency virus diseases: implications for therapy. Science 262:1011–1018.

359. Chun, T.W., D. Engel, S.B. Mizell, L.A. Ehler, A.S. Fauci. 1998. Induction of HIV-1 replication in latently infected CD4(+) T-cells using a combination of cytokines. J Exp Med 188:83–91.

360. Fultz, P.N., J.C. Gluckman, E. Muchmore, M. Girard. 1992. Transient increases in numbers of infectious cells in an HIV-infected chimpanzee following immune stimulation. AIDS Res Hum Retroviruses 8:313–317.

361. Goletti, D., D. Weissman, R.W. Jackson, N.M. Graham, D. Vlahov, R.S. Klein, S.S. Munsiff, L. Ortona, R. Cauda, A.S. Fauci. 1996. Effect of Mycobacterium tuberculosis on HIV replication. Role of immune activation. J Immunol 157:1271–1278.

362. Ostrowski, M.A., S.K. Stanley, J.S. Justement, K. Gantt, D. Goletti, A.S. Fauci. 1997. Increased in vitro tetanus-induced production of HIV type 1 following in vivo immunization of HIV type 1-infected individuals with tetanus toxoid. AIDS Res Hum Retroviruses 13:473–480.
363. Cheynier, R., S. Henrichwark, F. Hadida, E. Pelletier, E. Oksenhendler, B. Autran, S. Wain-Hobson. 1994. HIV and T cell expansion in splenic white pulps is accompanied by infiltration of HIV-specific cytotoxic T lymphocytes. Cell 78:373–387.
364. Grossman, Z., M.B. Feinberg, W.E. Paul. 1998. Multiple modes of cellular activation and virus transmission in HIV infection: a role for chronically and latently infected cells in sustaining viral replication. Proc Natl Acad Sci USA 95:6314–6319.
365. Choremi-Papadopoulou, H., V. Viglis, P. Gargalianos, T. Kordossis, A. Iniotaki-Theodoraki, J. Kosmidis. 1994. Downregulation of CD28 surface antigen on CD4+ and CD8+ T lymphocytes during HIV-1 infection. J AIDS 7:245–253.
366. Borthwick, N.J., M. Bofill, W.M. Gombert, A.N. Akbar, E. Medina, K. Sagawa, M.C. Lipman, M.A. Johnson, G. Janossy. 1994. Lymphocyte activation in HIV-1 infection. II. Functional defects of CD28− T-cells. AIDS 8:431–441.
367. Wolthers, K.C., S.A. Otto, S.M. Lens, R.A. Van Lier, F. Miedema, L. Meyaard. 1997. Functional B cell abnormalities in HIV type 1 infection: role of CD40L and CD70. AIDS Res Hum Retroviruses 13:1023–1029.
368. Hoxie, J.A., J.D. Alpers, J.L. Rackowski, K. Huebner, B.S. Haggarty, A.J. Cedarbaum, J.C. Reed. 1986. Alterations in T4 (CD4) protein and mRNA synthesis in cells infected with HIV. Science 234:1123–1127.
369. Garcia, J.V., A.D. Miller. 1991. Serine phosphorylation-independent downregulation of cell-surface CD4 by nef. Nature 350:508–511.
370. Willey, R.L., F. Maldarelli, M.A. Martin, K. Strebel. 1992. Human immunodeficiency virus type 1 Vpu protein induces rapid degradation of CD4. J Virol 66:7193–7200.
371. Schnittman, S.M., H.C. Lane, J. Greenhouse, J.S. Justement, M. Baseler, A.S. Fauci. 1990. Preferential infection of CD4+ memory T-cells by human immunodeficiency virus type 1: evidence for a role in the selective T-cell functional defects observed in infected individuals. Proc Natl Acad Sci USA 87:6058–6062.
372. Chun, T.-W., K. Chadwick, J. Margolick, R. Siliciano. 1997. Differential susceptibility of naive and memory CD4+ T cells to the cytopathic effects of infection with human immunodeficiency virus type 1 strain LAI. J Virol 71:4436–4444.
373. Spina, C.A., H.E. Prince, D.D. Richman. 1997. Preferential replication of HIV-1 in the CD45RO memory cell subset of primary CD4 lymphocytes in vitro. J Clin Invest 99:1774–1785.

374. Chirmule, N., S. Pahwa. 1996. Envelope glycoproteins of human immunodeficiency virus type 1: profound influences on immune functions. Microbiol Rev 60:386-406.
375. Oh, S.K., W.W. Cruickshank, J. Raina, G.C. Blanchard, W.H. Adler, J. Walker, H. Kornfeld. 1992. Identification of HIV-1 envelope glycoprotein in the serum of AIDS and ARC patients. J AIDS 5:251–256.
376. Amadori, A., G. De Silvestro, R. Zamarchi, M.L. Veronese, M.R. Mazza, G. Schiavo, M. Panozzo, A. De Rossi, L. Ometto, J. Mous, et al. 1992. CD4 epitope masking by gp120/anti-gp120 antibody complexes. A potential mechanism for CD4+ cell function down-regulation in AIDS patients. J Immunol 148:2709–2716.
377. Sunila, I., M. Vaccarezza, G. Pantaleo, A.S. Fauci, J.M. Orenstein. 1997. gp120 is present on the plasma membrane of apoptotic Cd4 cells prepared from lymph nodes of HIV-1-infected individuals: an immunoelectron microscopic study. AIDS 11:27–32.
378. Gupta, S., B. Vayuvegula. 1987. Human immunodeficiency virus-associated changes in signal transduction. J Clin Immunol 7:486–489.
379. Linette, G.P., R.J. Hartzman, J.A. Ledbetter, C.H. June. 1988. HIV-1-infected T cells show a selective signaling defect after perturbation of CD3/antigen receptor. Science 241:573–576.
380. Oyaizu, N., N. Chirmule, V.S. Kalyanaraman, W.W. Hall, R.A. Good, S. Pahwa. 1990. Human immunodeficiency virus type 1 envelope glycoprotein gp120 produces immune defects in CD4+ T lymphocytes by inhibiting interleukin 2 mRNA. Proc Natl Acad Sci USA 87:2379–2383.
381. Hivroz, C., F. Mazerolles, M. Soula, R. Fagard, S. Graton, S. Meloche, R. Sekaly, A. Fischer. 1993. Human immunodeficiency virus gp120 and derived peptides activate protein tyrosine kinase p56lck in human CD4 T lymphocytes. Eur J Immunol 23:600–607.
382. Liegler, T.J., D.P. Stites. 1994. HIV-1 gp120 and anti-gp120 induce reversible unresponsiveness in peripheral CD4 T lymphocytes. J AIDS 7: 340–348.
383. Tamma, S.M., N. Chirmule, T.W. McCloskey, N. Oyaizu, V.S. Kalyanaraman, S. Pahwa. 1997. Signals transduced through the CD4 molecule interfere with TCR/CD3-mediated ras activation leading to T cell anergy/apoptosis. Clin Immunol Immunopathol 85:195–201.
384. Cohen, D.I., Y. Tani, H. Tian, E. Boone, L.E. Samelson, H.C. Lane. 1992. Participation of tyrosine phosphorylation in the cytopathic effect of human immunodeficiency virus-1. Science 256:542–545.
385. Banda, N.K., J. Bernier, D.K. Kurahara, R. Kurrle, N. Haigwood, R.-P. Sekaly, T.H. Finkel. 1992. Crosslinking CD4 by human immunodeficiency virus gp120 primes T cells for activation-induced apoptosis. J Exp Med 176:1099–1106.

386. Westendorp, M.O., R. Frank, C. Ochsenbauer, K. Stricker, J. Dhein, H. Walczak, K.M. Debatin, P.H. Krammer. 1995. Sensitization of T cells to CD95-mediated apoptosis by HIV-1 Tat and gp120. Nature 375:497–500.
387. Cicala, C., J. Arthos, A. Rubbert, S. Selig, K. Wildt, O.J. Cohen, A.S. Fauci. 2000. HIV-1 envelope induces activation of caspase-3 and cleavage of focal adhesion kinase in primary human CD4(+) T cells. Proc Natl Acad Sci USA 97:1178–1183.
388. Weissman, D., R.L. Rabin, J. Arthos, A. Rubbert, M. Dybul, R. Swofford, S. Venkatesan, J.M. Farber, A.S. Fauci. 1997. Macrophage-tropic HIV and SIV envelope proteins induce a signal through the CCR5 chemokine receptor. Nature 389:981–985.
389. Misse, D., M. Cerutti, N. Noraz, P. Jourdan, J. Favero, G. Devauchelle, H. Yssel, N. Taylor, F. Veas. 1999. A CD4-independent interaction of human immunodeficiency virus-1 gp120 with CXCR4 induces their cointernalization, cell signaling, and T-cell chemotaxis. Blood 93:2454–2462.
390. Cefai, D., P. Debre, M. Kaczorek, T. Idziorek, B. Autran, G. Bismuth. 1990. Human immunodeficiency virus-1 glycoproteins gp120 and gp160 specifically inhibit the CD3/T-cell-antigen receptor phosphoinositide transduction pathway. J Clin Invest 86:2117–2124.
391. Goldman, F., W. Jensen, G. Johnson, L. Heasley, J. Cambier. 1994. gp120 ligation of CD4 induces p56lck activation and TCR desensitization independent of TCR tyrosine phosphorylation. J Immunol 153:2905–2917.
392. Cicala, C., J. Arthos, M. Ruiz, M. Vaccarezza, A. Rubbert, A. Riva, K. Wildt, O. Cohen, A.S. Fauci. 1999. Induction of phosphorylation and intracellular association of CC chemokine receptor 5 and focal adhesion kinase in primary human CD4+ T cells by macrophage-tropic HIV envelope. J Immunol 163:420–426.
393. Chirmule, N., T.W. McCloskey, R. Hu, V.S. Kalyanaraman, S. Pahwa. 1995. HIV gp120 inhibits T cell activation by interfering with expression of costimulatory molecules CD40 ligand and CD80 (B7–1). J Immunol 155:917–924.
394. Tamma, S.M.L., N. Chirmule, H. Yagura, N. Oyaizu, V. Kallyanaraman, S. Pahwa. 1997. CD4 cross-linking (CD4XL) induces RAS activation and tumor necrosis factor-alpha secretion in CD4+ T cells. Blood 90:1588–1593.
395. Davis, C.B., I. Dikic, D. Unutmaz, C.M. Hill, J. Arthos, M.A. Siani, D.A. Thompson, J. Schlessinger, D.R. Littman. 1997. Signal transduction due to HIV-1 envelope interactions with chemokine receptors CXCR4 or CCR5. J Exp Med 186:1793–1798.
396. Popovic, M., M. Sarngadharan, E. Read, R. Gallo. 1984. Detection, isolation, and continuous production of cytopathic retroviruses (HTLV-III) from patients with AIDS and pre-AIDS. Science 224:497–500.

397. Gallo, R., S. Salahuddin, M. Popovic, G. Shearer, M. Kaplan, B. Haynes, T. Palker, R. Redfield, J. Oleske, B. Safai, G. White, P. Foster, P.D. Markham. 1984. Frequent detection and isolation of cytopathic retroviruses (HTLV-III) from patients with AIDS and at risk for AIDS. Science 224: 500–503.
398. Levy, J.A., A.D. Hoffman, S.M. Kramer, J.A. Landis, J.M. Shimabukuro, L.S. Oshiro. 1984. Isolation of lymphocytopathic retroviruses from San Francisco patients with AIDS. Science 225:840–842.
399. Shaw, G.M., B.H. Hahn, S.K. Arya, J.E. Groopman, R.C. Gallo, F. Wong-Staal. 1984. Molecular characterization of human T-cell leukemia (lymphotropic) virus type III in the acquired immune deficiency syndrome. Science 226:1165–1171.
400. Schnittman, S.M., J.J. Greenhouse, M.C. Psallidopoulos, M. Baseler, N.P. Salzman, A.S. Fauci, H.C. Lane. 1990. Increasing viral burden in CD4+ T-cells from patients with human immunodeficiency virus (HIV) infection reflects rapidly progressive immunosuppression and clinical disease. Ann Intern Med 113:438–443.
401. Poznansky, M.C., B. Walker, W.A. Haseltine, J. Sodroski, E. Langhoff. 1991. A rapid method for quantitating the frequency of peripheral blood cells containing HIV-1 DNA. J AIDS 4:368–373.
402. Bagnarelli, P., S. Menzo, A. Valenza, A. Manzin, M. Giacca, F. Ancarani, G. Scalise, P.E. Varaldo, M. Clementi. 1992. Molecular profile of human immunodeficiency virus type 1 infection in symptomless patients and in patients with AIDS. J Virol 66:7328–7335.
403. Michael, N.L., M. Vahey, R.S. Burke, R.R. Redfield. 1992. Viral DNA and mRNA expression correlate with the stage of human immunodeficiency virus (HIV) type 1 infection in humans: evidence for viral replication in all stages of HIV disease. J Virol 66:310–316.
404. Connor, R.I., H. Mohri, Y. Cao, D.D. Ho. 1993. Increased viral burden and cytopathicity correlate temporally with CD4+ T-lymphocyte decline and clinical progression in human immunodeficiency virus type 1-infected individuals. J Virol 67:1772–1777.
405. Somasundaran, M., H.L. Robinson. 1988. Unexpectedly high levels of HIV-1 RNA and protein synthesis in a cytocidal infection. Science 242: 1554–1557.
406. Koga, Y., E. Lindstrom, E.M. Fenyo, H. Wigzell, T.W. Mak. 1988. High levels of heterodisperse RNAs accumulate in T cells infected with human immunodeficiency virus and in normal thymocytes. Proc Natl Acad Sci USA 85:4521–4525.
407. DeRossi, A., G. Franchini, A. Aldovini, A. DelMistro, L. Chieco-Bianchi, R.C. Gallo, F. Wong-Staal. 1986. Differential response to the cytopathic effects of human T-cell lymphotropic virus type III (HTLV-III) superin-

fection in T4+ (helper) and T8+ (suppressor) T-cell clones transformed by HTLV-1. Proc Natl Acad Sci USA 83:4297–4301.

408. Koga, Y., M. Sasaki, H. Yoshida, H. Wigzell, G. Kimura, K. Nomoto. 1990. Cytopathic effect determined by the amount of CD4 molecules in human cell lines expressing envelope glycoprotein of HIV. J Immunol 144:94–102.

409. Cao, J., I.W. Park, A. Cooper, J. Sodroski. 1996. Molecular determinants of acute single-cell lysis by human immunodeficiency virus type 1. J Virol 70:1340-1354.

410. Leonard, R., D. Zagury, I. Desportes, J. Bernard, J.F. Zagury, R.C. Gallo. 1988. Cytopathic effect of human mmunodeficiency virus in T4 cells is linked to the last stage of virus infection. Proc Natl Acad Sci USA 85: 3570–3574.

411. Lynn, W.S., A. Tweedale, M.W. Cloyd. 1988. Human immunodeficiency virus (HIV-1) cytotoxicity: perturbation of the cell membrane and depression of phospholipid synthesis. Virol 163:43–51.

412. Voss, T.G., C.D. Fermin, J.A. Levy, S. Vigh, B. Choi, R.F. Garry. 1996. Alteration of intracellular potassium and sodium concentrations correlates with induction of cytopathic effects by human immunodeficiency virus. J Virol 70:5447–5454.

413. Sodroski, J., W.C. Goh, K. Rosen, K. Campbell, W.A. Haseltine. 1986. Role of the IITLV-III/LAV envelope in syncytium formation and cytopathicity. Nature 322:470–474.

414. Lifson, J.D., G.R. Reyes, M.S. McGrath, B.S. Stein, E.G. Engleman. 1986. AIDS retrovirus induced cytopathology: giant cell formation and involvement of CD4 antigen. Science 232:1123–1127.

415. Lifson, J.D., M.B. Feinberg, G.R. Reyes, L. Rabin, B. Banapour, S. Chakrabarti, B. Moss, F. Wong-Staal, K.S. Steimer, E.G. Engleman. 1986. Induction of CD4-dependent cell fusion by the HTLV-III/LAV envelope glycoprotein. Nature 323:725–728.

416. Yoffe, B., D.E. Lewis, B.L. Petrie, C.A. Noonan, J.L. Melnick, F.B. Hollinger. 1987. Fusion as a mediator of cytolysis in mixtures of uninfected CD4+ lymphocytes and cells infected by human immunodeficiency virus. Proc Natl Acad Sci USA 84:1429–1433.

417. Sharer, L.R., E.S. Cho, L.G. Epstein. 1985. Multinucleated giant cells and HTLV-III in AIDS encephalopathy. Hum Pathol 16:760.

418. Maier, H., H. Budka, H. Lassmann, P. Pohl. 1989. Vacuolar myelopathy with multinucleated giant cells in the acquired immune deficiency syndrome (AIDS). Light and electron microscopic distribution of human immunodeficiency virus (HIV) antigens. Acta Neuropathol 78:497–503.

419. Burke, A.P., W. Benson, J.L. Ribas, D. Anderson, W.-S. Chu, J. Smialek, R. Virmani. 1993. Postmortem localization of HIV-1 RNA by in situ hy-

bridization in lymphoid tissues of intravenous drug addicts who died unexpectedly. Am J Pathol 142:1701–1713.

420. Burke, A.P., D. Anderson, P. Mannan, J.L. Ribas, Y.-H. Liang, J. Smialek, R. Virmani. 1994. Systemic lymphadenopathic histology in human immunodeficiency virus-1-seropositive drug addicts without apparent acquired immunodeficiency syndrome. Hum Pathol 25:248–256.
421. Teo, I., C. Veryard, H. Barnes, S.F. An, M. Jones, P.L. Lantos, P. Luthert, S. Shaunak. 1997. Circular forms of unintegrated human immunodeficiency virus type 1 DNA and high levels of viral protein expression: association with dementia and multinucleated giant cells in the brains of patients with AIDS. J Virol 71:2928–2933.
422. Golding, H., F.A. Robey, F.T. Gates, W. Linder, P.R. Beining, T. Hoffman, B. Golding. 1988. Identification of homologous regions in human immunodeficiency virus I gp41 and human MHC class II beta 1 domain. I. Monoclonal antibodies against the gp41-derived peptide and patient's sera react with native HLA class II antigens, suggesting a role for autoimmunity in the pathogenesis of acquired immune deficiency syndrome. J Exp Med 167:914–923.
423. Golding, H., G. Shearer, K. Hillman, P. Lucas, J. Manischewitz, R. Zajac, M. Clerici, R. Gress, R. Boswell, B. Golding. 1989. Common epitope in human immunodeficiency virus (HIV)1 gp41 and HLA class II elicits immunosuppressive autoantibodies capable of contributing to immune dysfunction in HIV 1-infected individuals. J Clin Invest. 83:1430–1435.
424. Metlas, R., V. Skerl, V. Veljkovic, A. Colombatti, S. Pongor. 1994. Immunoglobulin-like domain of HIV-1 envelope glycoprotein gp120 encodes putative internal image of some common human proteins. Viral Immunol 7:215–219.
425. Grassi, F., R. Meneveri, M. Gullberg, L. Lopalco, G. Rossi, P. Lanza, C. DeSantis, G. Brattsand, S. Butto, E. Ginelli, A. Beretta, A.G. Siccardi. 1991. Human immunodeficiency virus type 1 gp120 mimics a hidden monomorphic epitope borne by class I major histocompatibility complex heavy chains. J Exp Med 174:53–62.
426. Silvestris, F., R.C. Williams, F. Dammacco. 1995. Autoreactivity in HIV-1 infections: the role of molecular mimicry. Clin Immunol Immunopathol 75:197–205.
427. Zagury, J.F., H. Cantalloube, A. Achour, Y.Y. Cho, L. Fall, A. Lachgar, V. Chams, A. Astgen, D. Biou, O. Picard, et al. 1993. Striking similarities between HIV-1 Env protein and the apoptosis mediating cell surface antigen Fas. Role in the pathogenesis of AIDS. Biomed Pharmacother 47: 331–335.
428. Moukrim, Z., A. Achour. 1995. Cytotoxic T lymphocytes specific for the synthetic VEINCTR peptide, a sequence found within the Fas molecule

and env gp120 in the blood of HIV-1 seropositive individuals. Cell Mol Biol (Noisy-le-Grand) 41:439–444.
429. Grant, M.D., M.S. Weaver, C. Tsoukas, G.W. Hoffmann. 1990. Distribution of antibodies against denatured collagen in AIDS risk groups and homosexual AIDS patients suggests a link between autoimmunity and the immunopathogenesis of AIDS. J Immunol 144:1241–1250.
430. Cassani, F., L. Baffoni, E. Raise, L. Selleri, M. Monti, L. Bonazzi, F.M. Gritti, F.B. Bianchi. 1991. Serum non-organ specific autoantibodies in human immunodeficiency virus 1 infection. J Clin Pathol 44:64–68.
431. Muller, S., P. Richalet, A. Laurent-Crawford, S. Barakat, Y. Riviere, F. Porrot, S. Chamaret, J.P. Briand, L. Montagnier, A. Hovanessian. 1992. Autoantibodies typical of non-organ-specific autoimmune diseases in HIV-seropositive patients. AIDS. 6:933–942.
432. Grant, M.D., F.M. Smail, K.L. Rosenthal. 1994. Cytotoxic T-lymphocytes that kill autologous CD4+ lymphocytes are associated with CD4+ lymphocyte depletion in HIV-1 infection. J AIDS 7:571–579.
433. Weinhold, K.J., H.K. Lyerly, S.D. Stanley, A.A. Austin, T.J. Matthews, D.P. Bolognesi. 1989. HIV-1 GP120-mediated immune suppression and lymphocyte destruction in the absence of viral infection. J Immunol 142: 3091-3097.
434. Zarling, J.M., J.A. Ledbetter, J. Sias, P. Fultz, J. Eichberg, G. Gjerset, P.A. Moran. 1990. HIV-infected humans, but not chimipanzees, have circulating cytotoxic T lymphocytes that lyse uninfected CD4+ cells. J Immunol 144:2992–2998.
435. Manca, F., J.A. Habeshaw, A.G. Dalgleish. 1990. HIV envelope glycoprotein, antigen specific T-cell responses, and soluble CD4. Lancet 335:811–815.
436. Folks, T.M., S.W. Kessler, J.M. Orenstein, J.S. Justement, E.S. Jaffe, A.S. Fauci. 1988. Infection and replication of HIV-1 in purified progenitor cells of normal human bone marrow. Science 242:919–922.
437. Steinberg, H.N., C.S. Crumpacker, P.A. Chatis. 1991. In vitro suppression of normal human bone marrow progenitor cells by human immunodeficiency virus. J Virol 65:1765–1769.
438. Chelucci, C., J.H. Hassan, C. Locardi, D. Bulgarini, E. Pelosi, G. Mariani, U. Testa, M. Federico, M. Valtieri, C. Peschle. 1995. In vitro human immunodeficiency virus-1 infection of purified hematopoietic progenitors in single-cell culture. Blood. 85:1181–1187.
439. Deichmann, M., R. Kronenwett, R. Haas. 1997. Expression of the human immunodeficiency virus type-1 coreceptors CXCR-4 (fusin, LESTR) and CKR-5 in CD34+ hematopoietic progenitor cells. Blood. 89:3522–3528.
440. Carr, J.M., H.S. Ramshaw, P. Li, C.J. Burrell. 1998. CD34+ cells and their derivatives contain mRNA for CD4 and human immunodeficiency

virus (HIV) co-receptors and are susceptible to infection with M- and T-tropic HIV. J Gen Virol 79:71–75.
441. Ruiz, M.E., C. Cicala, J. Arthos, A. Kinter, A.T. Catanzaro, J. Adelsberger, K.L. Holmes, O.J. Cohen, A.S. Fauci. 1998. Peripheral blood-derived CD34+ progenitor cells: CXC chemokine receptor 4 and CC chemokine receptor 5 expression and infection by HIV. J Immunol 161: 4169–4176.
442. Stanley, S.K., S.W. Kessler, J.S. Justement, S.M. Schnittman, J.J. Greenhouse, C.C. Brown, L. Musongela, K. Musey, B. Kapita, A.S. Fauci. 1992. CD34+ bone marrow cells are infected with HIV in a subset of seropositive individuals. J Immunol 149:689–697.
443. Zauli, G., M.C. Re, G. Furlini, M. Giovannini, M. LaPlaca. 1991. Evidence for an HIV-1 mediated suppression of in vitro growth of enriched (CD34+) hematopoietic progenitors. J AIDS 4:1251–1253.
444. Zauli, G., M.C. Re, G. Furlini, M. Giovannini, M. LaPlaca. 1992. Human immunodeficiency virus type 1 envelope glycoprotein gp120-mediated killing of human haematopoietic progenitors (CD34+ cells). J Gen Virol 73:417–421.
445. Zauli, G., B.R. Davis, M.C. Re, G. Visani, G. Furlini, M. LaPlaca. 1992. Tat protein stimulates production of transforming growth factor-β1 by marrow macrophages: a potential mechanism for human immunodeficiency virus-1-induced hematopoietic suppression. Blood. 80:3036–3043.
446. Louache, F., A. Henri, A. Bettaieb, E. Oksenhendler, G. Raguin, M. Tulliez, W. Vainchenker. 1992. Role of human immunodeficiency virus replication in defective in vitro growth of hematopoietic progenitors. Blood 80:2991–2999.
447. DeLuca, A., L. Teofili, A. Antinori, M.S. Iovino, P. Mencarini, E. Visconti, E. Tamburrini, G. Leione, L. Ortona. 1993. Haemopoietic CD34+ progenitor cells are not infected by HIV-1 in vivo but show impaired clonogenesis. Br J Haematol 85:20–24.
448. Re, M.C., G. Zauli, D. Gibellini, G. Furlini, E. Ramazzotti, P. Monari, S. Raniere, S. Capitani, M. LaPlaca. 1993. Uninfected haematopoietic progenitor (CD34+) cells purified from the bone marrow of AIDS patients are committed to apoptotic cell death in culture. AIDS 7:1049–1055.
449. Zauli, G., M. Vitale, D. Gibellini, S. Capitani. 1996. Inhibition of purified CD34+ hematopoietic progenitor cells by human immunodeficiency virus 1 or gp120 mediated by endogenous transforming growth factor beta 1. J Exp Med 183:99–108.
450. Marandin, A., A. Katz, E. Oksenhendler, M. Tulliez, F. Picard, W. Vainchenker, F. Louache. 1996. Loss of primitive hematopoietic progenitors in patients with human immunodeficiency virus infection. Blood 88:4568–4578.

451. Schooley, R.T., J. Mladenovic, A. Sevin, S. Chiu, S.A. Miles, R.J. Pomerantz, T.B. Campbell, D. Bell, D. Ambruso, R. Wong, A. Landay, R.W. Coombs, L. Fox, M. Kamoun, J. Jacovini. 2000. Reduced mobilization of CD34+ stem cells in advanced human immunodeficiency virus type 1 disease. J Infect Dis 181:148–157.
452. Stanley, S., J. McCune, H. Kaneshima, J. Justement, M. Sullivan, E. Boone, M. Baseler, J. Adelsberger, M. Bonyhadi, J. Orenstein, A. Fauci. 1993. Human immunodeficiency virus infection of the human thymus and disruption of the thymic microenvironment in the SCID-hu mouse. J Exp Med 178:1151–1163.
453. Schnittman, S.M., K.H. Singer, J.J. Greenhouse, S.K. Stanley, L.P. Whichard, P.T. Le, B.F. Haynes, A.S. Fauci. 1991. Thymic microenvironment induces HIV expression. Physiologic secretion of IL-6 by thymic epithelial cells up-regulates virus expression in chronically infected cells. J Immunol 147:2553–2558.
454. Valentin, H., M.T. Nugeyre, F. Vuillier, L. Boumsell, M. Schmid, F. Barre-Sinoussi, R.A. Pereira. 1994. Two subpopulations of human triple-negative thymic cells are susceptible to infection by human immunodeficiency virus type 1 in vitro. J Virol 68:3041–3050.
455. Su, L., H. Kaneshima, M. Bonyhadi, S. Salimi, D. Kraft, L. Rabin, J.M. McCune. 1995. HIV-1-induced thymocyte depletion is associated with indirect cytopathogenicity and infection of progenitor cells in vivo. Immunity 2:25–36.
456. Ascher, M.S., H.W. Sheppard. 1990. AIDS as immune system activation. II. The panergic imnesia hypothesis. J AIDS 3:177–191.
457. Ameisen, J.C., A. Capron. 1991. Cell dysfunction and depletion in AIDS: the programmed cell death hypothesis. Immunol Today 12:102–105.
458. Laurent-Crawford, A.G., B. Krust, S. Muller, Y. Riviere, M.A. Rey-Cuille, J.M. Bechet, L. Montagnier, A.G. Hovanessian. 1991. The cytopathic effect of HIV is associated with apoptosis. Virology 185:829–839.
459. Terai, C., R.S. Kornbluth, C.D. Pauza, D.D. Richman, D.A. Carson. 1991. Apoptosis as a mechanism of cell death in cultured T lymphoblasts acutely infected with HIV-1. J Clin Invest 87:1710–1715.
460. Groux, H., G. Torpier, D. Monte, Y. Mouton, A. Capron, J.C. Ameisen. 1992. Activation-induced death by apoptosis in CD4+ T-cells from human immunodeficiency virus-infected asymptomatic individuals. J Exp Med 175:331–340.
461. Meyaard, L., S.A. Otto, R.R. Jonker, M.J. Mijnster, R.P.M. Keet, F. Miedema. 1992. Programmed death of T cells in HIV-1 infection. Science 257:217–219.
462. Oyaizu, N., T.W. McCloskey, M. Coronesi, N. Chirmule, V.S. Kalyanaraman, S. Pahwa. 1993. Accelerated apoptosis in peripheral blood mononu-

clear cells (PBMCs) from human immunodeficiency virus type-1 infected patients and in CD4 cross-linked PBMCs from normal individuals. Blood 82:3392–3400.

463. Gandhi, R.T., B.K. Chen, S.E. Straus, J.K. Dale, M.J. Lenardo, D. Baltimore. 1998. HIV-1 directly kills CD4+ T cells by a Fas-independent mechanism. J Exp Med 187:1113–1122.

464. Yagi, T., A. Sugimoto, M. Tanaka, S. Nagata, S. Yasuda, H. Yagita, T. Kuriyama, T. Takemori, Y. Tsunetsugu-Yokota. 1998. Fas/FasL interaction is not involved in apoptosis of activated CD4+ T cells upon HIV-1 infection in vitro. J Acquir Immune Defic Syndr Hum Retrovirol 18:307–315.

465. Berndt, C., B. Mopps, S. Angermuller, P. Gierschik, P.H. Krammer. 1998. CXCR4 and CD4 mediate a rapid CD95-independent cell death in CD4(+) T cells. Proc Natl Acad Sci USA 95:12556–12561.

466. Badley, A.D., J.A. McElhinny, P.J. Leibson, D.H. Lynch, M.R. Alderson, C.V. Paya. 1996. Upregulation of Fas ligand expression by human immunodeficiency virus in human macrophages mediates apoptosis of uninfected T lymphocytes. J Virol 70:199–206.

467. Badley, A.D., D.H. Dockrell, A. Algeciras, S. Ziesmer, A. Landay, M.M. Lederman, E. Connick, H. Kessler, D. Kuritzkes, D.H. Lynch, P. Roche, H. Yagita, C.V. Paya. 1998. In vivo analysis of Fas/FasL interactions in HIV-infected patients. J Clin Invest. 102:79–87.

468. Dockrell, D.H., A.D. Badley, J.S. Villacian, C.J. Heppelmann, A. Algeciras, S. Ziesmer, H. Yagita, D.H. Lynch, P.C. Roche, P.J. Leibson, C.V. Paya. 1998. The expression of Fas ligand by macrophages and its upregulation by human immunodeficiency virus infection. J Clin Invest 101: 2394–2405.

469. Zauli, G., D. Gibellini, P. Secchiero, H. Dutartre, D. Olive, S. Capitani, Y. Collette. 1999. Human immunodeficiency virus type 1 Nef protein sensitizes CD4(+) T lymphoid cells to apoptosis via functional upregulation of the CD95/CD95 ligand pathway. Blood. 93:1000–1010.

470. Xu, X.N., B. Laffert, G.R. Screaton, M. Kraft, D. Wolf, W. Kolanus, J. Mongkolsapay, A.J. McMichael, A.S. Baur. 1999. Induction of Fas ligand expression by HIV involves the interaction of Nef with the T-cell receptor zeta chain. J Exp Med 189:1489–1496.

471. Sloand, E.M., J.P. Maciejewski, T. Sato, J. Bruny, P. Kumar, S. Kim, F.F. Weichold, N.S. Young. 1998. The role of interleukin-converting enzyme in Fas-mediated apoptosis in HIV-1 infection. J Clin Invest 101:195–201.

472. Bartz, S.R., M. Emerman. 1999. Human immunodeficiency virus type 1 Tat induces apoptosis and increases sensitivity to apoptotic signals by upregulating FLICE/caspase-8. J Virol 73:1956–1963.

473. Li, C.J., D.J. Friedman, C. Wang, V. Metelev, A.B. Pardee. 1995. Induction of apoptosis in uninfected lymphocytes by HIV-1 Tat protein. Science 268:429–431.
474. Regamey, N., T. Harr, M. Battegay, P. Erb. 1999. Downregulation of Bcl-2, but not of Bax or Bcl-x, is associated with T lymphocyte apoptosis in HIV infection and restored by antiretroviral therapy or by interleukin 2. AIDS Res Hum Retroviruses. 15:803–810.
475. Meyaard, L., S.A. Otto, I.P. Keet, M.T. Roos, F. Miedema. 1994. Programmed death of T-cells in human immunodeficiency virus infection. No correlation with progression to disease. J Clin Invest 93:982–988.
476. Casella, C.R., E.L. Rapaport, T.H. Finkel. 1999. Vpu increases susceptibility of human immunodeficiency virus type 1- infected cells to fas killing. J Virol 73:92–100.
477. Muro-Cacho, C.A., G. Pantaleo, A.S. Fauci. 1995. Analysis of apoptosis in lymph nodes of HIV-infected persons. J Immunol 154:5555–5566.
478. Finkel, T.H., G. Tudor-Williams, N.K. Banda, M.F. Cotton, T. Curiel, C. Monks, T.W. Baba, R.M. Ruprecht, A. Kupfer. 1995. Apoptosis occurs predominantly in bystander cells and not in productively infected cells of HIV- and SIV-infected lymph nodes. Nat Med 1:129–134.
479. Rosok, B.I., J.E. Brinchmann, G. Stent, R. Bjerknes, P. Voltersvik, J. Olofsson, B. Asjo. 1998. Correlates of apoptosis of CD4+ and CD8+ T cells in tonsillar tissue in HIV type 1 infection. AIDS Res Hum Retroviruses 14:1635–1643.
480. Badley, A.D., D. Dockrell, M. Simpson, R. Schut, D.H. Lynch, P. Leibson, C.V. Paya. 1997. Macrophage-dependent apoptosis of CD4+ T lymphocytes from HIV-infected individuals is mediated by FasL and tumor necrosis factor. J Exp Med 185:55–64.
481. Herbein, G., C. Van Lint, J.L. Lovett, E. Verdin. 1998. Distinct mechanisms trigger apoptosis in human immunodeficiency virus type 1-infected and in uninfected bystander T lymphocytes. J Virol 72:660–670.
482. Wang, L., C.W. Robb, M.W. Cloyd. 1997. HIV induces homing of resting T lymphocytes to lymph nodes. Virology 228:141–152.
483. Wang, L., J.J. Chen, B.B. Gelman, R. Konig, M.W. Cloyd. 1999. A novel mechanism of CD4 lymphocyte depletion involves effects of HIV on resting lymphocytes: induction of lymph node homing and apoptosis upon secondary signaling through homing receptors. J Immunol 162:268–276.
484. Gougeon, M.-L., H. Lecoeur, A. Dulioust, M.-G. Enouf, M. Crouvoisier, C. Goujard, T. Debord, L. Montagnier. 1996. Programmed cell death in peripheral lymphocytes from HIV-infected persons. J Immunol 156:3509–3520.
485. Liegler, T.J., W. Yonemoto, T. Elbeik, E. Vittinghoff, S.P. Buchbinder,

W.C. Greene. 1998. Diminished spontaneous apoptosis in lymphocytes from human immunodeficiency virus-infected long-term nonprogressors. J Infect Dis 178:669–679.
486. Estaquier, J., T. Idziorek, F. DeBels, F. Barre-Sinoussi, B. Hurtrel, A.-M. Aubertin, A. Venet, M. Mehtali, E. Muchmore, P. Michel, Y. Mouton, M. Girard, J.C. Ameisen. 1994. Programmed cell death and AIDS: signficance of T-cell apoptosis in pathogenic and nonpathogenic primate lentiviral infections. Proc Natl Acad Sci USA 91:9431–9435.
487. Pantaleo, G., J.F. Demarest, H. Soudeyns, C. Graziosi, F. Denis, J.W. Adelsberger, P. Borrow, M.S. Saag, G.M. Shaw, R.P. Sekaly, A.S. Fauci. 1994. Major expansion of CD8+ T-cells with a predominant V beta usage during the primary immune response to HIV. Nature 370:463–467.
488. Wilson, J., G. Ogg, R. Allen, P. Goulder, A. Kelleher, A. Sewell, C. O'Callaghan, S. Rowland-Jones, M. Callan, A. McMichael. 1998. Oligoclonal expansions of CD8+ T cells in chronic HIV infection are antigen specific. J Exp Med 188:785–790.
489. Giorgi, J.V., R. Detels. 1989. T-cell subset alterations in HIV-infected homosexual men: NIAID Multicenter AIDS cohort study. Clin Immunol Immunopathol 52:10–18.
490. Giorgi, J.V., Z. Liu, L.E. Hultin, W.G. Cumberland, K. Hennessey, R. Detels. 1993. Elevated levels of CD38+CD8+ T cells in HIV infection add to the prognostic value of low CD4+ T cell levels: results of 6 years of follow-up. J AIDS 6:904–912.
491. Giorgi, J.V., H.-N. Ho, K. Hirji, C.-C. Chou, L.E. Hultin, S. O'Rourke, L. Park, J.B. Margolick, J. Ferbas, J.P. Phair. 1994. CD8+ Lymphocyte activation at human immunodeficiency virus type 1 seroconversion: development of HLA-DR+ CD38− CD8+ cells is associated with subsequent stable CD4+ cell levels. J Infect Dis 170:775–781.
492. Saukkonen, J.J., H. Kornfeld, J.S. Berman. 1993. Expansion of a CD8+CD28- cell population in the blood and lung of HIV-positive patients. J AIDS 6:1194–1204.
493. Brinchmann, J.E., J.H. Dobloug, B.H. Heger, L.L. Haaheim, M. Sannes, T. Egeland. 1994. Expression of costimulatory molecule CD28 on T cells in human immunodeficiency virus type 1 infection: functional and clinical correlations. J Infect Dis 169:730–738.
494. Caruso, A., A. Cantalamessa, S. Licenziati, L. Peroni, E. Prati, F. Martinelli, A.D. Canaris, S. Folghera, R. Gorla, A. Balsari, et al. 1994. Expression of CD28 on CD8+ and CD4+ lymphocytes during HIV infection. Scand J Immunol 40:485–490.
495. Fiorentino, S., M. Dalod, D. Olive, J.G. Guillet, E. Gomard. 1996. Predominant involvement of CD8+CD28- lymphocytes in human immunodeficiency virus-specific cytotoxic activity. J Virol 70:2022–2026.

496. Giorgi, J.V., M.A. Hausner, L.E. Hultin. 1999. Detailed immunophenotype of CD8+ memory cytotoxic T-lymphocytes (CTL) against HIV-1 with respect to expression of CD45RA/RO, CD62L and CD28 antigens. Immunol Lett 66:105–110.
497. Weekes, M.P., A.J. Carmichael, M.R. Wills, K. Mynard, J.G. Sissons. 1999. Human CD28-CD8+ T cells contain greatly expanded functional virus- specific memory CTL clones. J Immunol 162:7569–7577.
498. Vingerhoets, J.H., G.L. Vanham, L.L. Kestens, G.G. Penne, R.L. Colebunders, M.J. Vandenbruaene, J. Goeman, P.L. Gigase, M. De Boer, J.L. Ceuppens. 1995. Increased cytolytic T lymphocyte activity and decreased B7 responsiveness are associated with CD28 down-regulation on CD8+ T cells from HIV-infected subjects. Clin Exp Immunol 100:425–433.
499. Forte, M., G. Maartens, M. Rahelu, J. Pasi, C. Ellis, H. Gaston, D. Kumararatne. 1992. Cytolytic T-cell activity against mycobacterial antigens in HIV. AIDS 6:407–411.
500. Carmichael, A., X. Jin, P. Sissons, L. Borysiewicz. 1993. Quantitative analysis of the human immunodeficiency virus type 1 (HIV-1)-specific cytotoxic T lymphocyte (CTL) response at different stages of HIV-1 infection: differential CTL responses to HIV-1 and Epstein-Barr virus in late disease. J Exp Med 177:249–256.
501. Herbein, G., U. Mahlknecht, F. Batliwalla, P. Gregersen, T. Pappas, J. Butler, W.A. O'Brien, E. Verdin. 1998. Apoptosis of CD8+ T cells is mediated by macrophages through interaction of HIV gp120 with chemokine receptor CXCR4. Nature 395:189–194.
502. Meyaard, L., H. Schuitemaker, F. Miedema. 1993. T-cell dysfunction in HIV infection: anergy due to defective antigen-presenting cell function? Immunol Today 14:161–164.
503. Cheng-Mayer, C., R. Liu, N.R. Landau, L. Stamatatos. 1997. Macrophage tropism of human immunodeficiency virus type 1 and utilization of the CC-CKR5 coreceptor. J Virol 71:1657–1661.
504. Rana, S., G. Besson, D.G. Cook, J. Rucker, R.J. Smyth, Y. Yi, J.D. Turner, H.H. Guo, J.G. Du, S.C. Peiper, E. Lavi, M. Samson, F. Libert, C. Liesnard, G. Vassart, R.W. Doms, M. Parmentier, R.G. Collman. 1997. Role of CCR5 in infection of primary macrophages and lymphocytes by macrophage-tropic strains of human immunodeficiency virus: resistance to patient-derived and prototype isolates resulting from the delta ccr5 mutation. J Virol 71:3219–3227.
505. Di Marzio, P., J. Tse, N.R. Landau. 1998. Chemokine receptor regulation and HIV type 1 tropism in monocyte-macrophages. AIDS Res Hum Retroviruses 14:129–138.
506. He, J., Y. Chen, M. Farzan, H. Choe, A. Ohagen, S. Gartner, J. Busciglio, X. Yang, W. Hofmann, W. Newman, C.R. MacKay, J. Sodroski, D. Ga-

buzda. 1997. CCR3 and CCR5 are co-receptors for HIV-1 infection of microglia. Nature 385:645–649.

507. Verani, A., E. Pesenti, S. Polo, E. Tresoldi, G. Scarlatti, P. Lusso, A.G. Siccardi, D. Vercelli. 1998. CXCR4 is a functional coreceptor for infection of human macrophages by CXCR4-dependent primary HIV-1 isolates. J Immunol 161:2084–2088.
508. Gendelman, H.E., J.M. Orenstein, M.A. Martin, C. Ferrua, R. Mitra, T. Phipps, L.A. Wahl, H.C. Lane, A.S. Fauci, D.S. Burke, et al. 1988. Efficient isolation and propagation of human immunodeficiency virus on recombinant colony-stimulating factor 1-treated monocytes. J Exp Med 167: 1428–1441.
509. Perelson, A.S., P. Essunger, Y. Cao, M. Vesanen, A. Hurley, K. Saksela, M. Markowitz, D. Ho. 1997. Decay characteristics of HIV-1 infected compartments during combination therapy. Nature 387:188–191.
510. Schrager, L.K., M.P. D'Souza. 1998. Cellular and anatomical reservoirs of HIV-1 in patients receiving potent antiretroviral combination therapy. J Am Med Assoc 280:67–71.
511. Schnittman, S.M., M.C. Psallidopoulos, H.C. Lane, L. Thompson, M. Baseler, F. Massari, C.H. Fox, N.P. Salzman, A.S. Fauci. 1989. The reservoir for HIV-1 in human peripheral blood is a T cell that maintains expression of CD4. Science 245:305–308.
512. Weinberg, J.B., T.J. Mathhews, B.R. Cullen, M.H. Malim. 1991. Productive human immunodeficiency virus type 1 (HIV-1) infection of nonproliferating human monocytes. J Exp Med 174:1477–1482.
513. Valentin, A., A.V. Gegerfelt, S. Matsuda, K. Nilsson, B. Asjo. 1991. In vitro maturation of mononuclear phagocytes and susceptibility to HIV-1 infection. J Acquir Immune Defic Syndr Hum Retrovirol 4:751–759.
514. Armstrong, J., R. Horne. 1984. Follicular dendritic cells and virus-like particles in AIDS-related lymphadenopathy. Lancet ii:370–372.
515. Koenig, S., H.E. Gendelman, J.M. Orenstein, M.C. Dalcanto, G.H. Pezeshkpour, M. Yungbluth, F. Janotta, A.M. Aksamit, M.A. Martin, A.S. Fauci. 1986. Detection of AIDS virus in macrophages in brain tissue from AIDS patients with encephalopathy. Science 233: 1089–1093.
516. Orenstein, J., C. Fox, S. Wahl. 1997. Macrophages as a source of HIV during opportunistic infections. Science 276:1857–1861.
517. Ennen, J., I. Seipp, S.G. Norley, R. Kurth. 1990. Decreased accessory cell function of macrophages after infection with human immunodeficiency virus type 1 in vitro. Eur J Immunol 20:2451–2456.
518. Yoo, J., H. Chen, T. Kraus, D. Hirsch, S. Polyak, I. George, K. Sperber. 1996. Altered cytokine production and accessory cell function after HIV-1 infection. J Immunol 157:1313–1320.
519. Polyak, S., H. Chen, D. Hirsch, I. George, R. Hershberg, K. Sperber. 1997.

Impaired class II expression and antigen uptake in monocytic cells after HIV-1 infection. J Immunol 159:2177–2188.

520. Bender, B.S., F.A. Augor, T.C. Quinn, R. Redfield, J. Gold, T.M. Folks. 1986. Impaired antibody-dependent cell-mediated cytotoxic activity in patients with the acquired immunodeficiency syndrome. Clin Exp Immunol 64:166–172.

521. Baldwin, G.C., J. Fleischmann, Y. Chung, Y. Koyanagi, I.S. Chen, D.W. Golde. 1990. Human immunodeficiency virus causes mononuclear phagocyte dysfunction. Proc Natl Acad Sci USA 87:3933–3937.

522. Kent, S.J., G. Stent, S. Sonza, S.D. Hunter, S.M. Crowe. 1994. HIV-1 infection of monocyte-derived macrophages reduces Fc and complement receptor expression. Clin Exp Immunol 95:450–454.

523. Poli, G., B. Botazzi, R. Acero, L. Bergani, V. Rossi, M. Introna, A. Lazzarin, M. Galli, A. Mantovani. 1985. Monocyte function in intravenous drug abusers with lymphadenopathy syndrome and in patients with acquired immunodeficiency syndrome: selective impairment of chemotaxis. Clin Exp Immunol 62:136–142.

524. Muller, F., H. Rollag, S.S. Froland. 1990. Reduced oxidative burst responses in monocytes and monocyte-derived macrophages from HIV-infected subjects. Clin Exp Immunol 82:10–15.

525. Spear, G.T., H.A. Kessler, L. Rothberg, J. Phair, A.L. Landay. 1990. Decreased oxidative burst activity of monocytes from asymptomatic HIV-infected individuals. Clin Immunol Immunopathol 54:184–191.

526. Lafrenie, R.M., L.M. Wahl, J.S. Epstein, I.K. Hewlett, K.M. Yamada, S. Dhawan. 1996. HIV-1-Tat protein promotes chemotaxis and invasive behavior by monocytes. J Immunol 157:974–977.

527. Granelli-Piperno, A., B. Moser, M. Pope, D. Chen, Y. Wei, F. Isdell, U. O'Doherty, W. Paxton, R. Koup, S. Mojsov, N. Bhardwaj, I. Clark-Lewis, M. Baggiolini, R.M. Steinman. 1996. Efficient interaction of HIV-1 with purified dendritic cells via multiple chemokine coreceptors. J Exp Med 184:2433–2438.

528. Rubbert, A., C. Combadiere, M. Ostrowski, J. Arthos, M. Dybul, E. Machado, M.A. Cohn, J.A. Hoxie, P.M. Murphy, A.S. Fauci, D. Weissman. 1998. Dendritic cells express multiple chemokine receptors used as coreceptors for HIV entry. J Immunol 160:3933–3941.

529. Soto-Ramirez, L.E., B. Renjifo, M.F. McLane, R. Marlink, C. O'Hara, R. Sutthent, C. Wasi, P. Vithayasai, V. Vithayasai, C. Apichartpiyakul, P. Auewarakul, V. Pena Cruz, D.S. Chui, R. Osathanondh, K. Mayer, T.H. Lee, M. Essex. 1996. HIV-1 Langerhans' cell tropism associated with heterosexual transmission of HIV. Science 271:1291–1293.

530. Pope, M., S.S. Frankel, J.R. Mascola, A. Trkola, F. Isdell, D.L. Birx, D.S. Burke, D.D. Ho, J.P. Moore. 1997. Human immunodeficiency virus type

1 strains of subtypes B and E replicate in cutaneous dendritic cell-T-cell mixtures without displaying subtype-specific tropism. J Virol 71:8001–8007.

531. Dittmar, M.T., G. Simmons, S. Hibbitts, M. O'Hare, S. Louisirirotchanakul, S. Beddows, J. Weber, P.R. Clapham, R.A. Weiss. 1997. Langerhans cell tropism of human immunodeficiency virus type 1 subtype A through F isolates derived from different transmission groups. J Virol 71:8008–8013.
532. Reece, J.C., A.J. Handley, E.J. Anstee, W.A. Morrison, S.M. Crowe, P.U. Cameron. 1998. HIV-1 selection by epidermal dendritic cells during transmission across human skin. J Exp Med 187:1623–1631.
533. Macatonia, S.E., R. Lau, S. Patterson, A.J. Pinching, S.C. Knight. 1990. Dendritic cell infection, depletion and dysfunction in HIV-infected individuals. Immunology 71:38–45.
534. Cameron, P.U., U. Forsum, H. Teppler, A. Granelli-Piperno, R.M. Steinman. 1992. During HIV-1 infection most blood dendritic cells are not productively infected and can induce allogeneic CD4+ T cells clonal expansion. Clin Exp Immunol 88:226–236.
535. Grassi, F., A. Hosmalin, D. McIlroy, V. Calvez, P. Debre, B. Autran. 1999. Depletion in blood CD11c-positive dendritic cells from HIV-infected patients. AIDS 13:759–66.
536. Amadori, A., L. Chieco-Bianchi. 1990. B-cell activation and HIV-1 infection: deeds and misdeeds. Immunol Today 11:374–379.
537. Ginaldi, L., M. De Martinis, D.O. A, L. Marini, D. Quaglino. 1998. Changes in antigen expression on B lymphocytes during HIV infection. Pathobiology 66:17–23.
538. Conge, A.M., K. Tarte, J. Reynes, M. Segondy, J. Gerfaux, M. Zembala, J.P. Vendrell. 1998. Impairment of B-lymphocyte differentiation induced by dual triggering of the B-cell antigen receptor and CD40 in advanced HIV-1-disease. AIDS 12:1437–1449.
539. Glushakova, S., J.C. Grivel, W. Fitzgerald, A. Sylwester, J. Zimmerberg, L.B. Margolis. 1998. Evidence for the HIV-1 phenotype switch as a causal factor in acquired immunodeficiency. Nat Med 4:346–349.
540. Rieckmann, P., G. Poli, C.H. Fox, J.H. Kehrl, A.S. Fauci. 1991. Recombinant gp120 specifically enhances tumor necrosis factor-alpha production and Ig secretion in B lymphocytes from HIV-infected individuals but not from seronegative donors. J Immunol 147:2922–2927.
541. Macchia, D., F. Almerigogna, P. Parronchi, A. Ravina, E. Maggi, S. Romagnani. 1993. Membrane tumour necrosis factor-alpha is involved in the polyclonal B-cell activation induced by HIV-infected human T cells. Nature 363:464–466.
542. Berberian, L., L. Goodglick, T.J. Kipps, J. Braun. 1993. Immunoglobulin

VH3 gene products: natural ligands for HIV gp120. Science 261:1588–1591.

543. Chirmule, N., V.S. Kalyanaraman, C. Saxinger, F. Wong-Staal, J. Ghrayeb, S. Pahwa. 1990. Localization of B-cell stimulatory activity of HIV-1 to the carboxyl terminus of gp41. AIDS Res Hum Retroviruses 6: 299–305.
544. Monroe JG, Silberstein LE. 1995. HIV-mediated B-lymphocyte activation and lymphomagenesis. J Clin Immunol 15:61–68.
545. Schrager, L.K. 1988. Bacterial infections in AIDS patients. AIDS 2:S183–189.
546. Moir S, Lapointe R, Malaspina A, Ostrowski M, Cole CE, Chun TW, Adelsberger J, Baseler M, Hwu P, Fauci AS. 1999. CD40-Mediated induction of CD4 and CXCR4 on B lymphocytes correlates with restricted susceptibility to human immunodeficiency virus type 1 infection: potential role of B lymphocytes as a viral reservoir. J Virol 73:7972–7980.
547. Mertins, S.D., L. Ortona, R. Cauda. 1990. Role of polymorphonuclear leukocytes in infection by retroviruses with emphasis on the human immunodeficiency virus. Viral Immunol 3:173–194.
548. Torosantucci, A., P. Chiani, I. Quinti, C.M. Ausiello, I. Mezzaroma, A. Cassone. 1997. Responsiveness of human polymorphonuclear cells (PMNL) to stimulation by a mannoprotein fraction (MP-F2) of *Candida albicans*; enhanced production of IL-6 and tumour necrosis factor-alpha (TNF-alpha) by MP-F2-stimulated PMNL from HIV-infected subjects. Clin Exp Immunol 107:451–457.
549. Pitrak, D.L., H.C. Tsai, K.M. Mullane, S.H. Sutton, P. Stevens. 1996. Accelerated neutrophil apoptosis in the acquired immunodeficiency syndrome. J Clin Invest 98:2714–2719.
550. Munoz, J.F., S. Salmen, L.R. Berrueta, M.P. Carlos, J.A. Cova, J.H. Donis, M.R. Hernandez, J.V. Torres. 1999. Effect of human immunodeficiency virus type 1 on intracellular activation and superoxide production by neutrophils. J Infect Dis 180:206–210.
551. Monari, C., A. Casadevall, D. Pietrella, F. Bistoni, A. Vecchiarelli. 1999. Neutrophils from patients with advanced human immunodeficiency virus infection have impaired complement receptor function and preserved fcgamma receptor function. J Infect Dis 180:1542–1549.
552. Hu, P.F., L.E. Hultin, P. Hultin, M.A. Hausner, K. Hirji, A. Jewett, B. Bonavida, R. Detels, J.V. Giorgi. 1995. Natural killer cell immunodeficiency in HIV disease is manifest by profoundly decreased numbers of CD16+CD56+ cells and expansion of a population of CD16dimCD56- cells with low lytic activity. J Acquir Immune Defic Syndr Hum Retrovirol 10:331–340.
553. Ahmad A., Menezes J. 1996. Defective killing activity against gp120/

41-expressing human erythroleukaemic K562 cell line by monocytes and natural killer cells from HIV-infected individuals. AIDS 10:143–149.
554. Ullum, H., P.C. Gotzsche, J. Victor, E. Dickmeiss, P. Skinhoj, B.K. Pedersen. 1995. Defective natural immunity: an early manifestation of human immunodeficiency virus infection. J Exp Med 182:789–799.
555. Chehimi, J., J.D. Marshall, O. Salvucci, I. Frank, S. Chehimi, S. Kawecki, D. Bacheller, S. Rifat, S. Chouaib. 1997. IL-15 enhances immune functions during HIV infection. J Immunol 158:5978–5987.
556. Galiani, M.D., E. Aguado, R. Tarazona, P. Romero, I. Molina, M. Santamaria, R. Solana, J. Pena. 1999. Expression of killer inhibitory receptors on cytotoxic cells from HIV-1- infected individuals. Clin Exp Immunol 115:472–476.
557. Andre, P., C. Brunet, S. Guia, H. Gallais, J. Sampol, E. Vivier, F. Dignat-George. 1999. Differential regulation of killer cell Ig-like receptors and CD94 lectin-like dimers on NK and T lymphocytes from HIV-1-infected individuals. Eur J Immunol 29:1076–1085.
558. Cohen GB., Gandhi RT, Davis DM, Mandelboim O, Chen BK, Strominger BL, Baltimore D. 1999. The selective downregulation of class I major histocompatibility complex proteins by HIV-1 protects HIV-infected cells from NK cells. Immunity 10:661–671.

3

The Genetic Diversity of HIV-1 and Its Implications for Vaccine Development

Vladimir V. Lukashov, Jaap Goudsmit, and William A. Paxton

Academic Medical Center
University of Amsterdam
Amsterdam, The Netherlands

INTRODUCTION

The immense genetic variation of HIV-1 is one of the most striking characteristics of this virus: proteins among HIV-1 isolates can differ in more than 35% of amino acid positions and no two virus isolates are identical. HIV-1 variation is determined by multiple simultaneously acting virus and host factors. Traditionally, several levels of HIV-1 variation are considered. Within a single HIV-1–infected human host, HIV-1 population represents a complex mixture, or swarm, of mutant virus variants, in which all viruses are genetically related yet virtually every virus is unique (intrahost heterogeneity). Relative prevalence of various virus variants within this swarm is changing over time on almost a daily basis (intrahost evolution). Moreover, infected individuals within a human population harbor distinct viruses (interhost or populationwide heterogeneity). Finally, the global HIV-1 pandemic is composed of many local epidemics, which generally differ in human populations involved, risk factors for transmission, therapy availability, as well as virus genotypes in circulation (global variation).

One of the most pertinent questions relating to the variation seen in HIV-1 is whether or not an effective vaccine is plausible. For an HIV-1 prophylactic vaccine to be successful, it will have to provide sterilizing immunity against the circulating populations of HIV-1 as well as those that have yet to evolve, a formidable task. Even though complete sterilizing immunity may never be achieved, it may be possible to control viral replication after infection has occurred with a vaccine that has the capacity to enhance or expand an already effective anti-HIV immune response. Such a vaccine strategy may be simpler since the aim would be to boost an immune response already generated against the antigens of the actual infecting viral strain. Both of these vaccine strategies would have to remain effective in the face of constant viral variation. Ultimately, in order to maximize the success of a vaccine, prophylactic, or therapeutic, its design may have to be tailored to specific viral sequences, either for the infectious viral strain or for a consensus viral sequence of a particular geographical region, respectively.

The rate at which HIV-1 can escape effective anti-HIV-1 monotherapy, which can be as short as days, is daunting and highlights the challenge that lies ahead for vaccine development. There are, however, a few positive indicators to suggest that protection against viral transmission and/or disease progression may indeed be feasible. HIV-1 results in a chronic viral infection with the vast majority of infected individuals eventually progressing to disease. Those few individuals who can successfully control their viral replication and who have done so for more than 10–15 years may hold many of the answers to what is required of a HIV-1 vaccine. In the same way individuals who have been heavily exposed to HIV-1 but who have remained seronegative are also important individuals to study in order to decipher the natural mechanisms that can provide blocks to HIV-1 transmission. HIV-1 must keep many of its biological properties for survival, and this maintenance of phenotype may provide an advantage to the host. The less an HIV-1 virus changes, the less likely it is that that virus will evade an already established and effective anti-HIV-specific immune response since immune responses are based on the recognition of antigenic protein determinants.

As a way of introduction to the significance of viral variation, the reader should be familiar with some of the differences in HIV-1 biological phenotype that exist. It has been understood for many years that HIV-1 can carry various biological properties, such as cell-type tropism and replication phenotype, which have been associated with differences in disease status and rates of disease progression in infected individuals. Macrophage-tropic (M-tropic) viruses, otherwise known as non–syncytium inducing (NSI), are those associated with viral transmission and the early stages of disease, while T-cell line–tropic (T-tropic) or syncytium-inducing (SI) viruses are those predominantly associated with late-stage disease and fast progression. M-tropic viruses have the capacity to grow on macrophages and activated peripheral blood mononuclear cells (PBMCs) but not on T-cell lines, while the T-tropic viral isolates can grow on T-cell lines, and activated PBMCs but not macrophages. HIV-1 M-tropic viruses are regarded as the somewhat weaker and less pathogenic strains than the T-tropic strains, which are seen as more aggressive. Differences in the HIV-1 gp120 envelope amino acid sequences, especially in the V1-V2 and V3 variable loop regions, have been associated with the above biological phenotypes. It is now known that M-tropic viruses and T-tropic viruses utilize different coreceptors in conjunction with the CD4 molecule for their entry into cells. M-tropic viruses utilize predominantly the CCR5 chemokine receptor, while T-tropic viruses utilize mainly the chemokine receptor CXCR4. As an individual progresses in disease, the genetic sequence and phenotype of the virus will alter from using CCR5 to using CXCR4.

Not only is the immune response implicated in controlling HIV-1 infection and replication, but it has become apparent that multiple host genotypes can be associated with resistance to HIV-1 infection and altered rates of disease progression in infected individuals. These host factor restrictions to viral replication, largely based around coreceptors and their natural ligands, can function in a similar manner to controlling immune responses. In this chapter we wish to discuss viral variation and the effect that various immune responses and host factors have on driving HIV-1 sequence diversity and discuss the implications for vaccine development.

HIV-1 VARIATION AND EVOLUTION

Intrahost Variation of HIV-1: Transmission and Compartmentalization

HIV-1 replication is a highly error-prone process, mainly due to lack of proofreading activity of the reverse transcription. The rate of nucleotide substitutions introduced by reverse transcriptase is approximately 10^{-4} per nucleotide per cycle of replication (1–5), which means that, on average, every newly produced virus genome has one nucleotide substitution compared to the parental genome (the size of HIV-1 genome is approximately 9.7 Kb). In addition to nucleotide substitutions, other types of mutations, including insertions, deletions, duplications, and recombinations, contribute to genetic heterogeneity of HIV-1 (6–10). The extreme mutation rate of HIV, together with short replication time and high virus loads, are resulting in continual creation of random complex mixtures of antigenically and phenotypically different virus strains, which compete among themselves for survival. Although most of these mutants are replication defective or less adapted to the intrahost environment (less fit), some of them will, by chance, have a higher fitness and preferentially outgrow. Subsequent outgrowth of a certain virus strain is largely determined by its replicative properties, cellular tropism, ability to escape from host immune response and antiretroviral therapy as well as by stochastic processes like population bottleneck events. In addition to selective forces that arise within host and include receptor availability, cell permissiveness, immune and drug pressures, the virus populations is also shaped by events occurring during host-to-host transmission, which may depend on the transmission route and the dose of the inoculum.

From the documented cases of HIV-1 transmission, it has become apparent that HIV-1 populations in newly infected individuals are relatively homogeneous and may represent a major or a minor virus subpopulation present in the donors (11–18). Although these observations are evident for a limitation of virus heterogeneity occurring during transmission, the mechanisms of this process are not yet fully understood. The main question that remains to be answered is whether the nature of this process is random, and the probability of any virus strain present in the donor to be transmitted to the recipient by chance is similar, or a specific selection is operational during transmission, and only viruses with certain phenotype could establish infections in new hosts. The understanding of the mechanism of selection during transmission is especially difficult since these mechanisms could differ for different transmission routes (13,19–21).

Clearly massive random population bottlenecks are occurring during transmission, since the inoculum never contains the whole repertoire of virus strains present in the donor. On the other hand, selection of virus phenotype during transmission is supported by observations that the NSI viruses are present in the majority of infected individuals during the early stages of the HIV-1 infection following vertical, sexual, and parenteral transmission, even after transmission of a phenotypically mixed SI/NSI virus population (16,22,23). However, these observations could be strongly influenced by a fact that SI viruses are only present in HIV-infected individuals who are at the latest stages of the disease and do not cause the majority of new infections. Moreover, due to the peculiarities of experimental methods, even in individuals who are characterized as carrying the SI phenotype, the majority of clonal viruses in the bulk isolate (up to 95%) could indeed have the NSI phenotype (24).

In addition to HIV-1 diversity in serum and blood cells, HIV-1 strains in other tissues contribute to the intrahost heterogeneity of the virus. HIV-1 compartmentalization within hosts is essential to consider in studying virus transmission, since new infections could be caused by viruses originating from various donor tissue reservoirs. HIV-1 is present in a variety of human organs and tissues, and multiple studies have shown that HIV-1 populations in blood generally differ from those derived simultaneously from other tissues, including spleen, the central nervous system, semen, vaginal secretion, lung lavage, intestinal tissues, etc. (13,25–29). Yet, because of their cross-sectional design, most of the studies could not address the main question of whether the differences between tissue-specific virus populations are the results of independent evolution during virus adaptation to particular tissues or the consequences of random founder effects and time-related uneven distribution of virus strains within the host. Although independent HIV-1 evolution in different tissues and existence of tissue-specific genotypic patterns of HIV-1 have been hypothesized in some studies, the data on these issues are inconsistent. A longitudinal study of serum- and intestinum-derived viruses obtained over a period of several years from three individuals has revealed that virus strains that are present in the intestinum and are absent in serum at a certain time point could be found in serum at another time point (L. van der Hoek, V.V. Lukashov, and J. Goudsmit, unpublished). This indicates that differences in HIV-1 populations between different tissue compartments (at least between serum and intestinum) may be largely determined by random founder effects and sampling biases.

Immune-Mediated Factors

No HIV-1–infected individual has yet been shown to eradicate the virus from his or her system, with the majority progressing to disease. One of the complexities with HIV-1 infection is that HIV-specific, as well as nonspecific, immune responses are eventually diminished in infected people. Whether the development of immune dysfunction is a result of mechanisms such as cell lysis and/or induced T-cell anergy, or whether the virus has evolved to evade an effective controlling immune response is a hotly debated issue. There are worrying implications for the development of an HIV-1 vaccine if individuals who progress in their disease do so because the virus has evolved and escaped an effective immune response. There are numerous examples of infectious agents utilizing mechanisms that allow them to evade an effective immune response. The influenza virus, for example, can dramatically alter its immune recognition profile through a process termed antigenic shift and drift, which is reassortment and mutation of a segmented genome with new viral strains emerging periodically with devastating public health consequences (30,31). Another example is with the trypanosome parasites, which have developed a system whereby their variant surface glycoprotein (VSG) coats can be changed by a genetic recombination event which places a new and variant gene into a unique transcriptionally active site (32). The parasites carry an extensive array of different VSG genes, which code for VSGs that are immunologically distinguishable from each other and can be randomly recombined into the active expression site when the parasite comes under immune-induced stress. When this exchange occurs, the parasite alters its surface protein beyond sufficient immunological recognition by the host and thereby escapes an effective immune-mediated response and once again thrives. HIV-1 with its high replication rate and highly error-prone reverse transcription life-cycle stage is another example of how an infectious organism can help evade the immune response by dramatically altering its protein sequence.

The immune responses generated against HIV-1 antigens are presumably as varied and complex as against any other infectious agent. Neutralizing antibody responses, cytotoxic T-lymphocyte (CTL) responses, and T-lymphocyte helper

(Th) responses have all been extensively analyzed in both HIV-1–infected and exposed but uninfected individuals and are extensively reviewed in other chapters of this book and elsewhere (33). Monitoring individuals through acute infection suggests that the host immune response brings the viral load down to its postacute setpoint and continues to control virus replication for the duration of the asymptomatic period, which is highly variant dependent on the individual (34–36). What then results in the rapid rise in viral load, subsequent drop in CD4+ cell count, and progression to disease that is observed in most individuals. In a chronic infection like HIV-1, the immune response must have the capacity to alter so as to eradicate the new viruses that evolve during natural progression. Not only does the immune recognition have to be maintained, but effective immune function also has to be kept in the face of viral evolution. The development of a therapeutic vaccine for HIV-1 will therefore benefit from the better understanding of the correlates of protection against disease progression. The stronger the initial immune suppression by the host, the less chance there is of an escape mutation arising. This may help explain why individuals with the lower viral loads at setpoint tend to do better in disease than those with the higher loads. The existence of long-term survivors—individuals who have been infected with HIV-1 for more than 10–15 years and who have maintained high CD4 counts, low to undetectable viral loads, and who have not progressed to disease—suggests that immune responses can control infection. These individuals have been shown to develop neutralizing antibody responses, high CTL responses against a broad spectrum of antigens/epitopes as well as having strong HIV-1 Th responses against an array of antigens (37–40), the point being that strong immune responses and low viral loads are correlated with longer disease-free periods (34–36,41,42). Conversely, individuals who progress rapidly to disease within a short period of time after infection have been shown to have low HIV-1–neutralizing antibody responses, narrowly directed anti-HIV-1 CTL responses, and low levels of Th-cell responses (40,43). An analogy can be drawn here with anti-HIV-1 drug therapy, where the individuals with the higher levels of viral suppression tend to resist developing drug-resistant virus longer.

There is now evidence to show that vaccination with HIV-1 antigens, such as REMUNE, after HIV-1 antiretroviral drug therapy and viral suppression can be beneficial to the maintenance and enhancement of anti-HIV-1 immune responses (44). It has also been demonstrated that the periodic reemergence of virus in therapy-disrupted individuals can help boost an established anti-HIV-1 immune response that has the ability to subsequently control viral replication (45). These results indicate that a therapeutic interventive vaccine is indeed plausible for HIV-1, but the length of time that this enhanced immune response can be maintained while remaining effective is still not known. Below we will review different facets of the immune system that can influence viral variation and discuss how HIV-1 can evolve to specifically curtail their effectiveness. Obviously, every area of the immune system cannot be covered in one chapter, but we will discuss using specific examples just how viral adaptation and evolution may effect HIV-1 vaccine development.

Antibodies

The B cells of the immune system generate antibodies specific for the native structure of foreign protein with which they are presented. Therefore, minor alterations in either amino acid composition or protein modification patterns, such as glycosylation profiles, would be expected to greatly influence the antibody (Ab) responses generated against the virus. Antibodies function either by directly binding to virus particles and neutralizing their infectivity or by recruiting effector mechanisms such as the complement cascade or antibody-dependent cellular cytotoxicity pathways, where viruses and infected cells are recognized and destroyed, respectively (46). All strategies rely on a process of B-cell affinity maturation where the affinity, and ultimately effectiveness, of an antibody is improved over time. However, if the virus undergoes constant modification, this process will be limited and a proper and effective neutralizing antibody response may never mature.

The gp120 protein of HIV-1 provides a good example of how a protein can create poor immunological recognition. The gp120 viral protein is complex and composed of constant as well as variable regions, all of which can be heavily O- or N-linked glycosylated (contributing to approximately 50% of the envelope mass) (47,48). The recent elucidation of a modified envelope, in conjunction with a stabilizing monoclonal Ab mimicking CD4 binding has revealed many of the structural properties of the envelope, which provides some of the answers to structure-function questions (49,50). The hypervariable regions of the envelope, namely V1-V2 and V3, are believed to heavily influence the viral coreceptor requirement while at the same time masking the actual chemokine coreceptor binding site from antibody recognition and hence neutralization (51–54). Previous studies have also revealed through the mapping of monoclonal antibody binding epitopes (MAb) that the actual coreceptor binding site is situated close to the CD4 binding region and not the variable regions themselves (54). Glycosylation patterns within the V3 region have also been reported to alter the neutralization potential of viruses with deglycosylated V3 viruses showing more sensitivity to in vitro neutralization (55). There is supporting evidence for the significance of envelope glycosylation patterns in the simian immunodeficiency virus (SIV) model system where the mere deletion of *N*-linked glycosylation sites in the V1 region can greatly influence the in vivo neutralization potential of a virus (56). The gp120 envelope may also limit the recognition of some significant neutralization sites by forming oligomeric structures, thereby restricting the surface area of the molecule available to immune surveillance (57). However, given all this modification potential for the HIV-1 envelope, the protein has to retain some structural integrity, since all viruses have to ultimately bind and utilize the CD4-coreceptor complex to remain viable. Viruses that have been multiply passaged through T-cell lines have been shown to become sensitive to a wide array of neutralizing monoclonal antibodies and human sera, suggesting that the envelope has in someway been modified to expose neutralizing epitopes that were previously nonaccessible (46). It is also of interest to note that in a number of the monomeric gp120 vaccine trials to date, many of the sera from the vaccine recipients are perfectly capable of neutralizing T-cell line–adapted viruses but not primary isolates in vitro (58,59). Many groups are now working on ways to manipulate and modify the gp120 protein so that the neutralizing epitopes are exposed in order to help provide for the induction of broader and more effective neutralizing antibody responses.

Whether or not neutralization antibodies will be successful in limiting initial viral infectivity or subsequent viral replication, given the complex nature of cell-to-cell transmission by the virus, has still to be determined. There is mounting evidence, however, that anti-HIV-1 vaginal secretory IgA responses can be correlated with resistance to infection in a cohort of women who have been exposed to HIV-1 through multiple unsafe sexual exposures (60–62). This provides strong evidence that a prophylactic vaccine against HIV-1 that incorporates the induction of Ab responses may indeed be successful in limiting viral transmission. Determining the epitopes that these antibody responses are directed against will be significant for the development of an effective HIV-1 vaccine.

T-Cell Responses

Unlike the B cells that recognize the native protein structure, the T cells of the immune system recognize antigens that have been processed and presented by the major histocompatability complex (MHC) proteins. The MHC class I molecule presents processed antigen to CD8+ T lymphocytes, which includes the cytotoxic T lymphocytes (CTLs), while MHC class II molecule presents processed antigen to CD4+ T lymphocytes, which incorporates the Th cells (63–67). The two presentation pathways differ, and class I presentation usually requires endogenous protein synthesis while class II presentation only requires protein uptake and processing. Given these restrictions to presentation, the induction of CTL responses therefore requires active viral replication, while Th responses can be induced by native protein alone. These restrictions to antigenic presentation will also apply to vaccine candidates designed to stimulate anti-HIV-1 cellular immune responses. Class I epitopes are commonly 9–11 amino acids in length and have specific amino acid requirements, namely anchor residues at set positions that bind the peptide to the MHC molecule (68–70). For class II presentation, the epitope is usually longer and carries its own specific amino acid requirements for binding. Single amino acid changes within class I and II peptides have been shown to successfully eradicate peptide binding to MHC molecules (71–74). Not only can mutations affect the binding of the peptide to the MHC molecule, but other mutations in the peptide may inhibit the T-cell receptor on the T cell from recognizing the MHC-antigen complex.

Variation within a given epitope can affect recognition by the T lymphocytes and therefore lead to escape from an effective immune response (75). Even though immune escape can occur, alterations within viral antigenic sequences will create altered epitopes that other T cells within the total repertoire will recognize. These newly stimulated T cells would therefore become functional against the virus, and it does not necessarily follow that viral variation is detrimental to the infected host. CTL epitopes have been shown to be dominant or weak, suggesting that fluctuations in immune competence will occur with viral variation. From numerous studies with rapidly progressing and long-term surviving individuals, it seems evident that both the strength and breadth of the CTL response correlate with disease progression (43). For vaccine purposes, this does raise a problem, since most vaccines will carry a limited array of epitopes that cannot be representative of all the possible challenge viral sequences. The extreme heterogeneity of the MHC complex within the human population also carries significance in this regard, since no two individuals carry the exact same MHC profile, therefore a dominant epitope in one individual will not necessarily be dominant in another.

There has been considerable discussion in the past as to whether a strong CTL response can actually select for the emergence of escape mutations within the recognized epitope, thereby diminishing an effective anti-HIV-1 immune response. Recent evidence in MHC-matched monkeys has convincingly demonstrated that effective CTL responses can be evaded through CTL epitope selection and that this can be correlated with disease induction (76). This undoubtedly has implications for the development of a therapeutic vaccine in that the induction of a strong CTL response will place pressure on the virus to quickly escape immune control. Another possible complication with the development of vaccines that are capable of inducing powerful CTL responses is the concept of original antigenic sin (77). In this phenomenon, the variant form of a strong CTL epitope will be weakly recognized even though that epitope has the capacity to be highly effective. The induction of a strong CTL response may therefore limit the ability of the immune system to mount a good CTL response against any of the variant epitope sequences it may thereafter encounter and thereby limit CTL function and control. Preexposure to CTL epitopes therefore may be detrimental overall to the vaccine recipient since it will dampen any CTL responses against similar epitopes.

As with the B-cell responses, strong T-cell responses, both CD8+ and CD4+, have been demonstrated in cohorts of exposed but uninfected individuals (33). Again, the significance for prophylactic vaccine development is the identification that heavily exposed but uninfected commercial sex workers in Africa carry CTL activity, suggesting that protective immunity may be generated that protects against all viruses to which these individuals are exposed (78,78). Of more significance is the identification of strong cross-subtype epitope recognition in some of these individuals (79–83), which shows that the high degree of viral variation observed between HIV-1 subtypes does not necessarily lead to immune escape.

Although the HIV-1 envelope protein is the most obvious antigenic candidate for the induction of B-cell responses, the antigenic processing and presentation of T-cell epitopes indicates that all HIV-1 proteins should be considered as potential vaccine candidates. The obvious advantage of utilizing antigens other than the envelope is that these proteins may have more structural-functional constraints. The accessory protein Tat is a good example; this protein has been shown to carry conserved immunogenic epitopes. The significance of Tat as a potential anti-HIV-1 vaccine candidate has recently become apparent with a study demonstrating that the protein in recombinant form, when given to cymologus monkeys, provides protection against SHIV transmission (84). One of the strongest correlates associated with protection was an enhanced Tat CTL-specific immune response, even though the Tat protein was given as a recombinant antigen and therefore not undergoing the optimal presentation to the class I molecule. The Tat protein has also been shown to be associated with a reduced in vitro HIV-1 replication phenotype (85), therefore this protein may indeed turn out to be an interesting player in the development of an effective HIV-1 vaccine, be it either prophylactic or therapeutic.

Host Factors

The breadth and depth of the immune responses generated against HIV-1 are undoubtedly significant for HIV-1 infection and the control of viral replication. However, the last few years has seen an increase in the understanding of the importance that host factors play in the control of HIV-1 infectivity. The discovery that the CC-chemokine molecules RANTES, MIP-1α and MIP-1β can inhibit the replication of M-tropic viral strains of HIV, but not T-tropic strains, was a major breakthrough (86). Since the initial discovery that CCR5 and CXCR4 could function as viral coreceptors, many 7-transmembrane proteins have been identified with HIV-1 coreceptor function, but CCR5 and CXCR4 are still regarded as the most significant for HIV-1 pathogenesis (87,88). This may well be an oversimplification, and there are cases contradicting this central dogma, but for the purposes of this chapter we focus on CCR5 and CXCR4. The apparent requirement for HIV-1 to switch its coreceptor usage from CCR5 to CXCR4 during disease progression has both advantages and disadvantages for the virus as well as the host.

Much of the evidence implicating chemokines in the control of HIV-1 replication comes from the association between numerous chemokine/chemokine receptor genetic alleles with HIV-1 transmission and/or disease progression (88). The first such allele to be described, and probably the most dramatic, was the 32bp deletion within the coding region of the CCR5 receptor gene (Δ32) (89,90). This mutation results in a truncated protein that cannot be transported to the cell surface and therefore lacks both normal physiological function and the ability to be used by HIV-1 for entry into cells (90). Individuals homozygous for the Δ32 allele are highly protected against transmission of HIV, again highlighting the restriction to the transmission of predominantly CCR5 (M-tropic)–using viruses (91,92). Heterozygous individuals for the CCR5 deletion, although not protected against HIV-1 transmission, are more likely to develop lower viral loads, have slower rates of CD4 cell decline, and progress slower in their disease than CCR5 wild-type individuals (91–94). An array of other chemokine, chemokine receptor, and promotor mutations have now been associated with altered rates of HIV-1 disease progression, supporting the idea that levels of chemokine and/or chemokine receptor expression can influence viral replication (95–98).

The CC-chemokines RANTES, MIP-1α, and MIP-1β being the natural ligands for the CCR5 receptor can inhibit M-tropic viral replication by competing for receptor binding (99,100). These CC-chemokines are secreted from numerous cell types, including macrophages and CD4+ and CD8+ lymphocytes, and can therefore be seen as an extension of the HIV-1–specific mediated immune response since they themselves can limit M-tropic viral replication (86,101). Correlations have been found in vitro between CC-chemokine secretion levels from CD4+ lymphocytes and their infectability with M-tropic viral strains, and activated HIV-specific CTLs have been shown to secrete high levels of CC-chemokines (102). There have now been numerous reports describing a link between the in vivo levels of these chemokines and the control of disease progression and viral load measurements, with higher production levels from activated PBMCs being associated with individuals who do better in their disease or who are protected from infection (103,104). The significance of the CC-chemokine responses in providing protection against viral transmission has been best demonstrated in SIV or HIV-1 antigen–vaccinated macaques where high chemokine production was associated with protection against SIV or SHIV challenge, respectively (105,106). More recently it has been demonstrated that women allo-immunized with PBMCs elicit a strong CD8+ lymphocyte chemokine response, which can provide protection against in vitro viral replication (107). These results strongly indicate that the upregulation of CC-chemokines or a reduction in chemokine receptor expression levels by an HIV-1 vaccine may be beneficial. How and indeed whether an HIV-1 vaccine could maintain such an environment is still not known.

The emergence of CXCR4-using viruses is usually followed by a rapid rise in viral load measurement and a rapid fall in the CD4+ lymphocyte count. A virus that has lost its CCR5 usage will have lost sensitivity to the blocking effects of CC-chemokines, in the same way that a virus can gain resistance to either anti

HIV-1 drugs or an effective immune response. The natural ligand for the CXCR4 receptor, SDF-1α, is secreted by stromal derived stem cells and is present at low concentrations in vivo and so is less likely to be suppressing T-tropic viral replication in comparison to the CC-chemokine molecules. The CXCR4 receptor is expressed on a greater percentage of CD4+ lymphocytes and to higher levels than CCR5, which may help explain the rapid rise in viral load measurements seen during disease progression following the switch in receptor usage (102,108). Why solo CCR5-utilizing viruses are those preferentially transmitted is still not known, but one explanation is that a bottleneck in viral transmission exists and only the CCR5 viruses can initially replicate in the host and CXCR4 viruses have to evolve from this CCR5-using pool. An alternative explanation is that a swarm of viruses can establish infection but that the immune response generated can control T-tropic viral replication better than M-tropic viruses and as the immune system fails during disease progression the more promiscuous T-tropic viruses flourish. Given the few amino acid substitutions required for a virus to change phenotype and the diversity of the immune system involved, it seems unlikely that in all individuals M-tropic viruses would be better controlled than T-tropics. This initial requirement and restriction for CCR5 receptor usage may well be beneficial in the development of a vaccine.

Many regions of the HIV-1 gp120 envelope have been implicated in coreceptor usage, with mainly the variable regions V1-V2 and V3 being involved (57). As mentioned earlier, these regions are not thought to be the actual direct binding sites for the coreceptors, but they can greatly influence which receptor or receptors are used. The V3 region and its overall charge has been strongly implicated in determining the sensitivity of HIV-1 to the blocking effects of CC-chemokines, with the more positively charged V3 regions showing less blockage (109,110). Many studies have demonstrated that the positive charge of the V3 region increases during disease progression and this correlates with the replicative phenotype of the virus and towards that of the T-tropic phenotype and CXCR4 usage (111,112). These results suggest that the heavy suppression of viral replication early in infection, before alterations in the envelope can arise that allow the CCR5-to-CXCR4 switch to occur, will keep viral levels low. This biological constraint on viral transmission provides an ideal opportunity in vaccine development since the Env sequence of the viruses that are transmitted are limited.

All HIV-1 subtypes have been shown to possess this initial requirement for CCR5 usage, suggesting that a chemokine-based vaccine may be of universal significance (101,113,114). However, HIV-1 subtype C provides an interesting scenario in that it is becoming apparent that a lower percentage of individuals show a switch to CXCR4 usage than is seen for the other subtypes, even though they do progress to disease and have similar viral loads (115). Why these individuals should progress to disease when CCR5 usage is maintained remains to be answered.

The Role of HIV-1 Evolution in Virus Pathogenesis

Natural infection of HIV-1 is characterized by a highly variable incubation period between the moment of infection and the development of AIDS, which can last from several months or a few years in fast progressors to 10–15 years and more in slow or nonprogressors. HIV-1 load in plasma or serum is one of decisive factors in AIDS progression: the higher it is, the faster the virus causes immunodeficiency and AIDS (34–36,41,42). The level of virus production in a host is a reflection of the efficiency of a continuous virus adaptation to the versatile intrahost environment, including virus escape from the immune response. Therefore, HIV-1 variation is a factor that is involved in virus pathogenesis.

Early hypotheses considered virus variability, as reflected by a number of antigenically different virus strains simultaneously present in the host at a given time point, as a direct cause of disease progression. However, experimental data revealed that virus variability (ability to produce mutants) is the same in progressors and nonprogressors, yet the variation (evolution), which reflects the probability of new mutants to be fixed in the population, is different (116). These observations are inconsistent with earlier thoughts and led to a principle reconsideration of the role of HIV-1 variation in AIDS progression, which has recently been recapitulated in the model of continuous virus adaptation (117). The main feature of this model is its reevaluation of the weight of the respective contribution of host-specific versus virus-specific factors in the development of AIDS. The model considers a diverse virus population as a (passive) consequence of the host immune competence, rather than a factor leading to the development of AIDS, and explains the development of AIDS as a longitudinal process of the deterioration of the immune system caused by the virus, during which persistent virus production and continuous virus adaptation to the changing environment is taking place (117).

HIV-1 GLOBAL VARIATION AND VACCINE DEVELOPMENT

Phylogenetic analyses of globally collected HIV-1 strains have revealed that the vast majority of virus sequences can be separated into genetic subtypes A–J (12,118–125). Nucleotide distances among env gene sequences within one subtype are below 15–20%, while distances between sequences from different subtypes are 25–30% and more. The HIV-1 subtypes A–J belong to the group M (major) of HIV-1 and cause together more than 99.9% of all HIV-1 infections worldwide. A few more distantly related to subtypes A–J HIV-1 sequences, which compose HIV-1 groups O (outlier) and N, have also been identified. Many viruses have been shown to have mosaic genomes, in which different genes or gene regions are related to and probably derived from distinct HIV-1 subtypes (10,126). In many instances, HIV-1 genomic mosaicism could be a result of recombinations between parental sequences belonging to different subtypes. Most mosaic viruses have been found only in one human individual each, but some have taken off and caused epidemics, like the originally classified subtype A virus with complex mosaic genome (IbNG-like viruses) in Africa, subtype B/C mosaic virus in China, and subtype A/B mosaic virus in Russia (127–129). Of the mosaic virus in Russia, both subtypes A and B parental strains have been identified, which proves the recombinant nature of this virus (129); the evolutionary history of many other mosaic viruses is still under discussion.

Numerous molecular epidemiological studies have revealed that HIV-1 group M subtypes are unevenly distributed worldwide, and not all of them contribute equally to the global HIV-1 epidemic. In terms of geography, the most globally prevalent is HIV-1 subtype B, which is associated with most HIV-1 epidemics in the developed world, including those in North and South America, virtually all European countries, Australia, and several Asian countries. Yet all of these epidemics together account only for a small portion of global HIV-1 cases, and therefore HIV-1 subtype B is not the most predominant virus subtype in terms of number of infections caused. The epicenters of the HIV-1 pandemic is sub-Saharan Africa and South/Southeast Asia, which are estimated to account for 62% and 23% of global HIV-1 cases, respectively. In these regions, HIV-1 subtypes other than B are dominant. Among them, HIV-1 subtypes A (in Africa), C (in Africa and Asia), and E (in Asia) have been shown to be associated with great and rising numbers of infections in many countries, while expansion of other HIV-1 subtypes, including D, F, and G, is currently more limited. Other HIV-1 subtypes (H, I, and J) have each been found in only a few human individuals so far. In Africa, the largest variety of HIV-1 subtypes in circulation is observed in Central Africa, where all subtypes are found, with subtype A being predominant. Subtype A is also predominant in East (together with subtypes C and D) and West Africa, while epidemics among heterosexuals in northern and southern Africa are caused by HIV-1 subtype C (130).

The uneven distribution of HIV-1 subtypes worldwide can be attributed to a whole array of circumstances. Since the early epidemic in the developed world has been primarily associated with male-to-male and parenteral transmissions, while the epidemic in Africa is caused primarily by heterosexual transmissions, it has been suggested that the difference in HIV-1 subtypes circulating in developed versus developing countries could be due to adaptation of HIV-1 subtypes to certain transmission routes. However, the many studies conducted so far have not found significant biological differences between HIV-1 subtypes, all of which cause AIDS by the same mechanism, infect the same types of target cells by using the same primary and secondary receptors, etc. Moreover, a growing number of subtype B infections in developed countries is associated with heterosexual transmission of this subtype (131). On the other hand, newly arising epidemics among traditionally subtype B risk groups could be associated with HIV-1 subtypes other than B. A most recent example is an epidemic among injecting drug users (IDUs) in the former Soviet Union, where up to 100,000 IDUs have been infected since 1995 by HIV-1 subtype A (127–129,132,133). Taken together, these data suggest that the uneven global distribution of HIV-1 subtypes is caused by phenomena other than pure biological ones. Recently, it is becoming more clear that global distribution of HIV-1 subtypes has been strongly influenced by and is largely a result of multiple founder effects during HIV-1 migration among social networks (131).

SUMMARY

In this chapter, we have discussed many of the major implications and problems posed by the genetic variation seen with the human immunodeficiency virus towards the successful development of a vaccine. We have described the host and immune-mediated constraints that are placed on HIV-1 and argued that these can be both beneficial as well as detrimental to the host and the efforts to develop a vaccine. We should remain encouraged by the fact that some individuals can adequately control their own infection while others can remain uninfected. It is the belief in these individuals and their correlates of protection that suggest that an effective HIV vaccine is indeed achievable and a goal well worth pursuing. What influence the immense variation seen between the many different populations and subtypes of HIV-1 will have on the success of a vaccine is not known but will undoubtedly be answered by the many vaccine trials now in progress or planned for the future.

REFERENCES

1. Roberts, J.D., K. Bebenek, T.A. Kunkel. 1988. The accuracy of reverse transcriptase from HIV-1. Science 242:1171–1173.
2. Bebenek, K., J. Abbotts, J.D. Roberts, S.N. Wilson, T.A. Kunkel. 1989. Specificity and mechanism of error-prone replication by human immunodeficiency virus-1 reverse transcriptase. J Biol Chem 264(28):16948–16956.
3. Roberts, J.D., B.D. Preston, L.A. Johnston, A. Soni, L.A. Loeb, T.A. Kunkel. 1989. Fidelity of two retroviral reverse transcriptases during DNA-dependent DNA synthesis in vitro. Mol Cell Biol 9:469–476.
4. Preston, B.D., B.J. Poiesz, L.A. Loeb. 1988. Fidelity of HIV-1 reverse transcriptase. Science 242:1168–1171.
5. Ricchetti, M., H. Buc. 1990. Reverse transcriptases and genomic variability: the accuracy of DNA replication is enzyme specific and sequence dependent. EMBO J 9(5):1583–1593.
6. Hu, W.-S., H.M. Temin. 1990. Retroviral recombination and reverse transcription. Science 250:1227–1233.
7. Pathak, V.K., H.M. Temin. 1990. Broad spectrum of in vivo forward muta-

tions, hypermutations and mutational hotspots in a retroviral shuttle vector after a single replication cycle: substitutions, frameshifts, and hypermutations. Proc Natl Acad Sci USA 87:6019–6023.
8. Pulsinelli, G.A., H.M. Temin. 1991. Characterization of large deletions occurring during a single round of retrovirus vector replication: novel deletion mechanism involving errors in strand transfer. J Virol 65:4786–4797.
9. Hu, W.-S., H.M. Temin. 1990. Retroviral recombination and reverse transcription. Science 250:1227–1233.
10. Robertson, D.L., P.M. Sharp, F.E. McCutchan, B.H. Hahn. 1995. Recombination in HIV-1. Nature 374:124–126.
11. Wolfs, T.F.W., G. Zwart, M. Bakker, J. Goudsmit. 1992. HIV-1 genomic RNA diversification following sexual and parental virus transmission. Virology 189:103–110.
12. Zhu, T., H. Mo, N. Wang, D.S. Nam, Y. Cao, R.A. Koup, D.D. Ho. 1993. Genotypic and phenotypic characterization of HIV-1 in patients with primary infection. Science 261:1179–1181.
13. Zhu, T., N. Wang, A. Carr, D.S. Nam, R. Moor-Jankowski, D.A. Cooper, D.D. Ho. 1996. Genetic characterization of human immunodeficiency virus type 1 in blood and genital secretions: evidence for viral compartmentalization and selection during sexual transmission. J Virol 70:3098–3107.
14. Zhang, L.Q., P. MacKenzie, A. Cleland, E.C. Holmes, A.J. Leigh Brown, P. Simmonds. 1993. Selection for specific sequences in the external envelope protein of human immunodeficiency virus type 1 upon primary infection. J Virol 67:3345–3356.
15. Wolinsky, S.M., C.M. Wike, B.T.M. Korber, C. Hutto, W.P. Parks, L.L. Rosenblum, K.J. Kunstman, M.R. Furtado, J.L. Munoz. 1992. Selective transmission of human immunodeficiency virus type-1 variants from mothers to infant. Science 255:1134–1137.
16. Cornelissen, M., G. Mulder-Kampinga, J. Veenstra, F. Zorgdrager, C. Kuiken, S. Hartman, J. Dekker, L. van der Hoek, C. Sol, R. Coutinho, J. Goudsmit. 1995. Syncytium-inducing (SI) phenotype suppression at seroconversion after intramuscular inoculation of a non-syncytium-inducing/SI phenotypically mixed human immunodeficiency virus population. J Virol 69:1810–1818.
17. Mulder-Kampinga, G.A., C. Kuiken, J. Dekker, H.J. Scherpbier, K. Boer, J. Goudsmit. 1993. Genomic human immunodeficiency virus type 1 RNA variation in mother and child following intra-uterine virus transmission. J Gen Virol 74:1747–1756.
18. McNearney, T., Z. Hornickova, R. Markham, A. Birdwell, M. Arens, A. Saah, L. Ratner. 1992. Relationship of human immunodeficiency virus

type 1 sequence heterogeneity to stage of disease. Proc Natl Acad Sci USA 89:10247–10251.
19. Lukashov, V.V., J. Goudsmit. 1997. Founder virus population related to route of virus transmission: a determinant of intrahost human immunodeficiency virus type 1 evolution? J Virol 71:2023–2030.
20. Goudsmit, J., V.V. Lukashov, E.J. van Ameijden, F. Zorgdrager, R. van den Burg, M. Cornelissen. 1998. Impact of sexual versus parenteral transmission events on the evolution of the gag and env genes of HIV type 1. AIDS Res Hum Retroviruses 14:1483–1486.
21. Michelle, L.E., H.L. Martin, Jr., J.K. Kreiss, S.M. Rainwater, L. Lavreys, D.J. Jackson, J. Rakwar, K. Mandaliya, J. Overbaugh. 2000. Gender differences in HIV-1 diversity at time of infection. Nat Med 6:71–75.
22. Schuitemaker, H., N.A. Kootstra, R.E.Y. de Goede, F. de Wolf, F. Miedema, M. Tersmette. 1991. Monocytotropic human immunodeficiency virus type 1 (HIV-1) variants detectable in all stages of HIV-1 infection lack T-cell line tropism and syncytium-inducing ability in primary T-cell culture. J Virol 65:356–363.
23. Van 't Wout, A.B., N.A. Kootstra, G.A. Mulder-Kampinga, N.A. Albrecht-van Lent, H.J. Scherpbier, J. Veenstra, K. Boer, R.A. Coutinho, F. Miedema, H. Schuitemaker. 1994. Macrophage-tropic variants initiate human immunodeficiency virus type 1 infection after sexual, parenteral and vertical transmission. J Clin Invest 94:2060–2067.
24. Lukashov, V.V., J. Goudsmit. 1995. Increasing genotypic and phenotypic selection from the original genomic RNA populations of HIV-1 strains LAI and MN (NM) by peripheral blood mononuclear cell culture, B-cell-line propagation and T-cell-line adaptation. AIDS 9:1307–1311.
25. Cheng-Mayer, C., C. Weiss, D. Seto, J.A. Levy. 1989. Isolates of human immunodeficiency virus type 1 from the brain may constitute a special group of the AIDS virus. Proc Natl Acad Sci USA 86:8575–8579.
26. Epstein, L.G., C. Kuiken, B.M. Blumberg, S. Hartman, L.R. Sharer, M. Clement, J. Goudsmit. 1991. HIV-1 V3 domain variation in brain and spleen of children with AIDS: tissue-specific evolution within host-determined quasispecies. Virology 180:583–590.
27. Kuiken, C.L., J. Goudsmit, G.F. Weiller, J.S. Armstrong, S. Hartman, P. Portegies, J. Dekker, M. Cornelissen. 1995. Differences in human immunodeficiency virus type 1 V3 sequences from patients with and without AIDS dementia complex. J Gen Virol 76:175–180.
28. van der Hoek, L., C.J.A. Sol, J. Maas, V.V. Lukashov, C.L. Kuiken, J. Goudsmit. 1998. Genetic differences between human immunodeficiency virus type 1 subpopulations in faeces and serum. J Gen Virol 79:259–267.

29. van der Hoek, L., C.J.A. Sol, F. Snijders, J.F.W. Bartelsman, R. Boom, J. Goudsmit. 1996. Human immunodeficiency virus type 1 RNA populations in faeces with higher homology to intestinal populations than to blood populations. J Gen Virol 77:2415–2425.
30. Webster, R.G., W.G. Laver. 1971. Antigenic variation in influenza virus. Biology and chemistry. Prog Med Virol 13:271–338.
31. Webster, R.G., W.G. Laver, G.M. Air, G.C. Schild. 1982. Molecular mechanisms of variation in influenza viruses. Nature 296:115–121.
32. Borst, P., G.A. Cross. 1982. Molecular basis for trypanosome antigenic variation. Cell 29:291–303.
33. Paxton, W.A., R.A. Koup. 1997. Mechanisms of resistance to HIV infection. Springer Semin in Immunopathol 18:323–340.
34. Jurriaans, S., B. van Gemen, G.J. Weverling, D. van Strijp, P. Nara, R. Coutinho, M. Koot, H. Schuitemaker, J. Goudsmit. 1994. The natural history of HIV-1 infection: virus load and virus phenotype independent determinants of clinical course? Virology 204:223–233.
35. Mellors, J.W., C.R. Rinaldo, P. Gupta, R.M. White, J.A. Todd, L.A. Kingsley. 1996. Prognosis in HIV-1 infection predicted by the quantity of virus in plasma. Science 272:1167–1170.
36. Mellors, J.W., A. Munoz, J.V. Giorgi, J.B. Margolick, C.J. Tassoni, P. Gupta, L.A. Kingsley, J.A. Todd, A.J. Saah, R. Detels, J.P. Phair, C.R. Jr. Rinaldo. 1997. Plasma viral load and CD4+ lymphocytes as prognostic markers of HIV-1 infection. Ann Intern Med 126:946–954.
37. Harrer, T., E. Harrer, S.A. Kalams, P. Barbosa, A. Trocha, R.P. Johnson, T. Elbeik, M.B. Feinberg, S.P. Buchbinder, B.D. Walker. 1996. Cytotoxic T lymphocytes in asymptomatic long-term non-progressing HIV-1 infection. Breadth and specificity of the response and relation to in vivo viral quasispecies in a person with prolonged infection and low viral load. J Immunol 156:2616–2623.
38. Carotenuto, P., D. Looij, L. Keldermans, F. de Wolf, J. Goudsmit. 1998. Neutralizing antibodies are positively associated with CD4+ T-cell counts and T-cell function in long-term AIDS-free infection. AIDS 12:1591–1600.
39. Pontesilli, O., P. Carotenuto, S.R. Kerkhof-Garde, M.T. Roos, I.P. Keet, R.A. Coutinho, J. Goudsmit, F. Miedema. 1999. Lymphoproliferative response to HIV type 1 p24 in long-term survivors of HIV type 1 infection is predictive of persistent AIDS-free infection. AIDS Res Hum Retroviruses 15:973–981.
40. Rosenberg, E., J. Billingsley, A. Caliendo, S. Boswell, P. Sax, S. Kalams, B. Walker. 1997. Vigorous HIV-1-specific CD4+ T-cell responses associated with control of viremia. Science 278:1447–1450.
41. Mellors, J.W., L.A. Kingsley, C.R. Rinaldo, Jr., J.A. Todd, B.S. Hoo,

R.P.G.P. Kokka. 1995. Quantitation of HIV-1 RNA in plasma predicts outcome after seroconversion. Ann Intern Med 122:573–579.

42. Hogervorst, E., S. Jurriaans, F. de Wolf, A. van Wijk, A. Wiersma, M. Valk, M. Roos, B. van Gemen, R. Coutinho, F. Miedema, J. Goudsmit. 1995. Predictors for non- and slow progression in human immunodeficiency virus type 1 infection: low viral RNA copy numbers in serum and maintenance of high HIV-1 p24-specific, but not V3-specific antibody levels. J Infect Dis 171:811–821.
43. Hay, C.M., D.J. Ruhl, N.O. Basgoz, C.C. Wilson, J.M. Billingsley, M.P. DePasquale, R.T. D'Aquila, S.M. Wolinsky, J.M. Crawford, D.C. Montefiori, B.D. Walker. 1999. Lack of viral escape and defective in vivo activation of human immunodeficiency virus type 1-specific cytotoxic T lymphocytes in rapidly progressive infection. J Virol 73:5509–5519.
44. Valentine, F.T., A. Paolino, A. Saito, R.S. Holzman. 1998. Lymphocyte-proliferative responses to HIV antigens as a potential measure of immunological reconstitution in HIV disease. AIDS Res Hum Retroviruses 14(suppl 2):S161-S166.
45. Ortiz, G.M., D.F. Nixon, A. Trkola, J. Binley, X. Jin, S. Bonhoeffer, P.J. Kuebler,S.M. Donahoe, M.A. Demoitie, W.M. Kakimoto, T. Ketas, B. Clas, J.J. Heymann, L. Zhang, Y. Cao, A. Hurley, J.P. Moore, D.D. Ho, M. Markowitz. 1999. HIV-1-specific immune responses in subjects who temporarily contain virus replication after discontinuation of highly active antiretroviral therapy [comments]. J Clin Invest 104:R13–R18.
46. Parren, P.W.H.I., J.P. Moore, D.R. Burton, Q.J. Sattentau. 1999. The neutralization antibody response to HIV-1: viral evasion and escape from humoral immunity. AIDS 13(suppl A):S137-S162.
47. Bernstein, H.B., S.P. Tucker, E. Hunter, J.S. Schutzbach, R.W. Compans. 1994. Human immunodeficiency virus type 1 envelope glycoprotein is modified by O-linked oligosaccharides. J Virol 68:463–468.
48. Leonard, C.K., M.W. Spellman, L. Riddle, R.J. Harris, J.N. Thomas, T.J. Gregory. 1990. Assignment of intrachain disulfide bonds and characterization of potential glycosylation sites of the type 1 recombinant human immunodeficiency virus envelope glycoprotein (gp120) expressed in chinese hamster ovary cells. J Biol Chem 265:10373–10382.
49. Kwong, P.D., R. Wyatt, J. Robinson, R.W. Sweet, J. Sodroski, W.A. Hendrickson. 1998. Structure of an HIV gp120 envelope glycoprotein in complex with the CD4 receptor and a neutralizing human antibody. Nature 393:648–659.
50. Wyatt, R., P.D. Kwong, E. Desjardins, R.W. Sweet, J. Robinson, W.A. Hendrickson, J.G. Sodroski. 1998. The antigenic structure of the HIV gp120 envelope glycoprotein [comments]. Nature 393:705–711.

51. Wyatt, R., J. Sodroski. 1998. The HIV-1 envelope glycoproteins: fusogens, antigens, and immunogens. Science 280:1884–1888.
52. Wyatt, R., J. Moore, M. Accola, E. Desjardin, J. Robinson, J. Sodroski. 1995. Involvement of the V1/V2 variable loop structure in the exposure of human immunodeficiency virus type 1 gp120 epitopes induced by receptor binding. J Virol 69:5723–5733.
53. Wu, H., P.D. Kwong, W.A. Hendrickson. 1997. Dimeric association and segmental variability in the structure of human CD4. Nature 387:527–530.
54. Rizzuto, C.D., R. Wyatt, N. Hernandez-Ramos, Y. Sun, P.D. Kwong, W.A. Hendrickson, J. Sodroski. 1998. A conserved HIV gp120 glycoprotein structure involved in chemokine receptor binding. Science 280:1949–1953.
55. Back, N.K., L. Smit, J.J. de Jong, W. Keulen, M. Schutten, J. Goudsmit, M. Tersmette. 1994. An N-glycan within the human immunodeficiency virus type 1 gp120 V3 loop affects virus neutralization. Virology 199: 431–438.
56. Reitter, J.N., R.E. Means, R.C. Desrosiers. 1998. A role for carbohydrates in immune evasion in AIDS. Nature Med 4:679–684.
57. Ugolini, S., I. Mondor, Q.J. Sattentau. 1999. HIV-1 attachment: another look. Trends MicroBiol 7:144–149.
58. Mascola, J.R., S.W. Snyder, O.S. Weislow, S.M. Belay, R.B. Belshe, D.H. Schwartz, M.L. Clements, R. Dolin, B.S. Graham, G.J. Gorse, M.C. Keefer, M.J. Mcelrath, M.C. Walker, K.F. Wagner, J.G. McNeil, F.E. McCutchan, D.S. Burke. 1996. Immunization with envelope subunit vaccine products elicits neutralizing antibodies against laboratory-adapted but not primary isolates of human immunodeficiency virus type 1. The National Institute of Allergy and Infectious Diseases AIDS Vaccine Evaluation Group. J Infect Dis 173:340–348.
59. Matthews, T.J. 1994. Dilemma of neutralization resistance of HIV-1 field isolates and vaccine development. AIDS Res Hum Retroviruses 10:631–632.
60. Mazzoli, S., D. Trabattoni, C.S. Lo, S. Piconi, C. Ble, F. Meacci, S. Ruzzante, A. Salvi, F. Semplici, R. Longhi, M.L. Fusi, N. Tofani, Biasin, M.M.L. Villa, F. Mazzotta, M. Clerici. 1997. HIV-specific mucosal and cellular immunity in HIV-seronegative partners of HIV-seropositive individuals. Nature Med 3:1250–1257.
61. Kaul, R., D. Trabattoni, J.J. Bwayo, D. Arienti, A. Zagliani, F.M. Mwangi, C. Kariuki, E.N. Ngugi, K.S. MacDonald, T.B. Ball, M. Clerici, F.A. Plummer. 1999. HIV-1-specific mucosal IgA in a cohort of HIV-1-resistant Kenyan sex workers. AIDS 13:23–29.
62. Mazzoli, S., L. Lopalco, A. Salvi, D. Trabattoni, C.S. Lo, F. Semplici, M.

Biasin, C. Bl, A. Cosma, C. Pastori, F. Meacci, F. Mazzotta, M.L. Villa, A.G. Siccardi, M. Clerici. 1999. Human immunodeficiency virus (HIV)-specific IgA and HIV neutralizing activity in the serum of exposed seronegative partners of HIV-seropositive persons. J Infect Dis 180:871–875.

63. Byrne, J.A., M.B.A. Oldstone. 1984. Biology of cloned cytotoxic T lymphocytes specific for lymphocyte choriomeningitis virus: clearance of virus in vivo. J Virol 51:682–687.

64. Lukacher, A.E., V.L. Braciale, T.J. Braciale. 1984. In vivo effector function of influenza virus-specific cytotoxic T lymphocyte clones is highly specific. J Exp Med 160:814–820.

65. Sethi, K.K., Y. Omata, K.E. Schneweis. 1983. Protection of mice from fatal herpes simplex virus type 1 infection by adoptive transfer of cloned virus-specific and H-22-restricted cytotoxic T lymphocytes. J Gen Virol 64:443–447.

66. Yap, K.L., G.L. Ada. 1978. The recovery of mice from influenza A infection: adoptive transfer of immunity with influenza virus-specific cytotoxic T lymphocytes recognizing a common virion antigen. Scand J Immunol 8:413–420.

67. Schwarz, R.H. 1985. T-lymphocyte recognition of antigen in association with gene products of the major histocompatibility complex. Ann Rev Immunol 3:237–261.

68. Guo, H.C., T.S. Jardetzky, T.P. Garrett, W.S. Lane, J.L. Strominger, D.C. Wiley. 1992. Different length peptides bind to HLA-Aw68 similarly at their ends but bulge out in the middle. Nature 360:364–366.

69. Steel, C.M., C.A. Ludlam, D. Beatson, J.F. Peutherer, R.J. Cuthbert, P. Simmonds, H. Morrison, M. Jones. 1988. HLA haplotype A1 B8 DR3 as risk factor for HIV-related disease. Lancet 1:1185–1188.

70. Parker, K.C., M.A. Bednarek, L.K. Hull, U. Utz, B. Cunningham, H.J. Zweerink, W.E. Biddison, J.E. Coligan. 1992. Sequence motifs important for peptide binding to the human MHC class I molecule, HLA-A2. J. Immunol 149:3580–3587.

71. Goulder, P.J., R.E. Phillips, R.A. Colbert, S. McAdam, G. Ogg, M.A. Nowak, P. Giangrande, G. Luzzi, B. Morgan, A. Edwards, A.J. McMichael, S. Rowland-Jones. 1997. Late escape from an immunodominant cytotoxic T-lymphocyte response associated with progression to AIDS. Nature Med 3:212–217.

72. Borrow, P., H. Lewicki, X. Wei, M.S. Horwitz, N. Peffer, H. Meyers, J.A. Nelson, J.E. Gairin, B.H. Hahn, M.B.A. Oldstone, G.M. Shaw. 1997. Antiviral pressure exerted by HIV-1-specific cytotoxic T lymphocytes (CTLs) during primary infection demonstrated by rapid selection of CTL escape virus. Nature Med 3:205–211.

73. Pricc, D.A., P.J. Goulder, P. Klenerman, A.K. Sewell, P.J. Easterbrook,

M. Troop, C.R. Bangham, R.E. Phillips. 1997. Positive selection of HIV-1 cytotoxic T lymphocyte escape variants during primary infection. Proc Natl Acad Sci USA 94:1890–1895.

74. Klenerman, P., S. Rowland-Jones, S. McAdam, J. Edwards, S. Daenke, D. Lalloo, B. Koppe, W. Rosenberg, D. Boyd, A. Edwards. 1994. Cytotoxic T-cell activity antagonized by naturally occurring HIV-1 Gag variants. Nature 369:403–407.
75. Phillips, R.E., S. Rowland-Jones, D.F. Nixon, F.M. Gotch, J.P. Edwards, A.O. Ogunlesi, J.G. Elvin, J.A. Rothbard, C.R.M. Bangham, C.R. Rizza, A.J. McMichael. 1991. Human immunodeficiency virus genetic variation that can escape cytotoxic T-cell recognition. Nature 354:453–459.
76. Evans, D.T., D.H. O'Connor, P. Jing, J.L. Uris, J. Sidney, J. DaSiva, T.M. Allen, H. Horton, J.E. Venham, R.A. Rudersdorf, T. Vogel, C.D. Pauza, R.E. Bontrop, R. DeMars, A. Sette, A.L. Hughes, D.I. Watkins. 1999. Virus-specific cytotoxic T-lymphocyte responses select for amino-acid variation in simian immunodeficiency virus Env and Nef. Nat Med 5: 1270–1276.
77. Klenerman, P., R.M. Zinkernagel. 1998. Original antigenic sin impairs cytotoxic T lymphocyte responses to viruses bearing variant epitopes. Nature 394:482–485.
78. Rowland-Jones, S., J. Sutton, K. Ariyoshi, T. Dong, F. Gotch, S. McAdam, D. Whitby, S. Sabally, A. Gallimore, T. Corrah, M. Takiguchi, T. Schultz, A. McMichael, H. Whittle. 1995. HIV-specific cytotoxic T-cells in HIV-exposed but uninfected Gambian women. Nat Med 1:59–64.
79. Ferrari, G., W. Humphrey, M.J. Mcelrath, J.L. Excler, A.M. Duliege, M.L. Clements, L.C. Corey, D.P. Bolognesi, K.J. Weinhold. 1997. Clade B-based HIV-1 vaccines elicit cross-clade cytotoxic T lymphocyte reactivities in uninfected volunteers. Proc Natl Acad Sci USA 94:1396–1401.
80. Cao, H., P. Kanki, J.L. Sankale, A. Dieng-Sarr, G.P. Mazzara, S.A. Kalams, B. Korber, S. Mboup, B.D. Walker. 1997. Cytotoxic T-lymphocyte cross-reactivity among different human immunodeficiency virus type 1 clades: implications for vaccine development. J Virol 71:8615–8623.
81. Betts, M.R., J. Krowka, C. Santamaria, K. Balsamo, F. Gao, G. Mulundu, Luo, C,N. N'Gandu, H. Sheppard, B.H. Hahn, S. Allen, J.A. Frelinger. 1997. Cross-clade human immunodeficiency virus (HIV)-specific cytotoxic T-lymphocyte responses in HIV-infected Zambians. J Virol 71: 8908–8911.
82. McAdam, S., P. Kaleebu, P. Krausa, P. Goulder, N. French, B. Collin, T. Blanchard, J. Whitworth, A. McMichael, F. Gotch. 1998. Cross-clade recognition of p55 by cytotoxic T lymphocytes in HIV-1 infection. AIDS 12:571–579.
83. Lynch, J.A., M. deSouza, M.D. Robb, L. Markowitz, S. Nitayaphan, C.V.

Sapan, D.L. Mann, D.L. Birx, J.H. Cox. 1998. Cross-clade cytotoxic T-cell response to human immunodeficiency virus type 1 proteins among HLA disparate North Americans and Thais. J Infect Dis 178:1040–1046.
84. Cafaro, A., A. Caputo, C. Fracasso, M.T. Maggiorella, D. Goletti, Baroncelli, S.M. Pace, L. Sernicola, M.L. Koanga-Mogtomo, M. Betti, A. Borsetti, R. Belli, L. Akerblom, F. Corrias, S. Butto, J. Heeney, P. Verani, F. Titti, B. Ensoli. 1999. Control of SHIV-89.6P-infection of cynomolgus monkeys by HIV-1 Tat protein vaccine. Nature Med 5:643–650.
85. Zagury, D., A. Lachgar, V. Chams, L.S. Fall, J. Bernard, J.F. Zagury, Bizzini, B, A. Gringeri, E. Santagostino, J. Rappaport, M. Feldman, A. Burny, R.C. Gallo. 1998. Interferon alpha and Tat involvement in the immunosuppression of uninfected T-cells and C-C chemokine decline in AIDS. Proc Natl Acad Sci USA 95:3851–3856.
86. Cocchi, F., A.L. DeVico, A. Garzino-Demo, S.K. Arya, R.C. Gallo, P. Lusso. 1995. Identification of RANTES, MIP-1a, and MIP-1b as the major HIV suppressive factors produced by CD8+ T-cells. Science 270:1811–1815.
87. Unutmaz, D., V.N. KewalRamani, D.R. Littman. 1998. G protein-coupled receptors in HIV and SIV entry: new perspectives on lentivirus-host interactions and on the utility of animal models. Sem Immunol 10:225–236.
88. Paxton, W.A., S. Kang. 1998. Chemokine receptor allelic polymorphisms: relationships to HIV resistance and disease progression. Sem Immunol 10: 187–194.
89. Samson, M., F. Libert, B.J. Doranz, J. Rucker, C. Liesnard, C.-M. Farber, S. Saragosti, C. Lapoumroulie, J. Cogniaux, C. Forceille, G. Muyldermans, C. Verhofstede, G. Burtonboy, M. Georges, T. Imai, S. Rana, Y. Yi, R.J. Smyth, R.G. Collman, R.W. Doms, G. Vassart, M. Parmentier. 1996. Resistance to HIV-1 infection of Caucasian individuals bearing mutant alleles of the CCR5 receptor gene. Nature 382:722–725.
90. Liu, R., W.A. Paxton, S. Choe, D. Ceradini, S.R. Martin, R. Horuk, M.E. MacDonald, H. Stuhlmann, R.A. Koup, N.R. Landau. 1996. Homozygous defect in HIV-1 coreceptor accounts for resistance of some multiplyexposed individuals to HIV-1 infection. Cell 86:367–377.
91. Huang, Y., W.A. Paxton, S.M. Wolinsky, A.U. Neumann, L. Zhang, T. He, S. Kang, D. Ceradini, Z. Jin, K. Yazdanbakhsh, K. Kunstman, D. Erickson, E. Dragon, N.R. Landau, J. Phair, D.D. Ho, R.A. Koup. 1996. The role of a mutant CCR5 allele in HIV-1 transmission and disease progression. Nature Med 2:1240–1243.
92. Zimmerman, P.A., A. Buckler-White, G. Alkhatib, T. Spalding, J. Kubofcik, C. Combadiere, D. Weissman, O. Cohen, A. Rubbert, G. Lam, M. Vaccarezza, P.E. kennedy, V. Kumaraswami, J.V. Giorgi, R. Detels, J. Hunter, M. Chopek, E.A. Berger, A.S. Fauci, T.B. Nutman, P.M. Murphy.

1997. Inherited resistance to HIV-1 conferred by an inactivating mutation in CC chemokine receptor 5: studies in populations with contrasting clinical phenotypes, defined racial background, and quantified risk. Mol Med 3:23–36.

93. Michael, N.L., G. Chang, L.G. Louis, J.R. Mascola, D. Dondero, D.L. Birx, H.W. Sheppard. 1997. The role of viral phenotype and CCR-5 gene defects in HIV-1 transmission and disease progression. Nature Med 3: 338–340.

94. Roda Husman, A.M., M. Koot, M. Cornelissen, I.P. Keet, M. Brouwer, S.M. Broersen, M. Bakker, M.T. Roos, M. Prins, F. de Wolf, R.A. Coutinho, F. Miedema, J. Goudsmit, H. Schuitemaker. 1997. Association between CCR5 genotype and the clinical course of HIV-1 infection. Ann Intern Med 127:882–890.

95. Kostrikis, L.G., Y. Huang, J.P. Moore, S.M. Wolinsky, L. Zhang, Y. Guo, L. Deutsch, J. Phair, A.U. Neumann, D.D. Ho. 1998. A chemokine receptor CCR2 allele delays HIV-1 disease progression and is associated with a CCR5 promoter mutation. Nat Med 4:350–353.

96. Martin, M.P., M. Dean, M.W. Smith, C. Winkler, B. Gerrard, N.L. Michael, B. Lee, R.W. Doms, J. Margolick, S. Buchbinder, J.J. Goedert, T.R. O'Brien, M.W. Hilgartner, D. Vlahov, S.J. O'Brien, M. Carrington. 1998. Genetic acceleration of AIDS progression by a promoter variant of CCR5. Science 282:1907–1911.

97. Winkler, C., W. Modi, M.W. Smith, G.W. Nelson, X. Wu, M. Carrington, M. Dean, T. Honjo, K. Tashiro, D. Yabe, S. Buchbinder, E. Vittinghoff, J.J. Goedert, T.R. O'Brien, L.P. Jacobson, R. Detels, S. Donfield, A. Willoughby, E. Gomperts, D. Vlahov, J. Phair, S.J. O'Brien. 1998. Genetic restriction of AIDS pathogenesis by an SDF-1 chemokine gene variant. ALIVE Study, Hemophilia Growth and Development Study (HGDS), Multicenter AIDS Cohort Study (MACS), Multicenter Hemophilia Cohort Study (MHCS), San Francisco City Cohort (SFCC). Science 279:389–393.

98. Smith, M.W., M. Dean, M. Carrington, C. Winkler, G.A. Huttley, D.A. Lomb, J.J. Goedert, T.R. O'Brien, L.P. Jacobson, R. Kaslow, S. Buchbinder, E. Vitting hoff, D. Vlahov, K. Hoots, M.W. Hilgartner, Hemophilia Growth and Development Study (HGDS), Multicenter AIDS Cohort Study (MACS), Multicenter Hemophilia Cohort Study (MHCS), San Francisco City Cohort (SFCC), ALIVE Study, and S.J. O'Brien. 1997. Contrasting genetic influence of CCR2 and CCR5 variants on HIV-1 infection and disease progression. Science 277:959–965.

99. Trkola, A., T. Dragic, J. Arthos, J.M. Binley, W.C. Olson, G.P. Allaway, C. Cheng-Mayer, J. Robinson, P.J. Maddon, J.P. Moore. 1996. CD4-de-

pendent, antibody-sensitive interactions between HIV-1 and its coreceptor CCR-5. Nature 384:184–187.

100. Wu, L., N.P. Gerard, R. Wyatt, H. Choe, C. Parolin, N. Ruffing, A. Borsetti, A.A. Cardoso, E. Desjardin, W. Newman, C. Gerard, J. Sodroski. 1996. CD4-induced interaction of primary HIV-1 gp120 glycoproteins with the chemokine receptor CCR-5. Nature 384:179–183.
101. Zhang, L., Y. Huang, T. He, Y. Cao, D.D. Ho. 1996. HIV-1 subtype and second-receptor usage. Nature 383:768.
102. Paxton, W.A., R. Liu, S. Kang, L. Wu, T.R. Gingeras, N.R. Landau, C.R. Mackay, R.A. Koup. 1998. Reduced HIV-1 infectability of CD4+ lymphocytes from exposed- uninfected individuals: association with low expression of CCR5 and high production of beta-chemokines. Virology 244: 66–73.
103. Zagury, D., A. Lachgar, V. Chams, L.S. Fall, J. Bernard, J.F. Zagury, B. Bizzini, A. Gringeri, E. Santagostino, J. Rappaport, M. Feldman, S.J. O'Brien, A. Burny, R.C. Gallo. 1998. C-C chemokines, pivotal in protection against HIV type 1 infection. Proc Natl Acad Sci USA 95:3857–3861.
104. Garzino-Demo, A., R.B. Moss, J.B. Margolick, F. Gleghorn, A. Sill, W.A. Blattner, F. Cocchi, D. Carlo, A.L. DeVico, R.C. Gallo. 1999. Spontaneous and antigen-induced production of HIV-inhibitory beta-chemokines are associated with AIDS-free status. Proc Natl Acad Sci USA 96:11986–11991.
105. Heeney, J.L., V.J. Teeuwsen, M. van Gils, W.M. Bogers, M.C. De Giuli, A. Radaelli, S. Barnett, B. Morein, L. Akerblom, Y. Wang, T. Lehner, D. Davis. 1998. Beta-chemokines and neutralizing antibody titers correlate with sterilizing immunity generated in HIV-1 vaccinated macaques. Proc Natl Acad Sci USA 95:10803–10808.
106. Lehner, T., Y. Wang, M. Cranage, A. Bergmeier, E. Mitchell, L. Tao, G. Hall, M. Dennis, N. Cook, R. Brookes, L. Klavinskis, I. Jones, C. Doyle, R. Ward. 1996. Protective mucosal immunity elicited by targeted iliac lymph node immunization with a subunit SIV envelope and core vaccine in macaques. Nat Med 2:767–775.
107. Wang, Y., L. Tao, E. Mitchell, C. Bravery, P. Berlingieri, P. Armstrong, R. Vaughan, J. Underwood, T. Lehner. 1999. Allo-immunization elicits CD8+ T cell-derived chemokines, HIV suppressor factors and resistance to HIV infection in women. Nat Med 5:1004–1009.
108. Wu, L., W.A. Paxton, N. Kassam, N. Ruffing, J.B. Rottman, N. Sullivan, Choe, H, J. Sodroski, W. Newman, R.A. Koup, C.R. Mackay. 1997. CCR5 levels and expression pattern correlate with infectability by macrophage-tropic HIV-1, in vitro. J Exp Med 185:1681–1691.

109. Scarlatti, G., E. Tresoldi, A. Bjorndal, R. Fredriksson, C. Colognesi, Deng, HK, M.S. Malnati, A. Plebani, A.G. Siccardi, D.R. Littman, E.M. Fenyo, P. Lusso. 1997. In vivo evolution of HIV-1 co-receptor usage and sensitivity to chemokine-mediated suppression. Nat Med 3:1259–1265.
110. Cocchi, F., A.L. DeVico, A. Garzino-Demo, A. Cara, R.C. Gallo, P. Lusso. 1996. The V3 domain of the HIV-1 gp120 envelope glycoprotein is critical for chemokine-mediated blockade of infection. Nat. Med 2:1244–1247.
111. de Jong, J.J., A. de Ronde, W. Keulen, M. Tersmette, J. Goudsmit. 1992. Minimal requirements for the human immunodeficiency virus type 1 V3 domain to support the syncytium-inducing (SI) phenotype: analysis by single amino acid substitution. J Virol 66:6777–6780.
112. Fouchier, R.A.M., M. Groenink, N.A. Kootstra, M. Tersmette, H.G. Huisman, F. Miedema, H. Schuitemaker. 1992. Phenotype associated sequence variation in the third variable domain of the human immunodeficiency virus type 1 gp120 molecule. J Virol 66:3183–3187.
113. de Wolf, F., E. Hogervorst, J. Goudsmit, E.-M. Fenyö, H. Rübsamen-Waigmann, H. Holmes, B. Galvao-Castro, E. Karita, C. Wasi, S.D.K. Sempala, E. Baan, F. Zorgdrager, V. Lukashov, S. Osmanov, C. Kuiken, M. Cornelissen, and WHO Network on HIV Isolation and Characterization. 1994. Syncytium-inducing and non-syncytium-inducing capacity of human immunodeficiency virus type 1 subtypes other than B: phenotypic and genotypic characteristics. AIDS Res Hum Retroviruses 10:1387–1400.
114. Trkola, A., W.A. Paxton, S.P. Monard, J.A. Hoxie, M.A. Siani, D.A. Thompson, L. Wu, C.R. Mackay, R. Horuk, J. P. Moore. 1998. Genetic subtype-independent inhibition of human immunodeficiency virus type 1 replication by CC and CXC chemokines. J Virol 72:396–404.
115. Abebe, A., D. Demissie, J. Goudsmit, M. Brouwer, C.L. Kuiken, G. Pollakis, H. Schuitemaker, A.L. Fontanet, T.F. Rinke de Wit. 1999. HIV-1 subtype C syncytium- and non-syncytium-inducing phenotypes and coreceptor usage among Ethiopian patients with AIDS. AIDS 13:1305–1311.
116. Lukashov, V.V., C.L. Kuiken, J. Goudsmit. 1995. Intrahost human immunodeficiency virus type 1 evolution is related to length of the immunocompetent period. J Virol 69:6911–6916.
117. Lukashov, V.V., J. Goudsmit. 1998. HIV heterogeneity and disease progression in AIDS: a model of continuous virus adaptation. AIDS 12:S43-S52.
118. Hahn, B.H., M.A. Gonda, G.M. Shaw, M. Popovic, J.A. Hoxie, R.C. Gallo, F. Wong-Staal. 1985. Genomic diversity of the acquired immune deficiency syndrome virus HTLV-III: different viruses exhibit greatest divergence in their envelope genes. Proc Natl Acad Sci USA 82:4813–4817.

119. Wong-Staal, F., G.M. Shaw, B.H. Hahn, S.Z. Salahuddin, M. Popovic, P. Markham, R. Redfield, R.C. Gallo. 1985. Genomic diversity of human T-lymphotropic virus type III (HTLV-III). Science 229:759–762.
120. Kuiken, C.L., G. Zwart, E. Baan, R.A. Coutinho, J.A. R. van den Hoek, J. Goudsmit. 1993. Increasing antigenic and genetic diversity of the V3 variable domain of the human immunodeficiency virus envelope protein in the course of the AIDS epidemic. Proc Natl Acad Sci USA 90:9061–9065.
121. Kuiken, C.L., V.V. Lukashov, E. Baan, J. Dekker, J.A.M. Leunissen, J. Goudsmit. 1996. Evidence for limited within-person evolution of the V3 domain of the HIV-1 envelope in the Amsterdam population. AIDS 10: 31–37.
122. Kalish, M.L., C.-C. Luo, B.G. Weniger, K. Limpakarnjanarat, N. Young, C.-Y. Ou, G. Schochetman. 1994. Early HIV type 1 strains in Thailand were not responsible for the current epidemic. AIDS Res Hum Retroviruses 10:1573–1575.
123. Ou, C.-Y., Y. Takebe, B.G. Weniger, C.C. Luo, M.L. Kalish, W. Auwanit, S. Yamazaki, H.D. Gayle, N.L. Young, G. Schochetman. 1993. Independent introduction of two major HIV-1 genotypes into distinct high-risk populations in Thailand. Lancet 341:1171–1174.
124. Lukashov, V.V., M.T.E. Cornelissen, J. Goudsmit, M.N. Papuashvilli, P.G. Rytik, R.M. Khaitov, E.V. Karamov, F. de Wolf. 1995. Simultaneous introduction of distinct HIV-1 subtypes into different risk groups in Russia, Byelorussia and Lithuania. AIDS 9:435–439.
125. Lukashov, V.V., C.L. Kuiken, K. Boer, J. Goudsmit. 1996. HIV type 1 subtypes in The Netherlands circulating among women originating from AIDS endemic regions. AIDS Res Hum Retroviruses 12:951–953.
126. Cornelissen, M., G. Kampinga, F. Zorgdrager, J. Goudsmit, and the UNAIDS Network for HIV Isolation and Characterization. 1996. Human immunodeficiency virus type 1 subtypes defined by env show high frequency of recombinant gag genes. J Virol 70:8209–8212.
127. Lukashov, V.V., R. Huismans, A.G. Rakhmanova, Z.N. Lisitsina, N.A. Akhtyrskaya, N.N. Vlasov, O.B. Melnick, J. Goudsmit. 1999. Circulation of subtype A and gagA/envB recombinant HIV type 1 strains among injecting drug users in St. Petersburg, Russia, correlates with geographical origin of infections. AIDS Res Hum Retroviruses 15:1577–1583.
128. Bobkov, A., E. Kazennova, L. Selimova, M. Bobkova, T. Khanina, N. Ladnaya, A. Kravchenko, V. Pokrovsky, R. Cheingsong-Popov, J. Weber. 1998. A sudden epidemic of HIV type 1 among injecting drug users in the former Soviet Union: identification of subtype A, subtype B, and a novel gag A/env B recombinant. AIDS Res Hum Retroviruses 14:669–676.

129. Liitsola, K., I. Tashkinova, T. Laukkanen , G. Korovina, T. Smolskaja, O. Momot, N. Mashkilleyson, S. Chaplinskas, H. Brummer-Korvenkontio, J. Vanhatalo, P. Leinikki, M.O. Salminen. 1998. HIV-1 genetic subtype A/B recombinant strain causing an explosive epidemic in injecting drug users in Kaliningrad. AIDS 12:1907–1919.

130. van Harmelen, J., R. Wood, M. Lambrick, E.P. Rybicki, A.-L. Williamson, C. Williamson. 1997. An association between HIV-1 subtypes and mode of transmission in Cape Town, South Africa. AIDS 11:81–87.

131. Lukashov, V.V., E.L.M. Op de Coul, R.A. Coutinho, J. Goudsmit. 1998. HIV-1 strains specific for Dutch injecting drug users in heterosexually infected individuals in The Netherlands. AIDS 12:635–641.

132. Lukashov, V.V., E.V. Karamov, V.F. Eremin, L.P. Titov, J. Goudsmit. 1998. Extreme founder effect in an HIV type 1 subtype A epidemic among drug users in Svetlogorsk, Belarus. AIDS Res Hum Retroviruses 14:1299–1303.

133. Novitsky, V.A., M.A. Montano, M. Essex. 1998. Molecular epidemiology of an HIV-1 subtype A subcluster among injection drug users in the Southern Ukraine. AIDS Res Hum Retroviruses 14:1079–1085.

4

The Role of Cytotoxic T Lymphocytes in Protection Against HIV Infection and AIDS

Tomáš Hanke and Andrew J. McMichael

The Weatherall Institute of Molecular Medicine
The John Radcliffe
Oxford, England

DEVELOPMENT OF AN HIV VACCINE

Development of an effective human immunodeficiency virus (HIV) vaccine is one of the primary goals of global acquired immunodeficiency syndrome (AIDS) research. Despite progress in prevention of and powerful drug combinations to treat HIV infection, an estimated 16,000 people become infected every day. Over 90% of new infections occur in developing countries, in which recent medical advances are not immediately applicable or affordable. The best hope for these countries is the development of a safe, effective, accessible HIV vaccine. There is now growing optimism among scientists that an AIDS vaccine may be possible (1).

An ideal prophylactic vaccine should induce sterilizing immunity, so that after exposure the virus would not be detected in the body. However, this may be an unrealistic objective. Instead, what might be sought is a vaccine-induced immunity that results in a limited and transient virus replication, after which the virus becomes undetectable, there are no signs of disease and no transmission to other individuals. Alternatively, a potentially successful vaccine may induce immune responses that hold the virus in check at levels so low that both progression to AIDS and transmission are prevented.

Central to the evaluation of new vaccine strategies is the use of animal models, which allow testing of important aspects of vaccination in a relatively fast, inexpensive way and provide a basis for more effective planning of human clinical trials. For HIV infection and AIDS, infection of nonhuman primates with immunodeficiency viruses offers a spectrum of models in terms of disease severity and difficulty in preventing virus infection. These models range from the infection of chimpanzees with HIV-1 SF2, a model in which neutralizing antibodies (nAb) provide protection (2–4), to infection of rhesus macaques with simian immunodeficiency virus (SIV)mac, where a role for cell-mediated immune responses in partial or complete protection is strongly supported (5–8), although protection has been also achieved using very high levels of combined passively transferred nAb (9). It is important to bear in mind that to have a good chance of establishing infection in all control animals, monkey challenge doses are some 100- to 1000-fold higher that the estimated HIV doses infecting humans. Also, HIV in humans causes AIDS after some 10 years compared to 1–2 years for SIV infection of macaques. Therefore, the most important information from monkey experiments may be the immunogenicity of vaccines, because it is possible that some vaccines that fail to protect against experimental SIV challenges could still show a benefit in humans. Therefore, more vaccine approaches immunogenic in primates should be evaluated in humans and at an accelerating rate if an effective vaccine is to be developed soon. In turn, the results from these trials may indicate which of the monkey models is the closest to humans.

A prophylactic vaccine against HIV may have to induce both humoral and cell-mediated immune responses to achieve protection (10). Since HIV was isolated and sequenced, there has been a considerable effort to develop envelope-based vaccines that induce nAb. However, this has proved to be nearly impossible (11). Although some success was reported in inducing nAb against laboratory HIV strains (2,12), it has been extremely difficult to neutralize primary isolates (13,14). In follow-up of phase II human trials, at least 16 vaccinees immunized with recombinant gp120 subunit vaccines became infected (through sexual exposure) and did not handle the virus differently from placebo-vaccinated controls, nor were escape mutants selected (15).

An explanation for the first 15 years of frustration has come from the crystal structure of the core gp120, which revealed multiple mechanisms by which HIV prevents efficient induction of nAb (16,17). Thus, HIV sheds as a decoy monomeric gp120, on which the Ab response focuses. The relatively conserved part of the gp120 surface forms contacts in the naturally occurring homotrimer and is, therefore, not exposed on the virions, while the exposed areas are highly variable and the critical sites are masked by bulky polysaccharide structures, which are added by host cell enzymes. The CD4-binding site is buried deep in the molecule and can be more easily reached by an extended CD4 loop than antibodies. The chemokine coreceptor-binding site is hidden and becomes available only after the gp120 interaction with the CD4 receptor. Both of these sites are guarded by flexible and highly variable V1, V2, and V3 loops. Although some novel, promising approaches to induction of nAb are being developed (18,19), the emphasis of many vaccine designers has shifted to the induction of cell-mediated immune responses (11).

CYTOTOXIC T LYMPHOCYTES IN HIV INFECTION

Cytotoxic T lymphocytes (CTL) are usually CD8+ cells, the major function of which is to defend organisms against intracellular pathogens such as viruses. They do so through a recognition of 8- to 10-amino-acid-long peptides derived from viral proteins, which are presented in association with major histocompatibility complex (MHC) class I molecules (20). Upon recognition, CTL kill virus-infected cells and thus limit the production of new virions, and they secrete a variety of soluble factors that directly or indirectly contribute to the suppression of virus replication. These effector functions are adaptive, require a cascade of specific molecular and cellular interactions for their generation, and display a long-term memory.

A critical issue in determining the anti-HIV role of CTL is their reliable measurement. CTL are defined by their ability to lyse sensitized target cells in vitro, an activity determined for bulk lymphocyte cultures in a ^{51}Cr-release assay. This lytic activity can be in some cases measured not only after a prolong restimulation in vitro, i.e., expansion of CTL precursors, but also for freshly isolated peripheral blood mononuclear cells (PBMC), provided that the frequencies of specific effector CTL are in the order of 10^{-2} (21–24). Spectrotyping is a technique based on the lengths of polymerase chain reaction (PCR) products amplified across the highly variable complementarity determining regions of the T-cell receptor (TCR) Vβ chain repertoire, which estimates expansions of CTL clones during the generation of an immune response and has demonstrated large (>1% of CD8+ T cells in the peripheral blood) oligoclonal expansions in HIV-infected persons (25), which were antigen-specific (26). Other methods attempt to enumerate individual specific T cells. Limiting dilution assay (LDA) measures T cells that can divide 10–14 times and kill in a ^{51}Cr-release assay. The frequencies of HIV-specific CTL precursors in PBMC during the asymptomatic phase of HIV infection obtained by this method range from 10^{-3} to 10^{-5} and represent mainly long-term memory CTL (27–29). Enzyme-linked immunospot (ELISPOT) assay (30) detects cells secreting interferon (IFN)-γ or tumor necrosis factor-α upon epitope peptide stimulation of CD8+ T cells and gives frequencies in a chronic infection about fivefold higher than LDA. The limit of this method's sensitivity is about 1 in 100,000. However, not all antigen-specific cells produce IFN-γ and not all IFN-γ–producing cells are cytolytic. The use of fluorochrome-labeled soluble tetrameric MHC-peptide complexes in a FACS analysis allows direct enumeration of T cells bearing TCR reactive with a particular MHC-peptide complex in culture unexpanded cell populations. It gives the highest frequencies of HIV-specific cells during a chronic HIV infection of up to 10^{-1} with a sensitivity of about 1 in 5000. About 10% of tetramer-sorted cells from asymptomatic HIV patient can be cloned (31). However, antigenic stimulation downregulates surface expression of TCR and may render tetramer-reactive cells undetectable, and not all tetramer-reactive cells are necessarily fully functional (32,33). A big advantage of tetramer staining is that the reactive cells can be further characterized phenotypically for surface markers and/or intracellular cytokine or chemokine staining. These techniques have revealed a substantial heterogeneity and dynamism of tetramer-reactive cells, especially in terms of expressed immunomodulator and surface marker molecules, which most likely reflect multiple overlapping subpopulations at different states of maturation, activation, and/or time from the last antigen engagement (Fig. 1). In essence, each of the CTL-quantitation methods measures a different quality of CTL (or CD8+ cells), the frequencies these methods give correlate with each other reasonably well (34), and the relative ratio in the frequencies may depend on the antigenic load (i.e.,

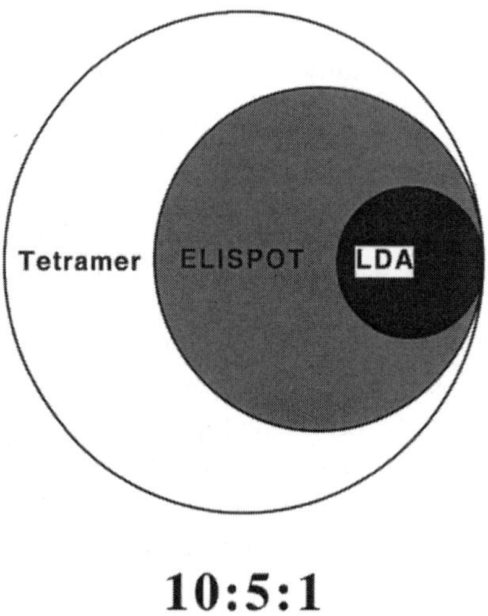

Figure 1 Subpopulations of antigen-specific CD8+ T lymphocytes determined by different assays.

may be different during the primary and chronic viral infections and when the antigen is cleared from the body completely). In the last situation, the frequencies of virus-specific T cells determined by each method may give similar results. These assays complement each other and together provide the best currently achievable picture of the status of the immune response.

There is growing evidence that CTL are an important component of the antiviral responses in both HIV-infected people and the SIV-infected macaque model of AIDS. Thus, during primary infection, occurrence of CTL rather than nAb correlated with the control of the acute infection (35–37), and depletion of CD8+ lymphocytes resulted in substantially higher virus loads (38). CTL activity was readily detected in many asymptomatic HIV+ individuals (21,39), and the frequency of circulating CTL was related inversely to plasma RNA virus loads in untreated infected patients (40). Depletion of CD8+ lymphocytes from macaques during chronic SIV infection caused a rapid increase in viremia that was again suppressed when the SIV-specific CD8+ T cells reappeared (38,41). The strongest indication that CTL can contain HIV replication is the isolation of CTL-escape mutants, which in some situations is associated with deterioration of the clinical status (35,42–48) and mother-to-child transmission (49). Loss of CTL function was correlated with the onset of AIDS (28,29,50).

At the same time, HIV persists in the face of vigorous HIV-specific CTL activity, which invariably fails to provide a life-long protection from progression to AIDS. Several mechanisms contribute. The error-prone reverse transcriptase (10^{-4} per base) together with rapid kinetics of HIV replication (10^{10} new virions per day) results in a quick accumulation of mutations, some of which may cause an escape from the CTL by altering epitopes so that they either cannot be recognized (35,42–48) or antagonize the index peptide-specific responses (51). Downregulation of MHC class I molecules is well described (52,53) but may be insufficient to prevent CTL killing (54,55). Upregulation of Fas ligand (CD95L) on HIV-infected cells has been demonstrated (56), which could induce apoptosis in approaching CTL. Selective loss of HIV-specific T-cell responses through exhaustion (28,57–59) and anergy (60) may occur. The rapid establishment of latently infected resting CD4+ T cells, which decay slowly with an estimated half-life of 6 months (61), gives an HIV reservoir safe from the CTL attack. The broad spectrum of cells that HIV infects (62), including those critically involved in proper functioning of the immune system, causes a progressive loss and impairment of CD4+ helper T-cell number and function.

Determination of the cause-and-effect relationship between the levels of CTL and HIV viremia is not straightforward. Primary HIV infection induces initial high CTL activity, which reduces substantially the replication, after which a dynamic equilibrium is established among CTL killing of HIV-infected cells, consequent reduction of the antigenic stimulation of CTL, and HIV suppression of CTL, which is direct or indirect through impairment of CD4+ helper T cells

(63). In essence, the more CTL, the less virus (40). NAb also impose a selective pressure on HIV (64), however, because of the ease with which HIV escapes, the antibody response is not generally believed to be very influential. The war is going on in connected, but spatially separated sites around the body in varying local environments of soluble factors, which can either inhibit or support both HIV replication and CTL, and be affected by other unrelated infection episodes. It has been shown that depletion of CTL results in increased viraemia (38), more CTL decreases temporarily the number of infected cells (65,66), suppressed virus replication is followed by a decrease in the CTL number (67), and an increase in HIV replication boosts CTL (64). However, when the effects of all of these interventions fade, both the HIV and CTL levels return to the pre-treatment equilibrium levels. With time, the CTL functions become more and more disabled and the equilibrium moves in favor of the virus until its precipitous collapse and development of AIDS.

Several observations raised the possibility that CTL may be able to protect against primary HIV infection. In the laboratory, CTL killed HIV-infected cells before these produced new virions (68) and released chemokines, which inhibited HIV infection (69–72). Thus, in vivo, CTL may be able to clear the initial small number of infected cells before HIV spreads further and establishes generalized infection (73,74). This might explain detection of HIV-specific CTL responses in exposed but uninfected commercial sex workers whose cells were fully susceptible to infection with HIV (75,76), in uninfected infants born to HIV-infected mothers (77), and in seronegative health care workers occupationally exposed to HIV-contaminated body fluids (78). CTL-mediated protection may depend on the levels of CTL present in the circulation (5), and specificity for proteins expressed early (regulatory proteins) rather than late (structural proteins) in the replication cycle (5,79,80) may be important. Broad CTL responses against multiple epitopes may be required for the control of replication (47,81,82).

Certain phenotypes of HLA class I and II molecules, and transporters associated with antigen processing (TAP) have been linked with the rate of progression to disease: fast progression (A1; A9; A11; A23; A28+TAP2.3; A29+TAP2.1; B8+DR3; B35+Cw4; DR2; and DR5) and slow progression (A9; A25+TAP2.3; A26, A32; B5; B14; B18; B27; B51; B57; Bw4; DR5; DR6; DR7; DRB1*0702+DQA1*0201; and DR13) (83). The HLA-dependent protection against HIV infection might result from a more efficient processing and presentation of HIV-derived peptides or selection of highly conserved epitopes. It has also been suggested that humoral and cellular immune responses to HLA antigens on the surface of virions or infected cells could offer protection (84,85). However, none of the above HLA associations has been conclusively proven.

One way to study the anti-HIV role of CTL more directly is to observe the effect of a strong CTL activity on the course of HIV infection in vivo. This can be attempted by an infusion of in vitro expanded CTL clones back into the patient's circulation. However, in contrast with the success of this CTL adoptive therapy in treating or preventing Epstein-Barr virus and cytomegalovirus diseases after bone marrow transplantation, so far the benefit of infusion of HIV-specific CTL into HIV-positive patients has been limited. This was due to a rapid selection of CTL escape mutants (indicating that the CTL were effective) (43), a loss of infused cells through immune responses directed to stably transformed gene markers (86) or apoptosis (87). Encouraging messages from the infusion studies are that the large amounts of cloned CTL were well tolerated, arguing against deleterious effects of CTL such as a major role in depleting CD4+ T cells suggested by some investigators (88,89), the CTL accumulated in lymph nodes in close contact with HIV-infected cells (66) and in some cases transiently increased the CD4+ cells counts (65) and decreased numbers of HIV-infected cells (66). It is possible that rather than transferring a large number of CTL, smaller numbers of CTL in a state of activation less susceptible to apoptosis, perhaps accompanied by T-helper cells (43,90,91), may show more benefit. Despite the limited value of this approach to therapy, the data so far support an important role for CTL in the control of HIV replication.

INDUCTION OF CYTOTOXIC T LYMPHOCYTES BY VACCINATION

Identification of immunization methods that induce strong CTL activity is a practical alternative to the more ‘‘academic’’ adoptive transfer of expanded CTL clones, which would provide not only a useful tool for studying CTL, but may also point the way towards an effective HIV vaccine. For practical and safety reasons, viral subunits rather than whole inactivated or attenuated HIV preparations are almost certain to be the choice for AIDS vaccines. The use of whole proteins is an obvious option for such vaccines. In the absence of any single HIV protein candidate that would induce strong protective cellular responses, multivalent vaccines constructed from several proteins delivered either individually or as a one-open-reading-frame (ORF) polyprotein seem to be the best start. An alternative approach for induction of CTL is to construct vaccines as a string of partially overlapping epitope peptides derived from viral proteins. It was shown that epitopes linked in this artificial way are in a majority of cases immunogenic (55,92–104). The disadvantage of this approach is that considerable prior knowledge about HLA types of the target population and the corresponding CTL epitopes is required. However, compared to whole proteins, the use of CTL epitopes reduces the amount of protein or genetic material that needs to be delivered during vaccination, enables focusing the immune responses towards important or conserved protein regions, overcomes the potential risk of undesired biological activities of whole proteins, makes the reversion to virulence impossible, and opens a possibility for a simple construction of multipathogen/clade/isolate vaccines. The polymorphism of HLA molecules causes each individual to present a different set of peptide epitopes to the T cells. It has been estimated that optimally selected peptides presented by only nine common HLA molecules would be required for coverage of a general population irrespective of ethnic origin (105). If more than one relevant epitope for each person were required, the complexity of a broadly efficacious epitope-based vaccine would increase, but still be feasible.

So how can CTL responses be efficiently and reliably induced? Antigens enter the MHC class I processing and presentation pathway most efficiently if they are synthesized within the target cell, although this may not be the case for so-called professional antigen-presenting cells essential for priming of immune responses (106). Therefore immunization vectors that deliver virus genes into the host cells are the most promising vaccine vehicles for induction of CTL. Before planning a human trial, the immunogenicity of a candidate vaccine should be tested in nonhuman primates that are closer to humans in size and immune responsiveness than, e.g., mice, and can be challenged with SIV. A relatively large number of vaccine approaches have been evaluated in primates, but only a few induced CTL activity, and yet fewer protected macaques against virus challenges. However, not all these approaches are applicable to humans for safety and/or large-scale production considerations. Examples of the subunit vaccines that have elicited detectable CTL responses in primates include a synthetic peptide in a mineral oil adjuvant (107), *Mycobacterium bovis* BCG-based vaccines alone (108) or in a combination with peptide (109), antigens incorporated into immune-stimulating complexes (ISCOMs) (110), mucosal or targeted lymph node immunization with a particulate SIV p27 protein (111), a CTL epitope fused with hepatitis B surface antigen as protein (112) or expressed from a DNA vector (113), DNA vaccines (114–116), poxvirus vectors (5,117–121) including modified vaccinia virus Ankara (MVA) (122), and bimodal DNA-vaccinia virus (123) or DNA-fowlpox virus (124,125) vaccine regimens.

So far, only live-attenuated virus vaccines have provided consistent protection against highly pathogenic challenges (7,8,126–128), but this approach carries a risk of a development of AIDS and is therefore not acceptable for human use (129,130). Protection with subunit vaccines has been harder to achieve and may depend on the route of immunization (131,132). Subunit DNA vaccines have protected chimpanzees from infection with HIV-1, which is nonpathogenic in this species (133), but subunit vaccine provided very limited protection against pathogenic SIV and nonpathogenic SIV/HIV chimera $(SHIV)_{HXBc2}$ challenges (134,135). Env protein boosting after DNA priming increased antibody, but not CTL responses and protected macaques against a nonpathogenic $SHIV_{HXBc2}$ challenge (136). Trivalent MVA immunization reduced postchallenge virus burden (137); recombinant vaccinia virus–based regimens gave some protection against an SIVmac challenge (5,138) and, in combination with DNA, significantly decreased virus loads after infection (123). Adjuvanted tat protein (79) and recombinant Semliki forest virus priming followed by MVA boosting delivering tat and rev (80) protected macaques against pathogenic challenges with $SHIV_{89.6PD}$ and SIVmacJ5, respectively. The most promising containment of challenge infections by subunit vaccines was achieved by i.d. DNA prime-recombinant fowlpox boost vaccinations, which held nonpathogenic HIV (124) and nonpathogenic $SHIV_{IIIB}$ (125) below the level of detection. In the latter study, two animals remained uninfected after a challenge with pathogenic $SHIV_{89.6P}$, a protection mediated by a nAb-independent mechanism. However, there is a real possibility that protective responses could have been boosted/induced by the two previous $SHIV_{IIIB}$ exposures. In none of the above studies were CTL correlated clearly and unequivocally with the protection mechanism, nevertheless, these results are very encouraging for the development of a safe vaccine for humans.

The significance of the extensive genetic diversity of the HIV isolates and its implication for vaccine design have been long debated. The predominant HIV-1 clade in Europe and North America is clade B, which is the most studied HIV clade with the most information including CTL epitopes available. In central and eastern Africa, the predominant circulating HIV-1 strain is clade A (139), while clade C dominates southern Africa, India, and China. Although there are some important differences between CTL epitopes of different HIV clades (76,140), there is a degree of cross-clade conservation in both HIV proteins due to structure/function constraints and many of the determined CTL epitopes (76,140–149). Some data suggested that cross-clade reactive CTL can be also induced by vaccination (150).

CTL may require "help" provided by CD4+ T cells for maintenance of their effector functions and even dendritic cells may be conditioned by CD4+ cells to provide sufficient costimulatory signals to CTL (151–153). In chronic HIV infection, vigorous gag-specific CD4+ T-cell responses were associated with the control of viremia (154) and correlated positively with levels of gag-specific CTL precursors and negatively with levels of plasma HIV-1 RNA (91). For CTL epitope-based vaccines, a long enough string of MHC class I–restricted epitopes will create novel helper epitopes presented by promiscuous MHC class II molecules and activate CD4+ T-cell responses. However, these CD4+ helper T cells induced by a prophylactic polyepitope vaccine will not be activated by incoming HIV. This could be an advantage. For a prophylactic vaccine, delay in CD4+ T-cell activation may slow the initial spread of HIV, because HIV replicates in activated CD4+ cells, and so gain important time in the race with HIV. No evidence of HIV-specific proliferative responses was detected in 20 individuals who had been repeatedly exposed sexually to HIV but remained uninfected (154). On the other hand, several studies found CD4+ T-cell responses in exposed seronegative individuals (155–157), which could suppress HIV replication by production of C-C chemokines (158). On the whole, the likely advantage of concomitant CD4+ T helper responses induced along with CTL probably outweighs the disadvantage of providing potential targets for virus replication. For a therapeutic vaccine (see below), one could also design an epitope peptide-based immunization for induction of CTL, where the help is provided without activation of CD4+ T cells through a parallel infusion of, e.g., anti-CD40L mAb (159,160).

A prophylactic AIDS vaccine has the best chance for controlling the HIV pandemic. However, there are close to 40 million already infected people around the world who should not be forgotten. Although powerful drug combinations are now available that have been effective in preventing serious complications and prolonging the life of many people, this treatment alone may not be able to clear HIV from the body (161) and do so before undesirable side effects require cessation of the treatment. Needless to say, prolonged intervention with the highly active antiretroviral therapy (HAART) is not affordable for the poorer countries. Thus, for HIV-positive people, a therapeutic vaccine may offer life. Unfortunately, there are some special issues connected with their application. In individuals chronically infected with HIV, immune stimulation through, e.g., opportunistic infections or an HIV-unrelated vaccination with a common recall antigen increased the patients' plasma virus load (162,163). Therefore, therapeutic vaccination should be applied together with HAART, which allows stimulation of HIV-specific CTL responses while holding HIV replication below detectable levels. Upon cessation of HAART, the induced CTL might suppress HIV replication, as was suggested in an SIV macaque model (164). Alternatively, CTL responses may be boosted by short discontinuations of HAART (64). As for prophylactic vaccines, efficient methods for induction of CTL and nAb are anxiously awaited.

OXFORD EXPERIMENTAL AIDS VACCINE

As a part of our team's long-term effort to develop an HIV vaccine, a prototype vaccine immunogen was constructed as a string of partially overlapping epitopes recognized by murine, macaque, and human CTL, which was delivered by vaccine vehicles that were safe and acceptable for use in humans—a DNA vector and MVA (97,98) (Fig. 2). The use of the mixed-species polyepitope greatly facilitated the preclinical development of these vaccines (165). Thus, in mice the most potent protocol for induction of CTL was found to be DNA priming followed by MVA boosting (99,166). A similar regimen showed an impressive protection of mice against a malaria challenge (166) and the construct shown in Figure 1 induced effectively SIV-specific CTL in rhesus macaques (55,167).

The DNA prime–MVA boost regimen may be efficient in induction of CTL for several reasons. First, priming using a DNA vaccine may focus the initial CTL responses on the recombinant immunogen as that is the only foreign protein expressed. Although MVA may be intrinsically more immunogenic than a DNA vaccine, MVA-infected cells produce a large number of MHC class I–restricted epitopes derived from at least 170 ORF of the vaccinia virus genome, all compet-

I. Immunogen * CROSS-SPECIES MULTI-CTL EPITOPE

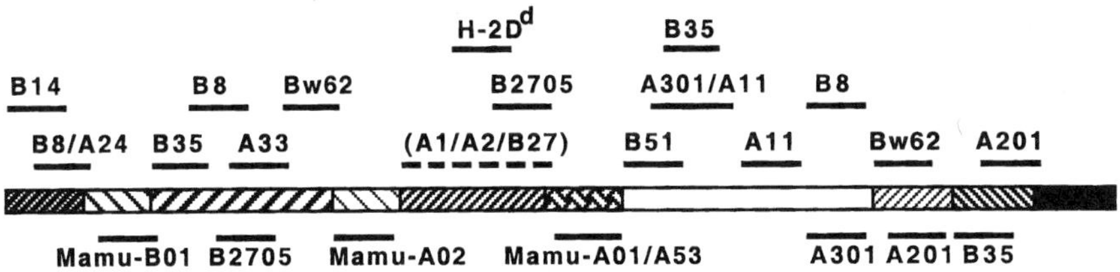

II. Vaccine Vehicles * DNA I.M. OR GENE GUN

* MVA ATTENUATED VACCINIA VIRUS

III. Regimen * DNA PRIME - MVA BOOST

IV. MICE ⟶ MACAQUES ⟶ HUMANS

Figure 2 Development of the Oxford HIV vaccines.

ing with the desired immunogen for immunodominance. Previous studies demonstrated that while vaccinees responded to poxvirus proteins, only 25–30% made CTL responses to the heterologous antigen (5,117–121). In the bimodal regimen, DNA priming first expands the immunogen-specific CTL precursors/memory, which the more immunogenic MVA further expands. This may also mean that there is no need for induction of high levels of CTL by the DNA vaccine as long as the CTL are primed (55). Second, dermis was chosen as the immunization route, which is considered to be a major immunological inductive site. This route delivered the multiepitope immunogen directly or indirectly to Langerhans cells, which upon activation migrate to the draining lymph nodes and serve as the most efficient initiators and modulators of immune reactions (106). In mice, the i.d. administration of vaccines was more immunogenic than the intramuscular needle injection (166). Third, MVA may be a more potent inducer of CTL than other vaccinia virus strains or poxviruses (166,168–170) possibly because of its genetic make-up, which was shaped by large deletions in the parental genome during the process of attenuation. The regions deleted include a number of genes coding for immunomodulators (171,172). However, a rigorous comparison of the immunogenicities of attenuated poxvirus vectors, especially in humans, is missing. Finally, as discussed above, there is a growing evidence that combined vaccination protocols induce more vigorous immune responses (55,99,101,124,125, 166,173,174).

The high immunogenicity of the multiepitope DNA and MVA vaccine approach in macaques has generated a hope that similar vaccines may induce efficiently cellular responses in humans. Phase I/II clinical trials in healthy low-risk volunteers in Oxford, United Kingdom, supported by the International AIDS Vaccine Initiative and MRC U.K. were scheduled to commence in the summer of year 2000. Provided the vaccines are shown to be safe and a satisfactory CTL immunogenicity is observed, phase I and II trials in Nairobi, Kenya, in a high-risk cohort will follow with a chance of an indication of efficacy in phase II. In particular, it may be possible to disprove the protective CTL hypothesis by careful study of ''breakthrough'' infections.

The Oxford vaccine (175) focuses on the induction of cellular immune responses mediated by the concerted action of CD4+ helper and CD8+ effector T lymphocytes. The immunogen, designated HIVA and delivered by DNA and MVA vectors, is tailor-designed for Nairobi. It is derived from the sequences of the predominant local HIV-1 clade A (139) and consists of about 73% of the gag protein fused to a string of 25 partially overlapping CTL epitopes (Fig. 3). The gag domain of HIVA contains p24 and p17 in an order reversed to the viral gag p17-p24-p15 polyprotein. This rearrangement prevents myristylation of the N-terminus of p17, which could direct the recombinant protein to the cell membrane and interfere with an efficient degradation into peptides necessary for the

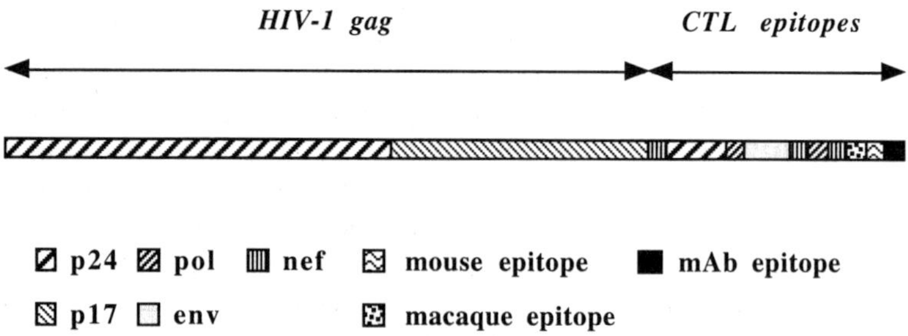

Figure 3 Schematic representation of the Oxford HIVA protein immunogen showing the origin of the HIV-1 sequences.

MHC class I presentation. The amino acid sequence of the gag domain was derived from the protein database consensus sequence of HIV-1 clade A (176). In the absence of available Kenyan strain sequences, regions without a strong amino acid clade A preference were biased towards Ugandan isolates. The HIV-1 gag protein contains not only important MHC class I–, but also class II–restricted epitopes, which stimulate CD4+ T helper cells (91,154).

The C-terminus of the HIVA protein is designed as a multi-CTL epitope. These epitopes were mostly identified in patients infected with HIV-1 clade A strains circulating in Africa and originate from the gag, pol, nef, and env proteins (76,140). Many of these epitopes are immunodominant and relatively conserved among other HIV-1 clades. They are presented by 17 different HLA alleles, which include both frequent African alleles as well as alleles common in most ethnic populations. Thus, given that majority of HIV-infected donors make good CTL responses to gag p17/p24, each vaccinee should have the potential to respond to at least two or three CTL epitopes present in the HIVA protein.

The HIVA polyepitope contains SIV gag and HIV env epitopes recognized by macaque and murine CTL, respectively, so that the quality, reproducibility and stability of the clinical batches can be easily assessed in a mouse (or macaque) potency assay. Both DNA and MVA vectors were shown to be highly immunogenic in mice (175).

The experimental HIVA vaccine does not contain the envelope glycoprotein and does not attempt to induce antibodies neutralizing HIV. The requirements for an efficient generation of such responses are quite different from those for the induction of CD8+ T cells and might compromise the T-cell immunogenicity of the current vaccination approach. Therefore, nAb may be better elicited separately when a reliable vaccine method for induction of nAb against primary HIV isolates is available. On the other hand, the absence of envelope in the vaccine has some advantages. Vaccination will not interfere with the anti-env antibody–based tests for HIV seropositivity, and, therefore, vaccination- and infection-induced immune responses can readily differentiated. It also offers the opportunity to add the env component to the vaccination protocol in the future without having to overcome the ''original-antigenic-sin'' phenomenon resulting from an immunization with a close, but different cross-reacting antigen (177).

This vaccine contrasts with the current AIDS vaccine efforts. So far more than 25 different HIV vaccines have entered human trials, very few of which have focused on the induction of CTL. The vast majority have focused on HIV clade B–derived antigens.

CONCLUDING REMARKS

Many basic immunological questions concerning CTL and CTL-inducing AIDS vaccines remain. What determines the immunodominance of CTL responses? Do vaccines need to take this into account, or can they establish new immunodominance based on conserved regions of HIV proteins? Is the induction of T-cell help desirable for a prophylactic HIV vaccine? Induction of which T-cell subtype(s) should be targeted—effector, memory, or both? At which site(s)—mucosal, local lymphoid organs, systemic, or all three—should the responses be induced, and which routes of vaccine delivery are best? Is the HIVA vaccine going to be equally immunogenic in Oxford and Nairobi given the differences in genetic background, nutritional status, and exposure to other infections of the target populations? How can longevity/maintenance of the T-cell responses be achieved? Persistence of vaccine antigens in the body is probably desirable for the maintenance of immunological memory but currently presents a major obstacle for the approval of clinical trials by regulatory authorities. All these considerations critically affect vaccine design, yet clear answers are not available. The scheduled Oxford/Nairobi and other ongoing clinical trials should help to shed light on at least some of these questions, as no animal model can replace a clinical assessment of an experimental vaccine.

ACKNOWLEDGMENTS

Grant supports from MRC U.K. and the International AIDS Vaccine Initiative are fully acknowledged.

REFERENCES

1. McMichael AJ, Hanke T. Is an HIV vaccine possible? Nat Med 1999; 5: 612–614.
2. Berman PW, Gregory TJ, Riddle L, Nakamura GR, Champe MA, Porter JP, Wurm FM, Hershberg RD, Cobb EK, Eichberg JW. Protection of chimpanzees from infection by HIV-1 after vaccination with recombinant glycoprotein gp120 but not gp160. Nature 1990; 345:622–625.
3. Girard M, Kieny M-P, Pinter A, Barré-Sinoussi F, Nara P, Kolbe H, Kusumi K, Chaput A, Reinhart T, Muchmore E, Ronco J, Kanczorek M, Gomard E, Gluckman J-P. Immunization of chimpanzee confers protection against challenge with human immunodeficiency virus. Proc Natl Acad Sci USA 1991; 88:542–546.
4. Emini EA, Schleif WA, Nunberg JH, Conley AJ, Eda Y, Tokiyoshi S, Putney SD, Matsushita S, Cobb KE, Jett CM, Eichberg JW, Murthy KK. Prevention of HIV-1 infection in chimpanzees by gp120 V3 domain-specific monoclonal antibody. Nature 1992; 355:726–730.
5. Gallimore A, Cranage M, Cook N, Almond N, Bootman J, Rud R, Silvera P, Dennis M, Corcoran T, Stott J, McMichael A, Gotch F. Early suppression of SIV replication by CD8+ nef-specific cytotoxic T cells in vaccinated animals. Nature Med 1995; 1:1167–1173.
6. Dittmer U, Hunsmann G. Long-term non-progressive human immunode-

ficiency virus infection: new insights from the simian immunodeficiency virus model. J Gen Virol 1997; 78:979–984.
7. Miller CJ, McChesney MB, Lu X, Dailey PJ, Chutkowski C, Lu D, Brosio P, Roberts B, Lu Y. Rhesus macaques previously infected with simian/human immunodeficiency virus are protected from vaginal challenge with pathogenic SIVmac239. J Virol 1997; 71:1911–1921.
8. Igarashi T, Ami Y, Yamamoto H, Shibata R, Kuwata T, Mukai R, Shinohara K, Komatsu T, Adachi A. Protection of monkeys vaccinated with vpr- and /or nef-defective simian immunodeficiency virus strain mac/human immunodeficiency virus type 1 chimeric viruses: a potential candidate live-attenuated human AIDS vaccine. J Gen Virol 1997; 78:985–989.
9. Mascola JR, Lewis MG, Stiegler G, Harris D, VanCott TC, Hayes D, Louder MK, Brown CR, Sapan CV, Frankel SS, Lu Y, Robb ML, Katinger H, Birx DL. Protection of macaques against pathogenic simian/human immunodeficiency virus 89.6PD by passive transfer of neutralizing antibodies. J Virol 1999; 73:4009–4018.
10. Salk J, Bretcher PA, Salk PL, Clerici M, Shearer GM. A strategy for prophylactic vaccination against HIV. Science 1993; 260:1270–1272.
11. Heilman CA, Baltimore D. HIV vaccines: where are we going? Nature Med 1998; 4(4 suppl):532–534.
12. Fultz PN, Nara P, Barré-Sinoussi F, Chaput A, Greenberg ML, Muchmore E, Kieny MP, Girard M. Vaccine protection of chimpanzies against challenge with HIV-1-infected peripheral blood mononuclear cells. Science 1992; 256:1687–1690.
13. Trkola A, Ketas T, Kewalramani VN, Endorf F, Binley JM, Katinger H, Robinson J, Littman DR, Moore JP. Neutralization sensitivity of human immunodeficiency virus type 1 primary isolates to antibodies and CD4-based reagents is independent of coreceptor usage. J Virol 1998; 72:1876–1885.
14. Haynes BF. HIV vaccine: where are we going? Lancet 1996; 34:933–937.
15. Connor RI, Korber BT, Graham BS, Hahn BH, Ho DD, Walker BD, Neumann AU, Vermund SH, Mestecky J, Jackson S, Fenamore E, Cao F, Kalams S, Kunstman KJ, McDonald D, McWilliams N, Trkola A, Moore JP, Wolinski SM. Immunological and immunological analyses of persons infected by human immunodeficiency virus type 1 while participating in trials of recombinant gp120 subunit vaccines. J Virol 1998; 72:1552–1576.
16. Wyatt R, Kwong, PD, Desjardins E, Sweet RW, Robinson J, Hendrickson WA, Sodroski JG. The antigenic structure of the HIV gp120 envelope glycoprotein. Nature 1998; 393:705–711.
17. Kwong PD, Wyatt R, Robinson J, Sweet RW, Sodroski J, Hendrickson WA. Structure of an HIV gp120 envelope glycoprotein in complex with

the CD4 receptor and a neutralizing human antibody. Nature 1998; 393: 638–659.

18. Chan DC, Kim PS. HIV entry and its inhibition. Cell 1998; 93:681–684.
19. LaCasse RA, Follis KE, Trahey M, Scarborough JD, Littman DR, Nunberg JH. Fusion-competent vaccines: broad neutralization of primary isolates of HIV. Science 1999; 283:357–362.
20. Zinkernagel RM, Doherty PC. Immunological surveillance against altered self components by sensitised T lymphocytes in lymphocytic choriomeningitis. Nature 1974; 251:547.
21. Walker BD, Chakrabarti S, Moss B, Paradis TJ, Flynn T, Durno AG, Blumberg RS, Kaplan JC, Hirsch MS, Schooley RT. HIV-specific cytotoxic T lymphocytes in seropositive individuals. Nature 1987; 328:345–348.
22. Walker BD, Flexner C, Paradis TJ, Fuller TC, Hirsch MS, Schooley RT, Moss B. HIV-1 reverse transcriptase is a target for cytotoxic T lymphocytes in infected individuals. Science 1988; 240:64–66.
23. Gotch FM, Nixon DF, Alp N, McMichael AJ, Borysiewicz LK. High frequency of memory and effector gag-specific cytotoxic T lymphocytes in HIV seropositive individuals. Int Immunol 1990; 2:707–712.
24. Johnson RP, Trocha A, Yang L, Mazzara GP, Panicali DL, Buchanan TM, Walker BD. HIV-1 gag-specific cytotoxic T lymphocytes recognize multiple highly conserved epitopes. Fine specificity of the gag-specific response defined by using unstimulated peripheral blood mononuclear cells and cloned effector cells. J Immunol 1991; 147:1512–1521.
25. Pantaleo G, Demarest JF, Schacker T, Vaccarezza M, Cohen OJ, Daucher M, Graziosi C, Schnittman SS, Quinn TC, Shaw GM, Perrin L, Tambussi G, Lazzarin A, Sekaly RP, Soudeyns H, Corey L, Fauci AS. The qualitative nature of the primary immune response to HIV infection is a prognosticator of disease progression independent of the initial level of plasma viremia. Nature 1994; 370:463–467.
26. Wilson JD, Ogg G.S, Allen RL, Goulder PJ, Kelleher A, Sewell AK, O'Callaghan CA, Rowland-Jones SL, Callan MF, McMichael AJ. Oligoclonal expansions of CD8+ T cells in chronic HIV infection and antigen-specific. J Exp Med 1998; 188:785.
27. Koup RA, Pikora CA, Luzuriaga K. Limiting dilution analysis of cytotoxic T lymphocytes to human immunodeficiency virus gag antigens in infected persons: in vitro quantitation of effector cell populations with p17 and p24 specificities. J Exp Med 1991; 174:1593–1600.
28. Carmichael A, Jin X, Sissons P, Borysiewicz L. Quantitative analysis of the human immunodeficiency virus type 1 (HIV-1)-specific cytotoxic T lymphocyte (CTL) response at different stages of HIV-1 infection: differ-

ential CTL responses to HIV-1 and Epstein-Barr virus in late disease. J Exp Med 1993; 177:249–256.

29. Klein MR, van Baalen CA, Holwerda AM, Kerkhof Garde SR, Bende RJ, Keet IPM, Eeftinck-Schattenkerk J-KM, Osterhaus ADME, Schuitemaker H, Miedema F. Kinetics of gag-specific cytotoxic T lymphocyte responses during the clinical course of HIV-1 infection: a longitudinal analysis of rapid progressors and long-term asymptomatics. J Exp Med 1995; 181: 1365–1372.
30. Miyahira Y, Murata K, Rodriguez D, Rodriguez JR, Esteban M, Rodrigues MM, Zavala F Quantification of antigen specific CD8+ T cells using an ELISPOT assay. J Immunol Methods 1995; 181:45–54.
31. Ogg GS, King AS, Dunbar PR, McMichael AJ. Isolation of HIV-1-specific cytotoxic T lymphocytes uaing human leukocyte antigen-coated beads. AIDS 1999; 13:1991–1993.
32. Zajac AJ, Blattman JN, Murali-Krishna K, Sourdive DJ, Suresh M, Altman JD, Ahmed R. Viral immune evasion due to persistence of activated T cells without effector function. J Exp Med 1998; 188:2205–2213.
33. Lee PP, Yee C, Savage PA, Fong L, Brockstedt D, Weber JS, Johnson D, Swetter S, Thompson J, Greenberg PD, Roederer M, Davis MM. Characterization of circulating T cells specific for tumor-associated antigens in melanoma patients. Nat Med 1999; 5:677–685.
34. Tan LC, Gudgeon N, Annels NE, Hansasuta P, O'Callaghan CA, Rowland-Jones S, McMichael AJ, Rickinson AB, Callan MF. A re-evaluation of the frequency of CD8+ T cells specific for EBV in healthy virus carriers. J Immunol 1999; 162:1827–1835.
35. Borrow P, Lewicki H, Hahn BE, Shaw GM, Oldstone MB. Virus-specific CD8+ CTL activity associated with control of viremia in primary HIV-1 infection. J Virol 1994; 68:6103–6110.
36. Koup RA, Safrit JT, Cao Y, Andrews CA, McLoed G, Borkowsky W, Farthing C, Ho DD. Temporal association of cellular immune responses with the initial control of viremia in primary human immunodeficiency virus type 1 syndrome. J Virol 1994; 68:4650–4655.
37. Kent SJ, Woodward A, Zhao A. Human immunodeficiency virus type 1 (HIV-1)-specific T cell responses correlate with the control of acute HIV-1 infection in macaques. J Infect Dis 1997; 176:1188–1197.
38. Schmitz JE, Kuroda MJ, Sasseville VG, Simon MA, Lifton MA, Racz P, Tenner-Racz K, Dalesandro M, Scallon BJ, Ghrayeb J, Forman MA, Montefiori DC, Rieber EP, Letvin NL, Reinmann KA. Control of viremia in simian immunodeficiency virus infection by CD8+ lymphocytes. Science 1999; 283:857–860.
39. Harrer T, Harrer E, Kalams SA, Elbeik T, Staprans SI, Feinberg MB, Cao

Y, Ho DD, Yilma T, Caliendo AM, Johnson RP, Buchbinder SP, Walker BD. Strong cytotoxic T cell and weak neutralizing antibody responses in a subset of persons with stable nonprogressing HIV type 1 infection. AIDS Res Hum Retroviruses 1996; 12:585–592.

40. Ogg GS, Jin X, Bonhoeffer S, Dunbar PR, Nowak MA, Monard S, Segal JP, Cao Y, Rowland-Jones SL, Cerundolo V, Hurley A, Markowitz M, Ho DD, Nixon DF, McMichael AJ. Quantitation of HIV-1-specific cytotoxic T lymphocytes and plasma load of viral RNA. Science 1998; 279: 2103–2106.
41. Jin X, Bauer DE, Tuttleton SE, Lewin S, Gettie A, Blanchard J, Irwin CE, Safrit JT, Mittler J, Weinberger L, Kostrikis LG, Zhang L, Perelson AS, Ho DD. Dramatic rise in plasma viremia after CD8(+) T cell depletion in simian immunodeficiency virus-infected macaques. J Exp Med 1999; 189:991–998.
42. Phillips RE, Rowland-Jones S, Nixon DF, Gotch FM, Edwards JP, Ogunlesi AO, Elvin JG, Rothbard JA, Bangham CR, Rizza CR, McMichael AJ. Human immunodeficiency virus genetic variation that can escape cytotoxic T cell recognition. Nature 1991; 354:453–459.
43. Koenig S, Conley AJ, Brewah YA, Jones GM, Leath S, Boots LJ, Davey V, Pantaleo G, Demarest JF, Carter C, et al. Transfer of HIV-1-specific cytotoxic T lymphocytes to an AIDS patient leads to selection for mutant HIV variants and subsequent disease progression. Nat Med 1995; 1:330–336.
44. Haas G, Plikat U, Debre P, Lucchiari M, Katlama C, Dudoit Y, Bonduelle O, Bauer M, Ihlenfeldt HG, Jung G, Maier B, Meyerhans A, Autran B. Dynamics of viral variants in HIV-1 Nef and specific cytotoxic T lymphocytes in vivo. J Immunol 1996; 157:4212–4221.
45. Wolinsky SM, Korber BT, Neumann, AU, Daniels M, Kunstman KJ, Whetsell AJ, Furtado MR, Cao Y, Ho DD, Safrit JT. Adaptive evolution of human immunodeficiency virus-type 1 during the natural course of infection. Science 1996; 272:537–542.
46. Price DA, Goulder PJ, Klenerman P, Sewell AK, Easterbrook PJ, Troop M, Bangham CR, Phillips RE. Positive selection of HIV-1 cytotoxic T lymphocyte escape variants during primary infection. Proc Natl Acad Sci USA 1997; 94:1890–1895.
47. Goulder PJR, Phillips RE, Colbert RA, McAdam S, Ogg G, Nowak MA, Giangrande P, Luzzi G, Morgan B, Edwards A, McMichael AJ, Rowland-Jones S. Late escape from an immunodominant cytotoxic T-lymphocyte response associated with progression to AIDS. Nat Med 1997; 3:212–217.
48. Borrow P, Lewicki H, Wei X, Horwitz MS, Peffer N, Meyers H, Nelson JA, Gairin JE, Hahn BH, Oldstone MBA, Shaw GM. Antiviral pressure

exerted by HIV-1-specific cytotoxic T lymphocytes (CTLs) during primary infection demonstrated by rapid selection of CTL escape virus. Nat Med 1997; 3:205–211.

49. Wilson CC, Brown RC, Korber BT, Wilkes BM, Ruhl DJ, Sakamoto D, Kunstman K, Luzuriaga K, Hanson IC, Widmayer SM, Wiznia A, Clapp S, Ammann AJ, Koup RA, Wolinsky SM, Walker BD. Frequent detection of escape from cytotoxic T-lymphocyte recognition in perinatal human immunodeficiency virus (HIV) type 1 transmission: the Ariel Project for the prevention of transmission of HIV from mother to infant. J Virol 1999; 73:3975–3985.
50. Rinaldo C, Huang XL, Fan ZF, Ding M, Beltz L, Logar A, Panicali D, Mazzara G, Liebmann J, Cottrill M, Gupta P. High levels of anti-human immunodeficiency virus type 1 (HIV-1) memory cytotoxic T-lymphocyte activity and low viral load associated with lack of disease in HIV-1 infected long-term nonprogressors. J Virol 1995; 69:5838–5842.
51. Klenerman P, Meier UC, Phillips RE, McMichael AJ. The effects of natural altered peptide ligands on the whole blood cytotoxic T lymphocyte response to human immunodeficiency virus. Nature 1995; 25:1927–1931.
52. Schwartz O, Marechal V, Le Gall S, Lemonnier F, Heard JM. Endocytosis of major histocompatibility complex class I molecules is induced by the HIV-1 Nef protein. Nat Med 1996; 2:338–342.
53. Howcroft TK, Strebel K, Martin MA, Singer DS. Repression of MHC class I gene promoter activity by two-exon Tat of HIV. Science 1993; 260:1320–1322.
54. Yang OO, Kalams SA, Rosenzweig M, Trocha A, Jones N, Koziel M, Walker BD, Johnson RP. Efficient lysis of human immunodeficiency virus type 1-infected cells by cytotoxic T lymphocytes. J Virol 1996; 70:5799–5806.
55. Hanke T, Samuel RV, Blanchard TJ, Neumann VC, Allen TM, Boyson JE, Sharpe AS, Cook N, Smith GL, Watkins DI, Cranage MP, McMichael A. Effective induction of simian immunodeficiency virus-specific cytotoxic T lymphocytes in macaques by using a multiepitope gene and DNA prime-modified vaccinia virus Ankara boost vaccination regimen. J Virol 1999; 73:7524–7532.
56. Xu X-N, Screaton GR, Gotch FM, Dong T, Tan R, Almond N, Walker B, Stebbings R, Kent K, Nagata S, Stott JE, McMichael AJ. Evasion of cytotoxic T lymphocyte (CTL) responses by nef-dependent induction of Fas ligand (CD95L) expression on simian immunodeficiency virus-infected cells. J Exp Med 1997; 186:7–16.
57. Pantaleo G, De Maria A, Koenig S, Butini L, Moss B, Baseler M, Lane HC, Fauci AS. CD8+ T lymphocytes of patients with AIDS maintain

normal broad cytolytic function despite the loss of human immunodeficiency virus-specific cytotoxicity. Proc Natl Acad Sci USA 1990; 87: 4818–4822.
58. Pantaleo G, Soudeyns H, Demarest JF, Vaccarezza M, Graziosi C, Paolucci S, Daucher M, Cohen OJ, Denis F, Biddison WE, Sekaly RP, Fauci AS. Evidence for rapid disappearance of initially expanded HIV-specific CD8+ T cell clones during primary HIV infection. Proc Natl Acad Sci USA 1997; 94:9848–9853.
59. Kersten MJ, Klein MR, Holwerda AM, Miedema F, van Oers MH. Epstein-Barr virus-specific cytotoxic T cell responses in HIV-1 infection: different kinetics in patients progressing to opportunistic infection or non-Hodgkin's lymphoma. J Clin Invest 1997; 99:1525–1533.
60. Miedema F, Petit AJ, Terpstra FG, Schattenkerk JK, de Wolf F, Al BJ, Roos M, Lange JM, Danner SA, Goudsmit J, et al. Immunological abnormalities in human immunodeficiency virus (HIV)-infected asymptomatic homosexual men. HIV affects the immune system before CD4+ T helper cell depletion occurs. J Clin Invest 1988; 82:1908–1914.
61. Zhang L, Ramratnam B, Tenner-Racz K, He Y, Vesanen M, Lewin S, Talal A, Racz P, Perelson AS, Korber BT, Markowitz M, Ho DD. Quantifying residual HIV-1 replication in patients receiving combination antiretroviral therapy. N Engl J Med 340:1605–1613 (1999).
62. Schuitemaker H, Miedema F. Viral and cellular determinants of HIV-1 replication in macrophages. AIDS 1996; 10(suppl A):S25-S32.
63. McMichael AJ, Ogg G, Wilson J, Callan M, Hambleton S, Appay V, Kelleher T, Rowland-Jones S. Memory CD8+ T cells in HIV infection. Philos Trans R Soc Lond, B Biol Sci 2000; 355:363–367.
64. Ortiz GM, Nixon DF, Trkola A, Binley J, Jin X, Bonhoeffer S, Kuebler PJ, Donahoe SM, Demoitie MA, Kakimoto WM, Ketas T, Clas B, Heymann JJ, Zhang L, Cao Y, Hurley A, Moore JP, Ho DD, Markowitz M. HIV-1-specific immune responses in subjects who temporarily contain virus replication after discontinuation of highly active antiretroviral therapy. J Clin Invest 1999; 104:R13–18.
65. Lieberman J, Skolnik PR, Parkerson GR, Fabry JA, Landry B, Bethel J, Kagan J. Safety of autologous, ex vivo-expanded human immunodeficiency virus (HIV)-specific cytotoxic T-lymphocyte infusion in HIV-infected patients. Blood 1997; 90:2196–2206.
66. Brodie SJ, Lewinsohn DA, Patterson BK, Jiyamapa D, Krieger J, Corey L, Greenberg PD, Riddell SR. In vivo migration and function of transferred HIV-1-specific cytotoxic T cells. Nat Med 1999; 5:34–41.
67. Ogg GS, Jin X, Bonhoeffer S, Moss P, Nowak MA, Monard S, Segal JP, Cao Y, Rowland-Jones S, Hurley A, Markowitz M, Ho DD, McMichael

AJ, Nixon DF. Decay kinetics of human immunodeficiency virus-specific effector cytotoxic T lymphocytes after combination antiretroviral therapy. J Virol 1999; 73:797–800.

68. Yang OO, Kalams SA, Trocha A, Cao H, Luster A, Johnson RP, Walker BD. Suppression of human immunodeficiency virus type 1 replication by CD8+ cells: evidence for HLA class I-restricted triggering of cytolityc and noncytolytic mechanisms. J Virol 1997; 71:3120–3128.
69. Zhang C, Cui Y, Houston S, Chang LJ. Protective immunity to HIV-1 in SCID/beige mice reconstituted with peripheral blood lymphocytes of exposed but uninfected individuals. Proc Natl Acad Sci USA 1996; 93: 14720–14725.
70. Wagner L, Yang OO, Garcia-Zepeda EA, Ge Y, Kalams SA, Walker BD, Pasternack, MS, Luster AD. Beta-chemokines are released from HIV-1-specific cytolytic T cell granules complexed to proteoglycans. Nature 1998; 391:908–911.
71. Price DA, Sewell AK, Dong T, Tan R, Goulder PJ, Rowland-Jones SL, Phillips RE. Antigen-specific release of beta-chemokines by anti-HIV-1 cytotoxic T lymphocytes. Curr Biol 1998; 8:355–358.
72. Stranford SA, Skurnick J, Louria D, Osmond D, Chang SY, Sninsky J, Ferrari G, Weinhold K, Lindquist C, Levy JA. Lack of infection in HIV-exposed individuals is associated with a strong CD8(+) cell noncytotoxic anti-HIV response. Proc Natl Acad Sci USA 1999; 96:1030–1035.
73. Nowak MA, Lloyd AL, Vasquez GM, Wiltrout TA, Wahl LM, Bischofberger N, Williams J, Kinter A, Fauci AS, Hirsch VM, Lifson JD. Viral dynamics of primary viremia and antiretroviral therapy in simian immunodeficiency virus infection. J Virol 1997; 71:7518–7525.
74. Wodarz D, Lloyd AL, Jansen VA, Nowak MA. Dynamics of macrophage and T cell infection by HIV. J Ther Biol 1999; 196:101–113.
75. Rowland-Jones S, Sutton J, Ariyoshi K, Dong T, Gotch F, McAdam S, Whitby D, Sabally S, Gallimore A, Corrah T, Takiguchi M, Schultz T, McMichael A, Whittle H. HIV-specific cytotoxic T-cells in HIV-exposed but uninfected Gambian women. Nature Med 1995; 1:59–64.
76. Rowland-Jones SL, Dong T, Fowke KR, Kimani J, Krausa P, Newell H, Blanchard T, Ariyoshi K, Oyugi J, Ngugi E, Bwayo JJ, MacDonald KS, McMichael AJ, Plummer FA. Cytotoxic T cell responses to multiple conserved epitopes in HIV-resistant prostitutes in Nairobi. J Clin Inv 1998; 102:1758–1765.
77. Rowland-Jones SL, Nixon DF, Aldhous MC, Gotch F, Ariyoshi K, Hallam N, Kroll JS, Froebel K, McMichael A. HIV-specific cytotoxic T-cell activity in an HIV-exposed but uninfected infant. Lancet 1993; 341:860–861.
78. Pinto LA, Sullivan J, Berzofsky JA, Clerici M, Kessler HA, Landay AL,

Shearer GM. Env-specific cytotoxic T lymphocytes in HIV seronegative health care workers occupationally exposed to HIV-contaminated body fluids. J Clin Invest 1995; 96:867–876.
79. Cafaro A, Caputo A, Fracasso C, Maggiorella MT, Goletti D, Baroncelli S, Pace M, Sernicola L, Koanga-Mogtomo ML, Betti M, Borsetti A, Belli R, Akerblom L, Corrias F, Butto S, Heeney J, Verani P, Titti F, Ensoli B. Control of SHIV-89.6P infection of cynomolgus monkeys by HIV-1 Tat protein vaccine. Nat Med 1999; 5:643–650.
80. Osterhaus AD, van Baalen CA, Gruters RA, Schutten M, Siebelink CH, Hulskotte EG, Tijhaar EJ, Randall RE, van Amerongen G, Fleuchaus A, Erfle V, Sutter G. Vaccination with Rev and Tat against AIDS. Vaccine 1999; 17:2713–2714.
81. Nowak MA, Anderson RM, Boerlijst MC, Bonhoeffer S, May RM, McMichael AJ. HIV-1 evolution and disease progression. Science 1996; 274: 1008–1011.
82. McMichael A. T cell responses and viral escape. Cell 1998; 93:673–676.
83. Levy, JA. HIV and the Pathogenesis of AIDS. Washington, DC: American Society for Microbiology, 1998.
84. Arthur LO, Bess JW, Urban RG, Strominger JL, Morton WR, Mann DL, Henderson LE, Benveniste RE. Macaques immunized with HLA-DR are protected from challenge with simian immunodeficiency virus. J Virol 1995; 69:3117–3124.
85. Chan WL, Rodgers A, Grief C, Almond N, Ellis S, Flanagan B, Silvera P, Bootman J, Stott J, Kent K, Bomford R. Immunization with class I human histocompatibility leukocytes antigen can protect macaques against challenge infection with SIVmac-23H. AIDS 1995; 9:223–228.
86. Riddell SR, Elliott M, Lewinsohn DA, Gilbert MJ, Wilson L, Manley SA, Lupton SD, Overell RW, Reynolds TC, Corey L, Greenberg PD. T-cell mediated rejection of gene-modified HIV-specific cytotoxic T lymphocytes in HIV-infected patients. Nature Med 1996; 2:216–223.
87. Tan R, Xu X, Ogg GS, Hansasuta P, Dong T, Rostron T, Luzzi G, Conlon CP, Screaton GR, McMichael AJ, Rowland-Jones S. Rapid death of adoptively transferred T cells in acquired immunodeficiency syndrome. Blood 1999; 93:1506–1510.
88. Zinkernagel RM. Are HIV-specific CTL responses salutary or pathogenic? Curr Opin Immunol 1995; 7:462–470.
89. Zinkernagel RM, Hengartner H. T-cell-mediated immunopathology versus direct cytolysis by virus: implications for HIV and AIDS. Immunol Today 1994; 15:262-268.
90. Hamann D, Baars PA, Rep MH, Hooibrink B, Kerkhof-Garde SR, Klein MR, van Lier RA. Phenotypic and functional separation of memory and effector human CD8+ T cells. J Exp Med 1997; 186:1407–1418.

91. Kalams SA, Buchbinder SP, Rosenberg ES, Billingsley JM, Colbert DS, Jones NG, Shea AK, Trocha AK, Walker BD. Association between virus-specific cytotoxic T-lymphocyte and helper responses in human immunodeficiency virus type 1 infection. J Virol 1999; 73:6715–6720.
92. Whitton JL, Sheng N, Oldstone MB, McKee TA. A ''string-of-beads'' vaccine, comprising linked minigenes, confers protection from lethal-dose virus challenge. J Virol 1993; 67:348–352.
93. Oldstone MB, Tishon A, Eddleston M, de la Torre JC, McKee T, Whitton JL. Vaccination to prevent persistent viral infection. J Virol 1993; 67: 4372–4378.
94. Thomson SA, Khanna R, Gardner J, Burrows SR, Coupar B, Moss DJ, Suhrbier A. Minimal epitopes expressed in a recombinant polyepitope protein are processed and presented to CD8+ cytotoxic T cells: implications for vaccine design. Proc Natl Acad Sci USA 1995; 92:5845–5849.
95. Thomson SA, Elliott SL, Sherritt MA, Sproat KW, Coupar BEH, Scalzo AA, Forbes CA, Ladhams AM, Mo XY, Tripp RA, Doherty PC, Moss DJ, Suhrbier A. Recombinant polyepitope vaccines for the delivery of multiple CD8 cytotoxic T cell epitopes. J Immunol 1996; 157:822–826.
96. Gilbert SC, Plebanski M, Harris SJ, Allsopp CEM, Thomas R, Layton GT, Hill AVS. A protein particle vaccine containing multiple malaria epitope. Nat Biotechnol 1997; 15:1280–1284.
97. Hanke T, Schneider J, Gilbert SC, Hill AVS, McMichael A. DNA multi-CTL epitope vaccines for HIV and *Plasmodium falciparum*: immunogenicity in mice. Vaccine 1998; 16:426-435.
98. Hanke T, Blanchard TJ, Schneider J, Ogg GS, Tan R, Becker M, Gilbert SC, Hill AVS, Smith GL, McMichael A. Immunogenicities of intravenous and intramuscular administrations of MVA-based multi-CTL epitope vaccine for HIV in mice. J Gen Virol 1998; 79:83–90.
99. Hanke T, Blanchard TJ, Schneider J, Hannan CM, Becker M, Gilbert SC, Hill AVS, Smith GL, McMichael A. Enhancement of MHC class I-restricted peptide-specific T cell induction by a DNA prime/MVA boost vaccination regime. Vaccine 1998; 16:439–445.
100. Thomson SA, Sherritt MA, Medveczky J, Elliott SL, Moss DJ, Fernando GJ, Brown LE, Suhrbier A. Delivery of multiple CD8 cytotoxic T cell epitopes by DNA vaccination. J Immunol 1998; 160:1717–1723.
101. Hanke T, Neumann VC, Blanchard TJ, Becker M, Sweeney P, Hill AVS, Smith GL, McMichael A. Effective induction of HIV-specific CTL by multi-epitope DNA using a gene gun in a combined vaccination regime. Vaccine 1999; 17:589–596.
102. Ishioka GY, Fikes J, Hermanson G, Livingston B, Crimi C, Qin M, France del Guercio M, Oseroff C, Dahlberg C, Alexander J, Chestnut RW, Sette A. Utilization of MHC class I transgenic mice for development of minigen

DNA vaccines encoding multiple HLA-restricted CTL epitopes. J Immunol 1999; 162:3915–3925.
103. Woodberry T, Gardner J, Mateo L, Eisen D, Medveczky J, Ramshaw I.A, Thomson SA, Ffrench RA, Elliott SL, Firat H, Lemonnier FA, Suhrbier A Immunogenicity of a human immunodeficiency virus (HIV) polytope vaccine containing multiple HLA A2 HIV CD8(+) cytotoxic T-cell epitopes. J Virol 1999; 73:5320–5325.
104. Mateo L, Gardner J, Chen Q, Schmidt C, Down M, Elliott SL, Pye SJ, Firat H, Lemonnier FA, Cebon J, Suhrbier A. An HLA-A2 polyepitope vaccine for melanoma immunotherapy. J Immunol 1999; 163:4058–4063.
105. Sidney J, Grey HM, Kubo RT, Sette A. Practical, biochemical and evolutionary implications of the discovery of HLA class I supermotifs. Immunol Today 1996; 17:261–266.
106. Banchereau J, Steinman RM. Dendritic cell and the control of immunity. Nature 1998; 392:245–252.
107. Yasutomi Y, Palker TJ, Gardner MB, Haynes BF, Letvin NL. Synthetic peptide in mineral oil adjuvant elicits simian immunodeficiency virus-specific CD8+ cytotoxic T lymphocytes in rhesus monkeys. J Immunol 1993; 151:5096–5105.
108. Yasutomi Y, Koenig S, Haun SS, Stover CK, Jackson RK, Conard P, Conley AJ, Emini EA, Fuerst TR, Letvin NL. Immunization with recombinant BCG-SIV elicits SIV-specific cytotoxic T lymphocytes in rhesus monkeys. J Immunol 1993; 150:3101–3107.
109. Yasutomi Y, Koenig S, Woods RM, Madsen J, Wassef NM, Alving CR, Klein HJ, Nolan TE, Boots LJ, Kessler JA, Emini EA, Conley AJ, Letvin NL. A vaccine-elicited, single viral epitope-specific cytotoxic T lymphocyte response does not protect against intravenous, cell-free simian immunodeficiency virus challenge. J Virol 1995; 69:2279–2284.
110. Hulskotte EG, Geretti AM, Siebelink KH, van Amerongen G, Cranage MP, Rud EW, Norley SG, de Vries P, Osterhaus AD. Vaccine-induced virus-neutralizing antibodies and cytotoxic T cells do not protect macaques from experimental infection with simian immunodeficiency virus SIVmac32H (J5). J Virol 1995; 69:6289–6296.
111. Klavinskis LS, Bergmeier LA, Gao L, Mitchell E, Ward RG, Layton G, Brookes R, Meyers NJ, Lehner T. Mucosal or targeted lymph node immunization of macaques with a particulate SIVp27 protein elicits virus-specific CTL in the genito-rectal mucosa and draining lymph nodes. J Immunol 1996; 157:2521–2527.
112. Schlienger K, Mancini M, Riviere Y, Dormont D, Tiollais P, Michel ML. Human immunodeficiency virus type 1 major neutralizing determinant exposed on hepatitis B surface antigen particles is highly immunogenic in primates. J Virol 1992; 66:2570–2576.

113. Le Borgne S, Mancini M, Le Grand R, Schleef M, Dormont D, Tiollais P, Riviere Y, Michel ML. In vivo induction of specific cytotoxic T lymphocytes in mice and rhesus macaques immunized with DNA vector encoding an HIV epitope fused with hepatitis B surface antigen. Virology 1998; 240:304–315.
114. Fuller DH, Murphey CM, Clements J, Barnett S, Haynes JR. Induction of immunodeficiency virus-specific immune responses in rhesus monkeys following gene gun-mediated DNA vaccination. J Med Primatol 1996; 25: 236–241.
115. Yasutomi Y, Robinson HL, Lu S, Mustafa F, Lekutis C, Arthos J, Mullins JI, Voss G, Manson K, Wyand M, Letvin NL. Simian immunodeficiency virus-specific cytotoxic T-lymphocyte induction through DNA vaccination of rhesus monkeys. J Virol 1996; 70:678–681.
116. Shiver JW, Davies ME, Yasutomi Y, Perry HC, Freed DC, Letvin NL, Liu MA. Anti-HIV env immunities elicited by nucleic acid vaccines. Vaccine 1996; 15:884–887.
117. Gotch FM, Hovell R, Delchambre M, Silvera P, McMichael AJ. Cytotoxic T-cell response to simian immunodeficiency virus by cynomolgus macaque monkeys immunized with recombinant vaccinia virus. AIDS 1991; 5:317–320.
118. Egan MA, Pavlat WA, Tartaglia J, Paoletti E, Weinhold KJ, Clements ML, Siliciano RF. Induction of human immunodeficiency virus type 1 (HIV-1)-specific cytolytic T lymphocyte responses in seronegative adults by a nonreplicating, host-range-restricted canarypox vector (ALVAC) carrying the HIV-1MN env gene. J Infect Dis 1995; 171:1623–1627.
119. Fleury B, Janvier G, Pialoux G, Buseyne F, Robertson MN, Tartaglia J, Paoletti E, Kieny MP, Excler JL, Riviere Y. Memory cytotoxic T lymphocyte responses in human immunodeficiency virus type 1 (HIV-1)-negative volunteers immunized with a recombinant canarypox expressing gp160 of HIV-1 and boosted with a recombinant gp160. J Infect Dis 1996; 174: 734–738.
120. Kent SJ, Hu SL, Corey L, Morton WR, Greenberg PD. Detection of simian immunodeficiency virus (SIV)-specific CD8+ T cells in macaques protected from SIV challenge by prior SIV subunit vaccination. J Virol 1996; 70:4941–4947.
121. Corey L, McElrath MJ, Weinhold K, Matthews T, Stablein D, Graham B, Keefer M, Schwartz D, Gorse G. Cytotoxic T cell and neutralizing antibody responses to human immunodeficiency virus type 1 envelope with a combination vaccine regimen. J Infect Dis 1998; 177:301–309.
122. Seth A, Ourmanov I, Kuroda MJ, Schmitz JE, Carroll MW, Wyatt LS, Moss B, Forman MA, Hirsch VM, Letvin NL. Recombinant modified vaccinia virus Ankara-simian immunodeficiency virus gag pol elicits cyto-

toxic T lymphocytes in rhesus monkeys detected by a major histocompatibility complex class I/peptide tetramer. Proc Natl Acad Sci USA 1998; 95:10112–10116.
123. Fuller DH, Simpson L, Cole KS, Clements JE, Panicali DL, Montelaro RC, Murphey-Corb M, Haynes JR. Gene gun-based nucleic acid immunization alone or in combination with recombinant vaccinia vectors suppresses virus burden in rhesus macaques challenged with a heterologous SIV. Immunol Cell Biol 1997; 75:389–396.
124. Kent SJ, Zhao A, Best SJ, Chandler JD, Boyle DB, Ramshaw I.A. Enhanced T-cell immunogenicity and protective efficacy of a human immunodeficiency virus type 1 vaccine regimen consisting of consecutive priming with DNA and boosting with recombinant fowlpox virus. J Virol 1998; 72:10180–10188.
125. Robinson HL, Montefiori DC, Johnson RP, Manson KH, Kalish ML, Lifson JD, Rizvi TA, Lu S, Hu S-L, Mazzara GP, Panicali DL, Herndon JG, Glickman R, Candido MA, Lydy SL, Wyand MS, McClure HM. Neutralizing antibody-independent containment of immunodeficiency virus challenges by DNA priming and recombinant pox virus booster immunizations. Nat Med 1999; 5:526–534.
126. Daniel MD, Kirchhoff F, Czajak SC, Sehgal PK, Desrosiers RC. Protective effects of a live attenuated SIV vaccine with a deletion in the nef gene. Science 1992; 258:1938–1941.
127. Cranage MP, Sharpe SA, Whatmore AM, Polyanskaya N, Norley S, Cook N, Leech S, Dennis MJ, Hall GA. In vivo resistance to simian immunodeficiency virus superinfection depends on attenuated virus dose. J Gen Virol 1998; 79:1935–1944.
128. Nilsson C, Makitalo B, Thorstensson R, Norley S, Binninger-Schinzel D, Cranage M, Rud E, Biberfeld G, Putkonen P. Live attenuated simian immunodeficiency virus (SIV)mac in macaques can induce protection against mucosal infection with SIVsm. AIDS 1998; 12:2261–2270.
129. Baba TW, Jeong Y.S, Pennick D, Bronson R, Greene MF, Ruprecht RM. Pathogenicity of live, attenuated SIV after mucosal infection of neonatal macaques. Science 1995; 267:1820–1825.
130. Ruprecht RM, Baba TW, Liska V. Attenuated HIV vaccine: caveats. Science 1996; 271:1790–1792.
131. Lehner T, Wang Y, Cranage M, Bergmeier LA, Mitchell E, Tao L, Hall G, Dennis M, Cook N, Brookes R, Klavinskis L, Jones I, Doyle C, Ward R. Protective mucosal immunity elicited by targeted iliac lymph node immunization with a subunit SIV envelope and core vaccine in macaques. Nat Med 1996; 2:767-775.
132. Lehner T, Wang Y, Ping L, Bergmeier L, Mitchell E, Cranage M, Hall

G, Dennis M, Cook N, Doyle C, Jones I. The effect of route of immunization on mucosal immunity and protection. J Infect Dis 1999; 179:S489-S492.

133. Boyer JD, Ugen KE, Wang B, Agadjanyan M, Gilbert L, Bagarazzi ML, Chattergoon M, Frost P, Javadian A, Williams WV, Refaeli Y, Ciccarelli RB, McCallus D, Coney L, Weiner DB. Protection of chimpanzees from high-dose heterologous HIV-1 challenge by DNA vaccination. Nat Med 1997; 3:526–532.

134. Boyer JD, Wang B, Ugen KE, Agadjanyan M, Javadian A, Frost P, Dang K, Carrano RA, Ciccarelli R, Coney L, Williams WV, Weiner DB. In vivo protective anti-HIV immune responses in non-human primates through DNA immunization. J Med Primatol 1996; 25:242–250.

135. Lu S, Arthos J, Montefiori DC, Yasutomi Y, Manson K, Mustafa F, Johnson E, Santoro JC, Wissink J, Mullins JI, Haynes JR, Letvin NL, Wyand M, Robinson HL. Simian immunodeficiency virus DNA vaccine trial in macaques. J Virol 1996; 70:3978–3991.

136. Letvin NL, Montefiori DC, Yasutomi Y, Perry HC, Davies M-E, Lekutis C, Alroy M, Freed DC, Lord CI, Handt LK, Liu MA, Shiver JW. Potent, protective anti-HIV immune responses generated by bimodal HIV envelope DNA plus protein vaccination. Proc Nat Acad Sci USA 1997; 94: 9378–9383.

137. Hirsch VM, Fuerst TR, Sutter G, Carroll MW, Yang LC, Goldstein S, Piatak M Jr, Elkins WR, Alvord WG, Montefiori DC, Moss B, Lifson JD. Patterns of viral replication correlate with outcome in simian immunodeficiency virus (SIV)-infected macaques: effect of prior immunization with a trivalent SIV vaccine in modified vaccinia virus Ankara. J Virol 1996; 70:3741–3752.

138. Daniel MD, Mazzara GP, Simon MA, Sehgal PK, Kodama T, Panicali DL, Desrosiers RC. High-titer immune responses elicited by recombinant vaccinia virus priming and particle boosting are ineffective in preventing virulent SIV infection. AIDS Res Hum Retroviruses 1994; 10:839–851.

139. Neilson JR, John GC, Carr JK, Lewis P, Kreiss JK, Jackson S, Nduati RW, Mbori-Ngacha D, Panteleeff DD, Bodrug S, Giachetti C, Bott MA, Richardson BA, Bwayo J, Ndinya-Achola J, Overbaugh J. Subtypes of human immunodeficiency virus type 1 and disease stage among women in Nairobi, Kenya. J Virol 1999; 73:4393–4403.

140. Dorrell L, Dong T, Ogg GS, McAdam S, Anzala O, Rostron T, Conlon C, McMichael AJ, Rowland-Jones SL. Distinct recognition of clade A HIV-1 epitopes by cytotoxic T lymphocytes generated from donors infected in Africa. J Virol 1999; 73:1708–1714.

141. Cao H, Kanki P, Sankale JL, Dieng-Sarr A, Mazzara GP, Kalams SA,

Korber B, Mboup S, Walker BD. Cytotoxic T lymphocyte cross-reactivity among different human immunodeficiency virus type 1 clades: implications for vaccine development. J Virol 1997; 71:8615–8623.
142. Betts MR, Krowka J, Santamaria C, Balsamo K, Gao F, Mulundu G, Luo C, N'Gandu N, Sheppard H, Hahn BH, Allen S, Frelinger JA. Cross-clade human immunodeficiency virus (HIV)-specific cytotoxic T-lymphocyte responses in HIV-infected Zambians. J Virol 1997; 71:8908–8911.
143. Lynch JA, deSouza, M, Robb, MD, Markowitz, L, Nitayaphan, S, Sapan, CV, Mann DL, Birx DL, Cox JH. Cross-clade cytotoxic T cell response to human immunodeficiency virus type 1 proteins among HLA disparate North Americans and Thais. J Infect Dis 1998; 178:1040–1046.
144. McAdam S, Kaleebu P, Krausa P, Goulder P, French N, Collin B, Blanchard T, Whitworth J, McMichael A, Gotch F. Cross-clade recognition of p55 by cytotoxic T lymphocytes in HIV-1 infection. AIDS 1998; 12:571–579.
145. Wilson SE, Pedersen SL, Kunich JC, Wilkins VL, Mann DL, Mazzara GP, Tartaglia J, Celum CL, Sheppard HW. Cross-clade envelope glycoprotein 160-specific CD8+ cytotoxic T lymphocyte responses in early HIV type 1 clade B infection. AIDS Res Hum Retroviruses 1998; 14: 1925–1937.
146. Buseyne F, Chaix ML, Fleury B, Manigard O, Burgard M, Blanche S, Rouzioux C, Riviere Y. Cross-clade-specific cytotoxic T lymphocytes in HIV-1-infected children. Virology 1998; 250:316–324.
147. Ogg GS, Dong T, Hansasuta P, Dorrell L, Clarke J, Coker R, Luzzi G, Conlon C, McMichael AJ, Rowland-Jones S. Four novel cytotoxic T-lymphocyte epitopes in the highly conserved major homology region of HIV-1 Gag, restricted through B*4402, B*1801, A*2601, B*70. AIDS 1998; 12:1561–1563.
148. Durali D, Morvan J, Letourneur F, Schmitt D, Guegan N, Dalon M, Saragosti S, Sicard D, Levy JP, Gomard E. Cross-reaction between cytotoxic T lymphocyte reponses of human immunodeficiency virus-infected African and European patients. J Virol 1998; 72:3547–3553.
149. Rowland-Jones SL, Dong T, Dorrell L, Ogg G, Hansasuta P, Krausa P, Kimani J, Sabally S, Ariyoshi K, Oyugi J, MacDonald KS, Bwayo J, Whittle H, Plummer FA, McMichael AJ. Broadly cross-reactive HIV-specific cytotoxic T-lymphocytes in highly-exposed persistently seronegative donors. Immunol Lett 1999; 66:9–14.
150. Ferrari G, Humphrey W, McElrath MJ, Excler JL, Duliege AM, Clements ML, Corey LC, Bolognesi DP, Weinhold KJ. Clade B-based HIV-1 vaccines elicit cross-clade cytotoxic T lymphocyte reactivities in uninfected volunteers. Proc Natl Acad Sci USA 1997; 94:1396–1401.
151. Bennett SR, Carbone FR, Karamalis F, Flavell RA, Miller JF, Heath WR.

Help for cytotoxic T-cell responses is mediated by CD40 signalling. Nature 1998; 393:478–480.
152. Ridge JP, Di Rosa F, Matzinger P. A conditioned dendritic cell can be a temporal bridge between a CD4+ T-helper and a T-killer cell. Nature 1998; 393:474–478.
153. Schoenberger SP, Toes RE, van der Voort EI, Offringa R, Melief CJ. T-cell help for cytotoxic T lymphocyte is mediated by CD40-CD40L interactions. Nature 1998; 393:480–483.
154. Rosenberg ES, Billingsley JM, Caliendo AM, Boswell SL, Sax PE, Kalams SA, Walker BD. Vigorous HIV-1-specific CD4+ T cell responses associated with control of viremia. Science 1997; 278:1447–1450.
155. Clerici M, Levin JM, Kessler HA, Harris A, Berzofsky JA, Landay AL, Shearer GM. HIV-specific T-helper activity in seronegative health care workers exposed to contaminated blood. JAMA 1994; 271:42–46.
156. Clerici M, Giorgi JV, Chou CC, Gudeman VK, Zack JA, Gupta P, Ho HN, Nishanian PG, Berzofsky JA, Shearer GM. Cell-mediated immune responses to human immunodeficiency virus (HIV) type 1 in seronegative homosexual men with recent sexual exposure. J Infect Dis 1992; 165: 1012–1019.
157. Kaul R, Trabattoni D, Bwayo JJ, Arienti D, Zagliani A, Mwangi FM, Kariuki C, Ngugi AN, MacDonald KS, Ball TB, Clerici M, Plummer FA. HIV-1 specific mucosal IgA in a cohort of HIV-1 resistant Kenyan sex workers. AIDS 1999; 13:23–29.
158. Furci L, Scarlatti G, Burastero S, Tambussi G, Colognesi C, Quillent C, Longhi R, Loverro P, Borgonovo B, Gaffi D, Carrow E, Malnati M, Lusso P, Siccardi AG, Lazzarin A, Beretta A. Antigen-driven C-C chemokine-mediated HIV-1 suppression by CD4(+) T cells from exposed uninfected individuals expressing the wild-type CCR-5 allele. J Exp Med 1997; 186: 455–460.
159. Diehl L, den Boer AT, Schoenberger SP, van der Voort EI, Schumacher TN, Melief CJ, Offringa R, Toes RE. CD40 activation in vivo overcomes peptide-induced peripheral cytotoxic T-lymphocyte tolerance and augments anti-tumor vaccine efficacy. Nat Med 1999; 5:774–779.
160. Sotomayor EM, Borrello I, Tubb E, Rattis FM, Bien H, Lu Z, Fein S, Schoenberger S, Levitsky HI. Conversion of tumor-specific CD4+ T-cell tolerance to T-cell priming through in vivo ligation of CD40. Nat Med 1999; 5:780–787.
161. Chun TW, Fauci AS. Latent reservoirs of HIV: obstacles to the eradication of virus. Proc Natl Acad Sci USA 1999; 96:10958–10961.
162. Stanley SK, Ostrowski MA, Justement JS, Gantt K, Hedayati S, Mannix M, Roche K, Schwartzentruber DJ, Fox CH, Fauci AS. Effect of immunization with a common recall antigen on viral expression in patients in-

fected with human immunodeficiency virus type 1. N Engl J Med 1996; 334:1222–1230.
163. Ostrowski MA, Stanley SK, Justement JS, Gantt K, Goletti D, Fauci AS. Increased in vitro tetanus-induced production of HIV type 1 following in vivo immunization of HIV type 1-infected individuals with tetanus toxoid. AIDS Res Hum Retroviruses 1997; 13:473–480.
164. Hel Z, Poudyal M, Tsai WP, Chougner C, Shearer G, Watkins DI, Woodworth R, Bischofberger, N, Altman J, Markham P, Tartaglia J, Franchini G. NYVAC-SIV vaccine-induced CD4 and CD8 T cell immune responses in SIV-infected macaques is dependent on the level of viremia. J Hum Virol 1999; 2:181.
165. Hanke T, McMichael A. Pre-clinical development of a multi-CTL epitope-based DNA prime-MVA boost vaccine for AIDS. Immunol Lett 1999; 66: 177–181.
166. Schneider J, Gilbert SC, Blanchard TJ, Hanke T, Robson KJ, Hannan CM, Becker M, Sinden, R, Smith GL, Hill AVS. Enhanced immunogenicity for CD8+ T cell induction and complete protective efficacy of malaria DNA vaccination by boosting with modified vaccinia virus Ankara. Nature Med 1998; 4:397–402.
167. Allen TM, Vogel TU, Fuller DH, Monthe BR, Steffen S, Boyson JE, Shipley T, Fuller J, Hanke T, Sette, A, Altman JD, Moss B, McMichael AJ, Watkins DI. An epitope-based DNA/MVA vaccine induces levels of antigen-specific CTL equivalent to those observed in acutely SIV-infected rhesus macaques. J Immunol 2000; 164:4968–4978.
168. Sutter G, Wyatt LS, Foley PL, Bennink JR, Moss B. A recombinant vector derived from the host range-restricted and highly attenuated MVA strain of vaccinia virus stimulates protective immunity in mice to influenza virus. Vaccine 1994; 12:1032–1040.
169. Moss B, Carroll MW, Wyatt LS, Bennink JR, Hirsch VM, Goldstein S, Elkins WR, Fuerst TR, Lifson JD, Piatak M, Restifo NP, Overwijk W, Chamberlain R, Rosenberg SA, Sutter G. Host range restricted, non-replicating vaccinia virus vectors as vaccine candidates. Adv Exp Med Biol 1996; 397:713.
170. Bender BS, Rowe CA, Taylor SF, Wyatt LS, Moss B, Small PAJ. Oral immunization with a replication-deficient recombinant vaccinia virus protects mice against influenza. J Virol 1996; 70:6418–6424.
171. Blanchard TJ, Alcami A, Andrea P, Smith GL. Modified vaccinia virus Ankara undergoes limited replication in human cells and lacks several immunomodulatory proteins: implications for use as a human vaccine. J Gen Virol 1998; 79:1159–1167.
172. Tough DF, Borrow, P, Sprent J. Induction of bystander T cell proliferation by viruses and type I interferon in vivo. Science 1996; 272:1947–1950.

173. Li S, Rodrigues M, Rodriguez D, Rodriguez JR, Esteban M, Palese P, Nussenzweig SR, Zavala F. Priming with recombinant influenza virus followed by administration of recombinant vaccinia virus induces CD8+ T-cell-mediated protective immunity against malaria. Proc Natl Acad Sci USA 1993; 90:5214–5218.
174. Sedegah M, Jones TR, Kaur M, Hedstrom R, Hobart P, Tine JA, Hoffman SL. Boosting with recombinant vaccinia increases immunogenicity and protective efficacy of malaria DNA vaccine. Proc Natl Acad Sci USA 1998; 95:7648–7653.
175. Hanke T, McMichael AJ. Design and construction of an experimental HIV-1 vaccine for a year-2000 clinical trial in Kenya. Nat Med 2000; 6: 951–955.
176. Korber B, Foley B, Leitner T, McCutchan F, Hahn B, Mellors JW, Myers G, Kuiken C. Human retroviruses and AIDS: a compilation and analysis of nucleic acid and amino acid sequences. Los Alamos, NM: Los Alamos National Laboratory, 1997.
177. Ivanyi J. Recall of antibody synthesis to the primary antigen following successive immunization with heterologous albumins: a two-cell theory of the original antigenic sin. Eur J Immunol 1972; 2:354–359.

5

Immune Reconstitution in HIV Infection

Guislaine Carcelain, Lucile Mollet, and Brigitte Autran

Hôpital Pitié-Salpétrière
Paris, France

INTRODUCTION

The introduction of highly active antiretroviral therapy (HAART) combining inhibitors of the HIV-1 reverse transcriptase and protease have dramatically modified the course of the HIV infection during the past 4 years. Despite some controversies about the extent to which the immune system can normalize, it is generally admitted nowadays that some immune reconstitution can be obtained in both asymptomatic HIV-infected individuals and AIDS patients and can confer host protection against opportunistic events (1–5). The best hallmark of such immune restoration is the massive decline in the mortality and morbidity related to AIDS that have been registered in all industrialized countries (6,7). Although these recent advances warrant optimism, the current HAART regimens are unable to eradicate the virus and restore an HIV-specific immunity (8,9), except when introduced immediately after virus contamination (10). Nevertheless, the immune reconstitution obtained with these antiretroviral drugs alone, even incomplete, has brought definitive evidences for the central role played by HIV itself in the massive immune alterations induced by such infection. We will review the improvements obtained in T-cell homeostasis, functions, and repertoires and the mechanisms currently proposed for such changes, which have provided better understanding of the pathophysiology of AIDS. We will also discuss the current limitations of immune restoration that emphasize the need for developing new immune-based therapeutic strategies.

THE REGENERATION OF A CD4 T-CELL COMPARTMENT WITH ANTIRETROVIRAL THERAPIES: ILLUSION OR REALITY?

Losses in peripheral CD4 T cells are thought to result from cumulative virus cell replication in the CD4 cell subpopulation either by direct virus pathogenicity and/or by CTL-mediated cytolysis, and from activation-induced cell death of ''innocent'' noninfected cells. In the meanwhile, compensation by newly produced T cells progressively diminishes during the course of the infection. A major controversy was raised as to whether the turnover of peripheral mature CD4+ T cells was massively enhanced (11). According to this hypothesis, an increased CD4 cell proliferation should take place to compensate cell losses and be responsible for the rapid increase of CD4 counts observed after reduction of viral replication with treatment. However, little evidence supports the hypothesis of a high replacement rate (12,13), and peripheral T-cell proliferation was shown to be severely limited during disease progression by the CD4 T-cell anergy and lack of IL-2 production (14). In addition thymic T-cell regeneration of naive CD4 T cells also decreases as a consequence of thymus involution with age and infection by HIV (15) and led to a preferential loss in naive CD4+ T cells co-expressing the CD45RA and the CD62L markers. In addition, to this low T-cell production, increased losses in peripheral mature T cells was related to an abnormal activation status assessed by an increased expression of activation cell markers (16): CD25, HLA-DR, CD38, and Fas, which enhance sensitivity to apoptosis, decreased expression of CD28 and CD7, markers associated with T-cell competence and T-helper differentiation (17,18). Function T-cell defects were assessed by a progressive loss in T helper-1 cell reactivity and IL-2 production by T cells against recall antigens and opportunistic pathogens (19). Normalizing these phenotypes and functions with antiretroviral drugs would thus require regeneration of full thymic function producing new naive T cells capable of protectecting against new pathogens and restoring memory T-cell functions and defenses against previously encountered pathogens.

Introduction of new antiretroviral drug regimens combining inhibitors of two HIV enzymes, the reverse transcriptase (RTI) and the protease (PI), opened a new era by inducing major and stable reduction in viral load accompanied by sustained CD4 cell increases (20–22) that had never been encountered previously with mono- or bitherapy with RTI. Such changes immediately raised the question of immune restoration and its mechanisms.

CD4 CELL REGENERATION UNDER HAART: ILLUSION OR REALITY?

A first study was conducted in 1996 on patients naive of any antiretroviral drugs who were treated with one PI and two nucleoside analogs in late disease stage (CD4 counts <250/mm^3). Our group demonstrated that the very early increase in CD4 counts was associated with a similar increment in CD8 counts (1). The early increase in CD4 cells was mostly composed of transiently activated memory CD4+ cells that lacked markers of cell proliferation. This was confirmed by various studies performed on lymph nodes and peripheral blood cells (4,5,23). Such findings suggested that the CD4 and CD8 T cells had been previously recruited in lymphoid tissues at time of active virus replication (24,25) and sequestered in an altered cytokine and chemokine milieu, as shown in animal models (26). The arrest of local virus production (27) in lymphoid tissues was indeed demonstrated and was proposed to allow the sequestered T cells to recirculate (28), thus increasing peripheral blood cell counts. Strong slopes of peripheral blood CD4 T cells of 1–5 CD4 cell/mm^3/day during the first 2 months (5) were observed concurrent with a rapid and major reduction in virus load of approximately 1 or 2 log of magnitude, contrasted in some cases with a modest virus reduction of less than 1 log (29,30). Since peripheral blood lymphocytes represent only 2% of the total lymphocyte compartment, a minimal virus reduction mobilizes enough CD4 cells from tissues to allow substantial increases in peripheral blood cell numbers at time of severe CD4 cell depletion.

According to cohort studies the kinetics of CD4 cell expansion is usually reduced after the second or third month of treatment and follows a slope of 10–15% each. A second phase of immune reconstitution appears to be correlated to the magnitude of the plasma viral load reduction and to its stability over time (31). In other words, a 4 log reduction in the plasma viral load can be associated with a 40% increment slope during the 2 years following HAART initiation, while a 1 log viral load reduction is usually associated with a 5% slope only. In contrast, the intensity of CD4 cell depletion at baseline plays only a minor role in such long term kinetics of CD4 cell recovery (31), suggesting that the immune system is repopulated at the same pace whatever the severity of the immune alterations that had taken place before introduction of HAART.

What are the mechanisms of such CD4 T-cell reconstitution? A biphasic process is usually observed. The first rapid wave of CD4 T cells is mostly composed of memory CD4 T cells bearing the CD45RO isoform. When treatment is initiated at early stages of the disease before the occurrence of a severe CD4 cell depletion, however, naive CD4 T cells, which do not display the CD45RO but the CD45RA isoform and the CD62L-selectin, are also present in this first step (32). These rapid changes are supposed to reflect redistribution of preexisting residual CD4 T cells from the tissues in which they were sequestered (1,5) rather than proliferation. Indeed, no (1) or a significant decrease in cell cycle markers can be observed in those cells (33,34), thus contrasting with the significant increases of CD4 T cells displaying the Ki67 cell cycle marker in peripheral blood and in tissues reported prior to administration of antiretroviral drugs (33,34). Therefore, the slight increase in CD4 cell production that was induced in vivo to compensate the losses in mature CD4 T cells at time of active virus production suddenly stops with efficient virus control. Such a phenomenon might not represent a net gain in total CD4 cell numbers during this first phase of immune reconstitution. The second step observed after 2 or 3 months of virus control is characterized by a slower rate of memory CD4 T-cell apparent peripheral expansion usually falling down slopes of approximately 10% (1,5). Despite its slower rate, this second phase of immune reconstitution is a true phase of long-term T-cell production. Indeed, in vivo evaluations of T-cell proliferation using either deuterated glucose incorporation (35) or Ki67 intracellular expression (36) are concordant and suggest a two- to threefold increase in the numbers of proliferating CD4 T cells after 6 months of treatment.

Regeneration of naive T-cell is now known to play the major role in the late reconstitution of the whole CD4 subset. Indeed, naive CD4 T cells increase significantly in both proportion and absolute numbers after the third month of treatment when introduced at late stages of CD4 cell depletion (1). These findings were confirmed by all subsequent studies (4,5). When treatment is introduced at earlier stages of the disease, or even at primary infection (32), slopes of naive CD4 cell recovery are indistinguishable from the memory CD4 T-cell ones, with a rapid and early increase indicating that naive CD4 T cells can be submitted, as memory T cells, to some sequestration/desequestration phenomenon. Such an increase in naive T cells, whatever its kinetics, was the most surprising observation in immune reconstitution in HIV-infected adults. Indeed, it contrasted with the very slow and weak regeneration in naive T cells observed in adults after chemotherapy or bone marrow transplantation (37) and suggested that HIV infection had not definitively impaired in adults the capacities of thymic production.

Considering the dogma of a thymic involution in adults that derived from postchemotherapy observations (37) and should be even more severe with HIV infection (15) together with the poor definition of naive T cells, the origin of such cells raised numerous questions. Was it assessing true regeneration of a thymic function? If yes, this finding would call into question the above-mentioned dogma of thymic involution or alternatively suggest that thymic alterations induced by HIV would be less definitive than the chemotherapy effects on the thymus. A negative answer would mean that regeneration was fake and only preexisting T cells that had escaped the HIV-induced destruction were capable of reappearing in a treated HIV-infected adult system.

Indeed, some memory T cells can revert their CD45 isoform from RO to RA (38), although such a phenomenon occurs mostly in the CD8 compartment. To overcome such difficulty, we assessed the naive cell status on the co-expression of the CD45RA and CD62L-selectin (1), the latter allowing naive cell penetration in lymph nodes (39), and further checked that the CD45RA+62L+CD4+ cells had functional characteristics of naive T cells that had not encountered antigens. Our results were confirmed by various studies (4,5) and strengthened the hypothesis of a preserved capacity to regenerate time naive cells in these settings that might differ from the massive thymic alterations induced by chemotherapy and irradiation in haematological malignancies (37).

Indeed, computed tomography showed the preservation of a thymic tissue in HIV-infected adults and its progressive increase in parallel to naive CD4 T-cell amplification during treatment (40). Direct evidence for a thymic participation and T-cell regeneration during antiretroviral therapy came only at the end of 1998 with the detection of markers of thymic origin in the increasing subset of naive T cells (41). Indeed, the DNA episomal circles produced within the thymus during rearrangements of the T-cell receptor (TCR) segments (38) do not replicate with the cell genome. Their detection in naive CD4 T cells indicate that those cells have not undergone multiple cycles of proliferation since leaving the thymus: populations of cells containing high proportions of these TCR rearrangement excision circles (TRECs) are called recent thymic emigrants (RTEs). However, the peripheral homeostasis of naive T cells is still poorly understood. Once a naive cell emigrates from the thymus it recirculates constantly in the periphery until it encounters a specific antigen, activates, proliferates, and converts into a memory T-cell. Intervals between two cell cycles in a naive cell might reach 10 years: thus, naive T cells that have not proliferated for 8–10 years still contain their TREC copies and are defined as "RTE"! Although inappropriately defined as a marker of "recent" thymic production, TREC proportions provide a good estimate of peripheral T-cell turnover. Their relative proportions within the CD4 cell subsets fit with the phenotypic definition of naive and memory T cells. TREC proportions also decline with age and HIV infection (41). These defects are corrected under potent antiretroviral therapy, resulting in a rapid and sustained increase in TREC proportions in the majority of patients, i.e., in comparison to the naive T-cell subset increases. Other studies confirmed the ability of the thymus at replenish the immune repertoire of the CD4 T cells (42,43).

These findings indicate a contribution of the thymus in the reconstitution of normal CD4 cell numbers and homeostasis, thus ensuring restoration of a naive T-cell repertoire diversity. However, thymic regeneration alone might not be responsible for this reconstitution. The decrease in abnormal T-cell activation and consumption of memory T cells might also reduce the consumption of the naive cell compartment and help restore it in the context of a functional thymus. Nevertheless, these overall studies have introduced unique insight into immunology dogmas and a new era in the investigation of thymus function.

RECONSTITUTION OF THE T-CELL REPERTOIRE: THE CONTROVERSIES

An enormous diversity of T-cell clones, approximately 10^{13}–10^{15}, is produced during intra-thymic maturation by the diversity of recombination in the gene fragments encoding for T-cell receptor (TCR), to antigen each TCR providing the specificity for a given antigen. Each antigen transforms the corresponding naive T cells into specific memory T cells, which proliferate. The TCR diversity is maximal in naive T cells of thymic origin and is reduced in the memory cell compartment, which represents an antigen-driven selection from the naive cell compartment. The overall diversity of the T-cell repertoire decreases with age and chronic exposure to antigens. Such a process is accelerated during HIV infection, particularly in the CD8 subset, but also in the CD4 subset during of AIDS when residual immune defenses against opportunistic pathogens need to be mobilized. CTL clones are permanently activated to limit virus dissemination (2,44) while the thymus input decreases with disease progression (41). A first study of the T-cell repertoire was conducted 3–6 months following antiretroviral therapy failed to demonstrate corrections of TCR repertoire abnormalities (42). On the contrary, the perturbed CD4 T-cell repertoire was shown by Gorochov et al. To slowly rediversify after the sixth month of highly active antiretroviral treatment (2). This process occurred once the activation status of memory CD4 cells had been normalized and after the increase in naive T cells numbers took place. The same phenomenon occurred in the CD8 compartment, though more slowly (2).

Thus, the diversity of the T-cell clone repertoire is restored during HAART. Regeneration of naive T cells certainly plays a major role in this process, but as discussed above for the TREC numbers, interpretation calls for caution. The rapid decrease in the number of T cells bearing markers of cell cycle described above together with the decreased levels of abnormal T-cell activation described below should also help prevent expansions of particular T-cell clones and biases in T-cell diversity. Therefore, normalization of T-cell repertoires reflects both increased production of a naive diverse T-cell repertoire and decreased turnover of T-cell clones that were previously mobilized against various pathogens once the virus is controlled. The enormous plasticity of the central and peripheral immune system prevents constitution of definitive holes in host defenses and allows restoration of a durable reservoir of T-cell clones capable of reacting against the wide spectrum of antigens an individual might encounter throughout his life.

REDUCTION OF IMMUNE ACTIVATION

Chronic immune activation is a hallmark of immune alterations observed during the natural course of HIV infection. One of our first observations of immune reconstitution was a rapid and remarkable reduction in the cell surface expression of various T-cell activation markers, such as HLA-DR, CD38 or CD25, the IL-2 receptor, both on CD4 and on CD8 T cells (1). The proportions of activated T cells significantly decreased in parallel to the reduction of the plasma virus load. The strong correlation coefficient ($r = 0.8$) observed between both phenomena indicate the responsibility of the virus itself for such abnormal activation (1). Other groups reported a similar decrease in soluble markers of immune activation, such as the inflammatory cytokines TNF-α and IL-6 (4,47). In addition, a reduction in the Fas-Fas-ligand cell surface expression was also observed resulting in a decreased T-cell sensitivity to apoptosis (46). Both phenomena, reduced Fas expression and TNF-α levels, certainly help to limit the abnormal rate of cell death observed in HIV infection and to restore normal numbers in the T-cell compartments. They also have an important impact on other immune cells, such as B cells or polymorphonuclear cells.

These changes occur very early after virus begins to be controlled, in both the peripheral blood and the lymphoid tissues (23,27,47,48). Reduced immune activation is also associated with decreased cell surface expression of adhesion molecules (47), which certainly contributes to cell recirculation.

Altogether, reduction in the various expressions of abnormal immune activation might be one of the key phenomena that allow, or at least contribute to, immune reconstitution. Indeed, as discussed above, reduced activation, losses, and turnover in the memory T-cell compartment reduce the consumption of naive T cells and help restore their numbers, reducing biases in T-cell repertoires. Thus, antiretroviral drugs, by blocking virus production, reduce virus-driven immune activation and play a potent anti-inflammatory role in the peripheral immune system. Overall, such anti-inflammatory effects might be as important as de novo thymic production for immune recovery.

RECONSTITUTION OF HOST DEFENSES DURING HAART: SUCCESSES

One of the major questions raised by physicians and patients was whether restoring CD4 cell numbers would mean restoration of the host defenses that had been lost with AIDS. These defects in host defenses were mediated by depletion in naive T cells, and anergy of memory T cells reflecting Th1 defects and abnormal activation. The phenotypic improvements reported above strongly suggested that the functional defects in the residual memory T cells would be corrected.

Indeed, such a restoration of CD4 T-cell function was observed after 3 months of HAART in AIDS patients who had previously lost their defenses against cytomegalovirus (CMV) and *Mycobacterium tuberculosis* the memory CD4 cell reactivities against these two opportunistic pathogens were restored and persisted over time when HAART was successful at controlling the virus load and at increasing CD4 memory cells (1,3). The regeneration of new naive T cells was not required in such a process, suggesting that the memory defenses against those pathogens had not been completely lost prior to treatment. Whether such a functional reconstitution was protective was rapidly called into question by some recurrence of CMV retinitis in the 3 months following introduction of HAART in AIDS patients (49,50). In fact, recurrence of CMV retinitis occurred during the first 3 months that followed introduction of HAART, i.e., once the memory CD4 T cells had been ''authorized'' to recirculate but before their over-activation had been reduced and their functionality had been restored. After this 3-month period, a solid protection was conferred against opportunistic pathogens as shown by the subsequent reduction in CMV viremia and CMV retinitis (51).

The clinical benefits of this restoration of immune defenses against opportunistic pathogens was rapidly confirmed by epidemiological surveys. Indeed, the incidence of opportunistic infections in treated patients recovering CD4 cell numbers $>200/mm^3$ was similar to the incidence observed $<200/mm^3$ in untreated patients (52). However, initiating treatment at very low CD4 counts leaves patients with a prolonged exposure to the risk of opportunistic infections in the lag time before they reach sufficient immune reconstitution. Finally, such expectation of immune reconstitution encouraged clinicians to discontinue secondary or even primary prophylactic treatments for opportunistic infections such as CMV (53,54) or *Pneumocystis carinii* (55–57). The lack of recurrence or onset of opportunistic infections in such recovering immune systems is currently some of the strongest evidence demonstrating that reconstituting CD4 cell numbers with antiretroviral therapies did indeed restore a protective immunity against pathogens.

Such restoration of immune competence requires a solid and durable control of HIV. Blocking HIV replication for only 3–6 months was not enough to restore a CMV- or a tuberculin-specific immunity (3). Memory T-cell responses were restored, however, against opportunistic pathogens that are highly prevalent in HIV-infected and AIDS patients but not against rare or vaccinal antigens (4). Artificial reexposure to these antigens during vaccination programs allows restoration of a vaccinal immunity (58), demonstrating once again that no gap had been introduced in immune repertoires and functions. Such findings also demonstrate the importance of antigen stimulation in the immune reconstitution processes and in T-cell homeostasis. Therefore, restoration of protective memory responses against pathogens appears to be antigen-driven. The slight increase in T-cell proliferation observed in vivo in the long term might represent such peripheral process of memory T-cell expansion, which is usually considered the main mechanism of T-cell homeostasis in adults.

LACK OF RESTORATION OF ANTI-HIV IMMUNITY: THE CURRENT LIMITATION OF IMMUNE RECONSTITUTION

No restoration of a CD4 cell reactivity against HIV itself was observed in parallel to the immune reconstitution described above (1,8,59,60). The CD4 helper cells specific for HIV were restored only when HAART was initiated at the time of primary infection (10) and appear to be deleted in chronic disease. A widely accepted hypothesis for such a lack of restoration is the lack of in vivo restimulation in the absence of antigen stimulation due to efficient virus control with treatment. We checked that those cells were not even sequestered in the tissues (T. S. Li, unpublished). The regeneration of new naive CD4 cells did not help at restoring such activity even after 2 or 3 years of fully suppressive treatments (9). However, the HIV-specific T-helper cells were not definitively deleted during chronic infection and persisted at very low frequencies (61). This question of T-helper cell activity against HIV appears of utmost importance considering the central role played by those cells in the generation and maintenance of the effector immune defenses mediated by cytotoxic T lymphocytes (CTLs) and antibodies (62,63). One of the best hallmarks of this unrestored immunity against HIV is the rebound of virus replication observed when HAART is stopped (64,65).

The effector arm of antiviral immunity, the HIV-specific CD8 cells, was known to persist at late stages of the disease, although it was progressively exhausted (66,67). The therapeutic control of HIV production not only does not restore strong numbers of HIV-specific CD8 T cells, it actually diminishes them (69–76). Indeed, frequencies of HIV tetramer-binding CD8 T cells (69,70,72,73), of CTLp (72,74), or of IFN-(producing CD8 cells as measured by ELISPOT (71,76) or flow cytometry (73) are concordant and show an exponential decay in the intensity of the HIV-specific CD8 T cells.

The dissociation between a strong and protective immunity rapidly restored against opportunistic pathogens and a waning immunity against HIV might be explained by the differences in the exposure to appropriate antigenic stimuli. Once the HIV antigens are withdrawn, even artificially with drugs, the immune system responds with a physiological elimination of dangerous effector killer cells. This phenomenon is responsible for the exponential decay in titers of virus-specific CD8 T cells that parallels plasma virus titers. Similarly high virus titers might be required to allow appropriate stimulation, proliferation, and reexpansion of HIV-specific CD4 T cells. The same phenomenon is reported for HIV-specific antibody titers which leads to lack of or a delayed seroconversion if treatment is introduced before seroconversion takes place (77).

The treated patients are thus left with a strong and protective immunity against any pathogen except HIV itself . Memory against HIV persists, however, even at very low levels, and is re-inducible (78).

Indeed, peaks of HIV-specific CD8 cell numbers have been registered during blips of virus replication when treatment fails or is interrupted (73,75,79). These observations led to the concept of structured therapeutic interruptions (STIs) which might reincrease HIV-specific immunity by transiently but recurrently re-exposing against virus particles during treatment windows. We reported that such reexpansions were usually transient and involved only the preexisting dominant HIV-specific CD8 cell clones in chronically infected patients (73). The situation might differ in patients treated at the time of primary infection where the peaks of HIV-specific CD8 T cells might be sustained over time and involve a broader spectrum of epitopes recognized than at treatment initiation (74,75). These latter observations are in line with the preservation of a T helper-1 cell response in primary infection that should help at enlarging the HIV-specific immune repertoire during successive reexposures to virus replication.

While STIs are currently being evaluated as a strategy to restore HIV-specific immunity in treated patients and to limit drug toxicity, another safer strategy proposed is to reimmunize treated patients against HIV with candidate vaccines. Inactivated virus particles have already been proven to be able to restore a CD4 T-cell response to HIV core proteins in treated patients (80), and recombinant viral vectors are currently being tested, such as canarypox (81). Whether the antigen doses and the immunogenicity of these compounds will be enough to restimulate a strong and protective anti-HIV immunity remains to be determined. One can indeed raise the argument that some HIV replication persists during the most suppressive antiviral regimens that should provide an antigenic exposure already above the level authorized by our most potent current vaccines. In addition, the ability of the antigen-presenting cell network to efficiently prime new naive CD4 and CD8 T cells during these reimmunization strategies might even be questioned. Indeed we could demonstrate that a defect in the frequencies of dendritic cells expressing the CD11c molecule, the ones supposed to produce IL-12, was not restored during treatment (82). Preliminary encouraging results suggest that cytokine such as IL-2 might help enhance the residual virus-specific immunity (83,84). Immune-based strategies aiming at restoring immunity against HIV might thus incorporate adjuvants enhancing the antigen-presenting cell functions and their capacity to generate protective Th1 and CD8 cell responses against HIV.

CONCLUSION

At whatever stage of the disease it is initiated, HAART allows immune restoration and protection against opportunistic pathogens. The single condition required for immune reconstitution is an efficient and durable inhibition of virus replication. These positive effects can be obtained at late stages of the disease even when patients have been heavily pretreated. These successes demonstrate that HIV does not definitively alter the lymphoid tissues or the immune defenses, even after years of infection and severe immune suppression. Initiating HAART in late versus in early disease might differ by 1) the time required to reach normalized immune functions and cell counts and 2) the lack of amplification of HIV-specific T cells in late disease. The delay to recovery or the lack of reconstitution of a solid immunity against HIV itself is currently raising the need for additive therapeutic strategies based upon immune interventions. Several immune therapies are currently being evaluated, such as periodic IL-2 infusions in order to accelerate and amplify immune reconstitution or therapeutic vaccinations to resuscitate immune responses to HIV. At a time when virus eradication does not appear plausible with the current drug regimens, the ultimate goal of HAART might be to help transform treated patients into long-term nonprogressors.

ACKNOWLEDGMENTS

The studies reported in this review could not have been performed without the valuable collaboration of Roland Tubiana, Hocine, and Pr. Christine Katlama in the Service des Maladies Infectieuses, at Hôpital Pitié-Salpétrière; with Dominique Mathez and Jacques Leibowitch, Laboratoire d'Immuno-virologie, Hôpital Raymond Poincaré, Garches; and with Guy Gorochov, Catherine Blanc, Marc Renaud, Fernanda Grassi, and Isabelle Porcher in the Laboratoire d'Immunologie Cellulaire, CNRS UMR 7627, directed by Pr. Patrice Debré at Hôpital Pitié-Salpétrière.

REFERENCES

1. Autran, B., G. Carcelain, T.S. Li, C. Blanc, D. Mathez, R. Tubiana, C. Katlama, P. Debre, J. Leibowitch. Positive effects of combined anti-retroviral therapy on CD4+ T-cell homeostasis and function in advanced HIV disease. Science 1997; 277:112–116.
2. Gorochov, G., A.U. Neumann, A. Kereveur, C. Parizot, T.S. Li, C. Katlama, M. Karmochkine, G. Raguin, B. Autran, P. Debre. Perturbation of CD4 and CD8 T-cell repertoires during progression to AIDS and influence of antiviral therapy. Nat Med 1998; 4(2):215–221.
3. Li, T.S., R. Tubiana, C. Katlama, V. Calvez, H.A. Mohand, B. Autran. Long lasting recovery in CD4+ T-cell function mirrors viral load reduction after highly active anti-retroviral therapy in patients with advanced HIV disease. Lancet 1998; 351:1682–1686.
4. Lederman, M.M., E. Connick, A. Landay, D.R. Kuritzkes, J. Spritzler, M. St Clair, B.L. Kotzin, L. Fox, M.H. Chiozzi, J.M. Leonard, F. Rousseau, M. Wade, J.D. Roe, A. Martinez, H. Kessler. Immunologic responses associated with 12 weeks of combination antiretroviral therapy consisting of Zidovudine, Lamivudine and Ritonavir: results of AIDS clinical trials group protocol 315. J Infect Dis 1998; 178:70–79.

5. Pakker, N.G., D.W. Notermans, R.J. De Boer, M.T.L. Roos, F. De Wolf, A. Hill, J.M. Leonard, S.A. Danner, F. Miedema, P.T.A. Schellekens. Biphasic kinetics of peripheral blood T cells after triple combination therapy in HIV-1 infection: a composite of redistribution and proliferation. Nat Med 1998; (4)2:208–214.
6. Hogg, R.S., M.W. O'Shaughnessy, N. Gataric, B. Yip, K. Craib, M.T. Schechter, J.S. Montaner. Decline in deaths from AIDS due to new antiretrovirals. Lancet 1997; 349:1294.
7. Palella, F.J., K.M. Delaney, A.C. Moorman, M.O. Loveless, J. Fuhrer, G.A. Satten, D.J. Aschman, S.D. Holmberg, and the HIV outpatient study investigators. Declining morbidity and mortality among patients with advanced human immunodeficiency virus infection. N Engl J Med 1998; 338(13): 853–860.
8. Plana, M., F. Garcia, T. Gallart, J.M. Miro, J.M. Gatell. Lack of T-cell proliferative response to HIV-1 antigens after 1 year of highly active antiretroviral treatment in early HIV-1 disease. Lancet 1998; 352:1194–1195.
9. Carcelain, G., R. Tubiana, T.S. Li, V. Calvez, N. Jouy, M. Jouan, M.A. Valantin, C. Olivier, P.M. Girard, P. Debré, C. Katlama, B. Autran. Long-term recovery in CD4+ T-cell function with highly efficient antiretroviral therapy. 6th Conference on Retrovirus and Oppotunistic Infections, Chicago, 1999.
10. Rosenberg, E.S, J.M. Billingsley, A.M. Caliendo, S.L. Boswell, P.E. Sax, S.A. Kalams, B.D. Walker. Vigorous HIV-1 specific CD4+ T-cell responses associated with control of viremie. Science 1997; 278:1447.
11. Ho, D., A.V. Neumann, A.S. Perelson, W. Chen, J.M. Leonard, M. Markowitz. Rapid turnover of plasma virions and CD4 lymphocytes in HIV-1 infection. Nature 1995; 373:123–126.
12. Wolthers, K.C, G. Bea, A. Wisman, S.A, Otto, A.M. de Roda Husman, N. Scaft N, F. de Wolf, J. Goudsmit, R.A. Counho, A.G. van der Zee, L. Meyaard, F. Miedema. T-cell telomere length in HIV-1 infection: no evidence for increased CD4+ T cell turnover. Science 1996; 274:1543–1547.
13. Tissot, O., J.P. Viard, C. Rabian, N. Ngo, M. Burgard, C. Rouzioux, C. Penit. No evidence for proliferation in the blood CD4+ T-cell pool during HIV-1 infection and triple combination therapy. AIDS 1998; 12:879–884.
14. Clerici, M., N.I. Stocks, R.A. Zajac, R.N. Boswell, D.R. Lucey, C.S. Via, G.M. Shearer. Detection of three distinct patterns of T helper cell dysfunction in asymptomatic, HIV-seropositive patients: Independence of CD4+ cell numbers and clinical staging. J Clin Invest 1989; 84:1892–1899.
15. Hellerstein, M.K., J.M. McCune. T-cell turnover in HIV-1 disease. Immunity 1997; 7:583–589.
16. Giorgi, J.V, J.L. Fahey, D.C. Smith, L.E. Hultin, H.L. Cheng, R.T. Mitsuy-

asu, R. Detels. Early effects of HIV on CD4 lymphocytes in vivo. J Immunol 1987; 138:3725–3730.

17. Autran, B., E. Legac, C. Blanc, P. Debré. THO/TH2 function of CD4+CD7− T lymphocyte subset in normal and HIV-seropositive individuals. J Immunol 1995; 154. 3:1408–1417.
18. Borthwick, N.J, M. Bofill, W.M. Gombert, A.N. Akbar, E. Medina, K. Sagawa, M.C. Lipman, M.A. Johnson, G. Janossy. Lymphocyte activation in HIV-1 infection II. Functional defects of CD28 T cells. AIDS 1994; 8:431–441.
19. Lane, H.C., H. Masur, E.P. Gelmann, D.L. Longo, R.G. Steis, T. Chused, G. Whalen, L.C. Edgar, A.S. Fauci. Correlation between immunologic function and clinical subpopulations of patients with the acquired immune deficiency syndrome. Am J Med 1985; 78:417–422.
20. Collier, A.C., R.W. Coombs, D.A. Schoenfeld, R.L. Bassett, J. Timpone, A. Baruch, J.M. Facey, C. Whitacre, V.J. McAuliffe, H.M. Friedman, T.C. Merigan, R.C. Reichman, C. Hooper, L. Corey. Treatment of human immunodeficiency virus infection with saquinavir zidovudine and zalcitabine. N Engl J Med 1996; 334:1011–1017.
21. Katzenstein, D.A., S.M. Hammer, M.D. Hugues, et al. The relation of virologic and immunologic markers to clinical outcomes after nucleoside therapy in HIV-infected adults with 200 to 500 CD4 cells per cubic millimeter. N Engl J Med 1996; 335:1091–1098.
22. Hammer, S.M., K.E. Squires, M.D. Hughes, J.M. Grimes, L.M. Demeter, J.S. Currier, J.J. Eron, J.E. Feinberg, H.H. Balfour, L.R. Deyton, J.A. Chodakewitz, M.A. Fischl, and the ACTG 320 study team. A controlled trial of two nucleoside analogues plus indinavir in persons with human immunodeficiency virus infection and CD4 cell counts of 200 per cubic millimeter or less. N Engl J Med 1997; 337(11):725–739.
23. Tenner-Racz, K., H.J. Stellbrink, J. van Lunzen, C. Schneider, J.P. Jacobs, B. Raschdorff G. Grosschupff, R.M. Steinman, P. Racz. The unenlarged lymph nodes of HIV-1-infected, asymptomatic patients with high CD4 T-cell counts are sites for virus replication and CD4 T-cell proliferation. The impact of highly active antiretroviral therapy. J Exp Med 1998; 187: 949–959.
24. Rosok, B.I., L. Bostad, P. Voltersvik, J. Olofsson, B. Asjö. Reduced CD4 cell counts in blood do not reflect CD4 cell depletion in tonsillar tissue in asymptomatic HIV-1 infection. AIDS 1996; 10:35–38.
25. Cheynier, R., S. Henrichwark, F. Hadida, E. Pelletier, E. Oksenhendler, B. Autran, S. Wain-Hobson. HIV and T-cell expansion in splenic white pulps is accompanied by infiltration of HIV-specific cytotoxic T lymphocytes. Cell 1994; 78:373–387.

26. Sprent, J., D.F. Tough. Lymphocyte life-span and memory. Science 1994; 265:1395–1400.
27. Cavert, W., D.W. Notermans, K. Staskus, S.W. Wietgrefe, M. Zupancic, K. Gebhard, K. Henry, Z.Q. Zhang, R. Mills, H. McDade, C.M. Schuwirth, J. Goudsmit, S.A. Danner, A.T. Haase. Kinetics of response in lymphoid tissues to antiretroviral therapy of HIV-1 infection. Science 1997; 176:960–964.
28. Wong, J.K., H.F. Gunthard, D.V. Havler, Z.Q. Zhang, A.T. Haase, C.C. Ignacio, S. Kwok, E. Emini, D.D. Richman. Reduction in HIV-1 in blood and lymph nodes following potent antiviral therapy and the virologic correlates of treatment failure. Proc Natl Acad Sci USA 1997; 94:12574–12579.
29. Kaufmann, D.D., G. Pantaleo, P. Sudre, A. Telenti. CD4-cell count in HIV-1-infected individuals remaining viraemic with highly active antiretroviral therapy (HAART). Lancet 1998; 333:723.
30. Piketty, C., P. Castiel, L. Belec, D. Batisse, A.S. Mohamed, J. Gilquin, G. Gonzales-Canali, M. Karmochkine, L. Weiss, J.P. Aboulker, M.D. Kazatchkine. Discrepant responses to triple combination antiretroviral therapy in advanced HIV disease. AIDS 1998; 12:745–750.
31. Renaud, M., C. Katlama, A. Mallet, V. Calvez, G. Carcelain, R. Tubiana, M. Jouan, E. Caumes, H. Agut, F. Bricaire, P. Debre, B. Autran. Determinants of paradoxical CD4 cell reconstitution after protease inhibitor containing antiretroviral regiment. AIDS 1999; 13:669–676.
32. Carcelain, G., C. Blanc , J. Leibowitch, P. Mariot, D. Mathez, V. Schneider, A.G. Saimot, F. Damont, F. Simon, P. Debre, B. Autran, P.M. Girard. T-cell changes after combined nucleoside analogue therapy in HIV primary infection. AIDS 1999; 13:1077–1081.
33. Sachsenberg, N., A.S. Perelson, S. Yerly, G.A. Schockmel, D. Leduc, B. Hirschel, L. Perrin. Turnover of CD4+ and CD8+ T lymphocytes in HIV-1 infection as measured by Ki-67 antigen. J Exp Med 1998; 187(8):1295–1303.
34. Fleury, S., R.B. de Boer, G.P. Rizzardi, K.C. Wolthers, S.A. Otto, C.C. Welbon, C. Grasiozi, C. Knabenhans, H. Soudeyns, P.A. Bart, S. Gallant, J.M. Corpataux, M. Gillet, P. Meylan, P. Schnyder, J.Y. Meuwly, W. Spreen, M. Glauser, F. Miedema, G. Pantaleo. Limited CD4+ T-cell renewal in early HIV-1 infection: effect of highly active antiretroviral therapy. Nat Med 1998; 4:794–801.
35. Hellerstein, M., M.B. Hanley, D. Cesar, S. Siler, C. Papageorgopoulos, E. Wieder, D. Schmidt, R. Hoh, R. Neese, D. Macallan, S. Deeks, J.M. McCune. Directly measured kinetics of circulating T lymphocytes in normal and HIV-1 infected humans. Nat Med 1999; 5:83–89.
36. Fleury, S., G.P. Rizzardi, A. Chapuis, G. Tambussi, C. Knabenhans, E. Simeoni, J. Meuwly, J. Corpataux, A. Lazzarin, F. Miedema, G. Pantaleo.

Long-term kinetics of T cell production in HIV-infected subjects treated with highly active antiretroviral therapy. Proc Natl Acad Sci USA 2000; 97:5393–5398.

37. Mackall, C.L., L. Granger, M.A. Sheard, R. Cepeda, R.E. Gress. T-cell regeneration after bone marrow transplantation: differential CD45 isoform expression on thymic-derived versus thymic-independent progeny. Blood 1993; 82:2585–2894.
38. Bell, E.S., S.M. Sparshott. Interconversion of CD45R of CD4 T cells in vivo. Nature 1990; 348:163–166.
39. Picker, L.J., J.R. Treer, D.B. Ferguson, P.A. Collins, D. Buck, L.W. Terstappen. Control of lymphocyte recirculation in man. I. Differential regulation of the peripheral lymph node homing receptor L-selection on T cells during the virgin to memory cell transition. J Immunol 1993; 150:1105–1121.
40. McCune, J.M., R. Loftus, D.K. Schmidt, P. Carrell, D. Webster, L.B. Swor-Yim, I.R. Francis, B.H. Gross, R.M. Grant. High prevalence of thymic tissue in adults with human immunodeficiency virus-1 infection. J Clin Invest 1998; 101:2301–2308.
41. Douek, D.C., R.D. McFarlard, P.H. Keiser, E.A. Gage, J.M. Massey, B.F. Haynes, M.A. Polis, A.T. Haase, M.B. Feinberg, J.L. Sullivan, B.D. Jamieson, J.A. Zack, L.J. Picker, R.A. Koup. Changes in thymic function with age and during the treatment of HIV infection. Nature 1998; 396:690–695.
42. Poulin, J.F., M.N. Viswanathan, J.M. Harris, K.V. Komanduri, E. Wieder, N. Ringuette, M. Jenkins, J.M. Mc Cune, R.P. Sekaly. Directe evidence for thymic function in adult humans. J Exp Med 1999; 190:479–486.
43. Zhang, L., S.R. Lewin, M. Markowitz, H.H. Lin, E. Skulsky, R. Karanicolas, Y. He, X. Jin, S. Tuttleton, M. Vesanen, H. Spiegel, R. Kost, J. van Lunzen, H.J. Stellbrink, S. Wolinsky, W. Borkowsky, P. Palumbo, L.G. Kostrikis, D.D. Ho. Measuring recent thymic emigrants in blood of normal and HIV-1-infected individuals before and after effective therapy. J Exp Med 1999; 190:725–732.
44. Pantaléo, G., J.F. Demarest, H. Soudeyns, C. Grasiozi, F. Denis, J.W. Adelsberger, P. Borrow, M.S. Saag, G.M. Shaw, R.P. Sekaly. Major expansion of CD8+ T cells with a predominant V(usage during the primary immune response to HIV. Nature 1994; 370:463–467.
45. Connors, M., J.A. Kovacs, S. Krevat, J.C. Gea-Banacloche, M.C. Sneller, M. Flanigan, J.A. Metcalf, R.E. Walker, J. Falloon, M. Baseler, R. Stevens, R.E. Feuerstein, H. Masur, H.C. Lane. HIV infection induces changes in CD4+ T-cell phenotype and depletion within the CD4+ T-cell repertoire that are not immediately restored by antiviral or immune based therapies. Nat Med 1997; 3:533–540.

46. Badley, A.D., D.H. Dockrell, A. Algeciras, S. Ziesmer, A. Landay, M.M. Lederman, E. Connick, D. Kuritzkes, D.H. Lynch, P. Roche, H. Yagita, C.V. Paya. In vivo analysis of Fas/Fas-L interactions in HIV-infected patients. J Clin Invest 1998; 102:79–87.
47. Bucy, R.P., R.D. Hockett, C.A. Derdeyn, M.S. Saag, K. Squires, M. Sillers, R.T. Mitsuyasu, J.M. Kilby. Initial increase in blood CD4(+) lymphocytes after HIV retroviral therapy reflects redistribution from lymphoid tissues. J Clin Invest 1999; 103:1391–1398.
48. Andersson, J., T.E. Fehniger, B.K. Patterson, et al. Early reduction of immune activation in lymphoid tissue following highly active HIV therapy. AIDS 1998; 12:F123–F129.
49. Miller, V., A. Mocroft, P. Reiss, C. Katlama, A.I. Papadopoulos, T. Katzenstein, J. van Lunzen, F. Antunes, A.N. Phillips, J.D. Lundgren, and the EuroSIDA group. Relations among CD4 lymphocyte count Nadir, antiretroviral therapy, and HIV-1 disease progression: results from the EuroSIDA study. Ann Intern Med 1999; 130:570–577.
50. Jacobson, M.A., M. Zegans, P.R. Pavan, et al. Cytomegalovirus retinitis after initiation of highly active antiretroviral therapy. Lancet 1997; 349: 1443–1445.
51. Gilquin, J., C. Piketty, U. Thomas, et al. Acute cytomegalovirus infection in AIDS patients with CD4 counts above $100x10^6$ cells/l following combination anti-retroviral therapy including protease inhibitors. AIDS 1997; 11: 1659–1660.
52. Li, T.S., R. Tubiana, A.M. Fillet, B. Autran, C. Katlama. Negativation of cytomegalovirus blood culture with restoration of CD4+ T-cell reactivity to CMV after HAART in an HIV-1 infected patient. J AIDS Hum Retrovirol 1999; 20:514–515.
53. Tural, C., J. Romeu, G. Sirera, D. Andreu, M. Conejero, S. Ruiz, A. Jou, A. Bonjoch, L. Ruiz, A. Arno, B. Clotet. Long-lasting remission of cytomegalovirus retinitis without maintenance therapy in humanimmunodeficiency virus-infected patients. J Infect Dis 1998; 177:1080–1083.
54. Jouan, M., M. Saves, R. Tubiana, G. Carcelain, C. Olivier, B. Autran, RESTIMOP (ANRS 078). A multicenter prospective study to evaluate the discontinuation of maintenance therapy for CMV retinitis in HIV-patients receiving HAART. Abstract 456. 6th Conference on Retrovirus and Oppotunistic Infections, Chicago, 1999.
55. Schneider, M.M., J.C. Borleffs, R.P. Stolk, C.A. Jaspers, A.I. Hoepelman. Discontinuation of prophylaxis for *Pneumocystis carinii* pneumonia in HIV-1-infected patients treated with highly active antiretroviral therapy. Lancet 1999; 353:201–203.
56. Weverling, G.J., A. Mocroft, B. Ledergerber, O. Kirk, J. Gonzales-Lahoz, A. d'Arminio Monforte, R. Proenca, A.N. Phillips, J.D. Lundgren, P. Reiss.

Discontinuation of *Pneumocystis carinii* pneumonia prophylaxis after start of highly active antiretroviral therapy in HIV-1 infection. EuroSIDA Study Group. Lancet 1999; 353:1293–1298.
57. Furrer, H., M. Egger, M. Opravil, E. Bernasconi, B. Hirschel, M. Battegay, A. Telenti, P.L. Vernazza, M. Rickenbach, M. Flepp, R. Malinverni. Discontinuation of primary prophylaxis against *Pneumocystis carinii* pneumonia in HIV-1-infected adults treated with combination antiretroviral therapy. Swiss HIV Cohort Study. N Engl J Med 1999; 340:1301–1306.
58. Valdez, H., K. Smith, M. Lederman, et al. Response to immunization with recall and neoantigens after 48 weeks of HAART [abstr]. 6th Conference on Retroviruses and Opportunistic Infections, Chicago, 1999.
59. Rinaldo, C.R., J.M. Liebman, X.L. Huang, Z. Fan, A.l. Shboul, D.K. McMahon D.K., et al. Prolonged suppression of human immunodeficiency virus type 1 (HIV-1) viremia in persons with advanced disease results in enhancement of CD4 T-cell reactivity to microbial antigens but not to HIV-1 antigens. J Infect Dis 1999; 179:329–336.
60. Pontselli, O., S. Kerkhof-Garde, D.W. Notermans, N.A. Foudraine, M.T. Roos, M.R. Klein et al. Functional T-cell reconstitution and human immunodeficiency virus-1-specific cell-mediated immunity during highly active antiretroviral therapy. J Infect Dis 1999; 180:76–86.
61. Pitcher, C.J., C. Quittner, D.M. Peterson, M. Connors, R.A. Koup, V.C. Maino, L.J. Picker. HIV-A-specific CD4+ T cells are detectable in most individuals with active HIV-1 infection, but decline with prolonged viral suppression. Nat Med 1999; 5:518–525.
62. Matloubian, M., R.J. Conception, R. Ahmed. CD4+ T cells are required to sustain CD8+ cytotoxic T-cell responses during chronic viral infection. J Virol 1994; 68:8056–8063.
63. Kalams S, Walker B. The critical need for CD4 help in maintaining effective cytotoxic T lymphocytes responses. J Exp Med 1998; 188:2199–2204.
64. De Jong MD, De Boeer RJ, De Wolf F. Overshoot of HIV-1 viraemia after early discontinuation of antiretroviral treatment. AIDS 1997; 11:F79-F84.
65. Neumann, A.U., R. Tubiana, V. Calvez, C. Robert, T.S. Li, H. Agut, B. Autran, C. Katlama and the Comet study group. HIV-1 rebound during interruption of HAART has no deleterious effect on reinitiated treatment. AIDS 1999; 13:677–683.
66. Hoffenbach A, L.-D. P., G. Dadaglio, E. Vilmer, F. Michel, C. Mayaud, B. Autran, F. Plata. Unusually high frequencies of HIV-specific cytotoxic T lymphocytes in humans. J Immunol 1998; 142:452–462.
67. Klein MR., C.A. Van Baalen, A.M. Holwerda, S.R. Kerkhof Garde, R.J. Bende, I.P. Keet, J.K. Eeftinck Schattenkerk, A.D. Osterhaus, H. Schuitemaker, F. Miedema. Kinetics of Gag-specific cytotoxic T lymphocyte responses during the clinical course of HIV-1 infection: a longitudinal analy-

sis of rapid progressors and long-term asymptomatics. J Exp Med 1995; 1365–1372.

68. Ogg, G.S., X. Jin, S. Bonhoeffer, P.R. Dunbar, M.A. Nowak, S. Monard, J.P. Segal, Y. Cao, S.I. Rowland-Jones, V. Cerundolo, A. Hurley, M. Markowitz, D.D. Ho, D.F. Nixon, A.J. McMichael. Quantitation of HIV-1-specific cytotoxic T lymphocytes and plasma load of viral RNA. Science 1998; 279:2103–2106.
69. Ogg, G.S., X. Jin, S. Bonhoeffer, P. Moss, M.A. Nowak, S. Monard, J.P. Segal, Y. Cao, S.l. Rowland-Jones, A. Hurley, M. Markowitz, D.D. Ho, A.J. McMichael, D.F. Nixon. Decay kinetics of human immunodeficiency virus-specific effector cytotoxic T lymphocytes after combination antiretroviral therapy. J Virol 1999; 73:797–800.
70. Dalod M, Harzic M, Pellegrin I, Dumon B, Hoen B, Sereni D, Deschemin JC, Levy P, Venet A, Gomard E. Evolution of cytotoxic T lymphocytes responses to HIV-1 in patients with symptomatic primary infection on antiretroviral triple therapy. J Infect Dis 1998; 178:61–69.
71. Gray CM, Lawrence J, Schapiro JM, Altman JD, Winters MA, Crompton M, Loi M, Kundu SK, Davis MM, Merigan TC. Frequency of class I HLA-restricted anti-HIV CD8+ T cells in individuals receiving highly active antiretroviral therapy (HAART). J Immunol 1999; 162:1780–1788.
72. Mollet, L., T.S. Li, A. Samri, C. Tournay, R. Tubiana, The Restim and Comet Study Groups, V. Calvez, P. Debre, C. Katlama, B. Autran. Dynamics of HIV-specific CD8+ T lymphocytes with changes in viral load. J Immunol. In press 2000.
73. Kalams, S.A., P.J. Goulder, A.K. Shea, N.G. Jones, A.K. Trocha, G.S. Ogg, B.D. Walker. 1999. Levels of human immunodeficiency virus type 1-specific cytotoxic T-lymphocyte effector and memory responses decline after suppression of viremia with highly active antiretroviral therapy. J Virol. 73:6721–6728.
74. Ortiz, G.M., D.F. Nixon, A. Trkola, J. Binley, X. Jin, S. Bonhoeffer, P.J. Kuebler, S.M. Donahoe, M.A. Demoitie, W.M. Kakimoto, T. Ketas, B. Clas, J.J. Heymann, L. Zhang, Y. Cao, A. Hurley, J.P. Moore, D.D. Ho, M. Markowitz. HIV-1-specific immune responses in subjects who temporarily contain virus replication after discontinuation of highly active antiretroviral therapy. J Clin Invest 1999; 104:R13–18.
75. Dalod, M., M. Dupuis, J.C. Deschemin, D. Sicard, D. Salmon, J.F. Delfraissy, A. Venet, M. Sinet, J.G. Guillet. Broad, intense anti-human immunodeficiency virus (HIV) ex vivo CD8(+) responses in HIV type 1-infected patients: comparison with anti-Epstein- Barr virus responses and changes during antiretroviral therapy. J Virol. 1999; 73:7108–16.
76. Morris, L., J.M. Binley, B.A. Clas, S. Bonhoeffer, T.P. Astill, R. Kost, A. Hurley, Y. Cao, M. Markowitz, D.D. Ho, J.P. Moore. HIV-1 antigen-

specific and -nonspecific B cell responses are sensitive to combination antiretroviral therapy. J Exp Med 1998; 188:233–245.

77. Gallimore, A., A. Glithero, A. Godkin, A.C. Tissot, A. Pluckthun, T. Elliott, H. Hengartner, R. Zinkernagel. Induction and exhaustion of lymphocytic choriomeningitis virus-specific cytotoxic T lymphocytes visualized using soluble tetrameric major histocompatibility complex class I-peptide complexes. J Exp Med 1998; 187:1383–1393.
78. Lisziewicz J, Rosenberg E, Lieberman J, Jessen H, Lopalco L, Siliciano R, Walker B, Lori F. Control of HIV despite the discontinuation of antiretroviral therapy. N Engl J Med 1999; 340:1683–1684.
79. Valentine F, De Gruttola V, and the Remune 316 study team. Immunological and virological evaluations of the effects of HAART compared to HAART plus an inactivated HIV immunogen after 32 weeks [abstr]. 6th Conference on Retrovirus and Opportunistic Infections, Chicago, 1999.
80. Kaslow, R.A., C. Rivers, P. Goepfert, J. Tang, R. El Habib, K. Weinhold, M.J. Mulligan. Association of HLA class I alleles with cytotoxic T lymphocyte (CTL) responses to Gag and Env in recipients of ALVAC-HIV canarypox vaccines [abstr]. 7th Conference on Retroviruses and Opportunistic Infections, San Francisco, 2000.
81. Grassi F, Hosmalin A, Mcilroy D, Calvez V, Debre P, Autran B. Depletion in blood CD11c-positive dendritic cells from HIV-infected patients. AIDS 1999; 13:7841.
82. Gougeon, M.L., C. Rouzioux, I. Liberman, M. Burgard, J.P. Viard, C. Capitant, J.F. Delfraissy, Y. Levy. Abstract: Immunological and virological efficacy of long-term IL-2 therapy in HIV-infected patients. 7th Conference on Retroviruses and Opportunistic Infections, San Francisco, 2000.
83. Katlama, C., C. Duvivier, C. Chouquet, A. Autran, G. Carcelain, L. de Sa M, Zagury, D. Costagliola, R. Tubiana. Abstract: ILSTIM (ANRS 082). A randomized comparative open-label study of interleukin (IL2) in patients with CD4 $<200/mm^3$ despiste effective HAART. 7th Conference on Retroviruses and Opportunistic Infections, San Francisco, 2000.

6

Design of Engineered Vaccines for HIV

Jay A. Berzofsky, Jeffrey D. Ahlers, and Igor M. Belyakov

National Cancer Institute
National Institutes of Health
Bethesda, Maryland

INTRODUCTION

Although natural infection with HIV-1 induces a multiarmed immune response, including neutralizing antibodies, helper T cells (Th), and cytotoxic T lymphocytes (CTL) (1–8), this response is not usually sufficient to prevent the progression of HIV-1–mediated disease to AIDS and ultimately death. Therefore, for a vaccine to be successful, it will have to do better than natural infection at eliciting an adequate immune response. That such a response is possible is suggested both by the protective immunity achieved in monkeys using live attenuated simian immunodeficiency (SIV) vaccines (9–11) and by the small number of individuals who, despite normal chemokine receptors, appear to be resistant to multiple exposures to HIV-1 or who are long-term nonprogressors after infection (2,5,12–15). Furthermore, it is not surprising that a virus that evolves to escape the immune response of its host would not necessarily be the most potent vaccine for inducing immunity against itself. Thus, it should be possible to design a vaccine that is more effective at eliciting protective immunity than is the virus infection itself. The challenge is to design such a vaccine.

In what ways might a vaccine improve on the ability of the virus to induce an appropriate immune response? One may need to increase the magnitude of the immune response, to broaden its specificity to include more epitopes presented by more major histocompatibility complex (MHC) molecules, such as subdominant epitopes that are less subject to escape mutation, or to increase the affinity of the effector molecules and cells. The need for high-affinity neutralizing antibodies is self-evident, but we will show that the affinity or avidity of CTL is also critical to their ability to eliminate virus. One may also need to alter the type of immune response induced, for example, Th1 and CTL rather than Th2 (4,7,16–20), and we will show that this skewing of the response can be achieved with cytokines incorporated into the vaccine. One may need to avoid epitopes that induce potentially harmful immune responses, such as enhancing antibodies (21,22) that facilitate uptake of virus through Fc or complement receptors, or autoimmune responses that might contribute to immunodeficiency (23–27). Thus, selective use of epitopes may be essential. The response may need to be focused on the site of entry of the virus, so for the natural route of mucosal transmission, mucosal immunity may be critical (28). Finally, for a prophylactic vaccine the response must be present or able to be expanded rapidly before the establishment of latent infection or the diversification of the virus.

The challenge, then, becomes one of engineering a vaccine that meets all of these objectives and is safe and effective against a wide range of HIV-1 isolates in a broad HLA-diverse population of humans. We have taken a reductionist approach, selecting individual epitopes, improving on them, and trying to address each of these goals one at a time in constructing a vaccine (27). This chapter summarizes our progress in several of these areas.

SELECTIVE USE OF EPITOPES

Epitope Selection

Many labs, including our own, have described helper-T-cell, CTL, and/or neutralizing antibody epitopes within different proteins of HIV (1–8,27,29–46). One goal of selecting particular epitopes is to avoid epitopes present in whole viral proteins, such as the envelope, that have been reported to elicit enhancing antibodies that facilitate virus uptake into cells via Fc or complement receptors (21,22) or autoimmune responses that might contribute to immunodeficiency (23–27). A second goal is to be able to focus the immune response on desirable epitopes even if they may be subdominant when the whole virus or a whole viral protein is used as immunogen. A third goal is to be able to enhance the efficacy of these epitopes by selective modification of the amino acid sequence in a process we call epitope enhancement, which we will describe in the next section.

One drawback of individual epitopes is that they are each presented by only one or a limited number of HLA molecules and so are not likely to work in the entire human population. The problem of HLA polymorphism is not, however, as vast as the breadth of polymorphism observed, because in any given population one can find about five class I HLA molecules that are sufficiently common that over 90% of the population carries at least one (47). Thus, a handful of epitopes may be sufficient.

We have approached this problem by identifying multideterminant regions in the HIV-1 envelope protein that contain several overlapping helper-T-cell epitopes that are presented by different class II MHC molecules in both mice and humans (34,38). We reasoned that if each epitope within a multideterminant region of sequence is presented by a different class II molecule, the whole region should be functional in individuals or mice of at least a number of MHC types. Thus, if we synthesized a slightly longer peptide spanning the region of overlapping epitopes, we might make an immunogen able to elicit T-cell help in a diverse population. We called such peptides cluster peptides because they contained a cluster of overlapping epitopes, and we found that, indeed, several of these were broadly recognized (38).

As an epitope to elicit effector arms of the response, we used a portion of the V3 loop of gp120 because it was not only a dominant neutralizing antibody epitope, as had been found by several labs (29–31,48), but also a CTL epitope, as we had first identified in mice of four different MHC types (35,49–51), as well as in humans of at least four different HLA types (39,52–54). Since many neutralizing antibodies recognize assembled topographic sites that require the intact folded conformation of the protein, for a short peptide vaccine it was important to select an epitope that induced neutralizing antibodies with only a short synthetic peptide (55,56). The ability to elicit CTL with the same epitope allowed construction of a shorter peptide that would elicit all three types of response: neutralizing antibodies, CTL, and helper T cells. The disadvantage of the V3 loop is its high variability, but this was not a limitation for its experimental use in developing a prototype vaccine to work out the principles for engineering an improved vaccine. Once those problems were solved, one could broaden the vaccine by incorporation of more conserved CTL epitopes and neutralizing antibody epitopes.

Requirement for Covalent Linkage of Helper and CTL Epitopes

One concern was the requirement for covalent linkage of the helper epitope to the antibody and CTL epitope. It had been known for decades that a hapten needed to be attached to a carrier protein for optimal induction of an antibody response (57), but it was not clear whether the same applied to linkage of helper and CTL epitopes. Classically, CTL were elicited by a live virus, live cells, or a tissue graft, so that it was not possible to separate the CTL epitope from the helper epitope. Further, the mechanism could not be the same, because linkage of hapten to carrier is required for the B cell specific for the hapten to take up the carrier as well, by receptor-mediated endocytosis of its surface immunoglobulin-bound antigen, to allow processing and presentation of the carrier epitopes on class II MHC molecules to helper T cells. Since murine T cells do not even express class II MHC molecules, the same mechanism could not apply to helper epitope-CTL linkage. Therefore, we tested whether the helper epitope needed to be linked to the CTL epitope to provide help for a CTL response. We mixed helper and CTL epitope peptides and compared the mixture to the covalently linked construct of the helper and CTL epitopes synthesized as one long continuous peptide and found that only the covalently linked construct elicited CTL in the absence of a mechanism to trap the two components together (58,59). In contrast, with an emulsion adjuvant that trapped the two unlinked petides in the same microdroplets of aqueous phase, we found that CTL could be elicited to some extent without the covalent linkage between the epitopes, and similar results were obtained by others (60,61). We concluded that some physical if not covalent association was needed, probably to assure that both epitopes were take up by the same antigen-presenting cells after they were injected into the recipient. Allowing them to be taken up in the same cell permitted this presenting cell to focus the helper and CTL precursors to the same site to interact and allowed the presenting cell to receive helper signals that activated it and made it more effective at stimulating the CTL. Recent evidence from several labs supports this explanation (62–65).

These covalent peptide vaccine constructs were found to elicit very high titers of neutralizing antibodies in mice when given s.c. in complete Freund's adjuvant (66), as well as to elicit strong CTL responses when given in QS21 (58). Similar HIV peptide vaccine constructs have also been found by others to induce neutralizing antibodies, Th, and CTL in mice and monkeys (67–72). To see if a single adjuvant would be effective in promoting both neutralizing antibody responses and CTL responses to these peptide, we compared several adjuvants and found that montanide ISA 51 (Seppic), a human clinical grade of incomplete Freund's adjuvant, was effective at eliciting all three responses: neutralizing antibodies, CTL, and helper T cells (73).

These two peptide constructs, PCLUS3–18MN and PCLUS6.1–18MN, representing two different Th epitope cluster peptides from the envelope protein linked to a CTL and neutralizing antibody epitope from the envelope V3 loop, have been used in a phase I trial of safety and immunogenicity in humans (74,75). No safety problems were observed, and the peptide in montanide ISA51 was able to elicit a new CTL response not previously present in at least one HIV-1–infected human, but detectable at multiple time points after immunization, and new helper T-cell responses and increases in neutralizing antibodies to the MN strain of HIV-1 in a number of individuals (75). This study showed both safety and the ability of a peptide vaccine to elicit such responses in humans infected with HIV-1. Another similar HIV-1 peptide vaccine was shown also to be safe and to elicit neutralizing antibody and Th responses in human volunteers (76). However, to improve on the immunogenicity and efficacy of such engineered vaccines, we turned to the development of second-generation vaccines in mouse models, described below.

EPITOPE ENHANCEMENT: SEQUENCE MODIFICATION TO IMPROVE EFFICACY

The sequences of viral proteins, as noted above, evolve primarily for function, and secondarily to evade the immune response, so if they contain epitopes that can be presented by class I or class II MHC molecules of the species they infect, this must be purely coincidental. These sequences may not necessarily be optimal for binding to these MHC molecules. Thus, there may frequently be room for improvement. Furthermore, since the antigenic peptide lies partly buried in the MHC groove and only one surface is exposed for interaction with the T-cell receptor (TCR), it is likely that one could replace amino acid residues that interface only with the MHC molecule without interfering with the surface exposed to the TCR, provided the substitutions do not alter the conformation of the bound peptide. Maintenance of the same recognition surface for the TCR is important because one is altering only the vaccine, not the virus, and thus must be able to induce helper T cells or CTL that still recognize the corresponding sequences from the natural virus. If such higher-affinity peptides could be achieved, one could make a vaccine that promised to be more potent than a corresponding construct expressing or containing the natural viral sequence. A related alternative approach is to improve binding to the TCR, when the response tended to be relatively consistently oligoclonal, or to induce T cells with TCRs capable of recognizing a broader array of viral variants. We proposed these approaches, collectively called ''epitope enhancement,'' in the early 1990s (25,26,77) based on our experiences with an HIV helper epitope T1 presented by a murine class II MHC molecule (78) and with an HIV CTL epitope peptide presented by a murine class I MHC molecule, for which more broadly cross-reactive CTL could be elicited by a chimeric peptide (79). Work from our lab and a number of others has shown that epitope enhancement can indeed generate more potent vaccines for viruses and cancer (80–84). The knowledge of sequence motifs for peptides binding to MHC molecules (85), in particular of the role of secondary anchor residues (86), has facilitated rational strategies to design such enhanced peptides.

Enhancement of T-Cell Help

In the course of studying three different amino acid substitutions at each of 12 positions in the first helper-T-cell epitope of HIV-1 described, called T1 [residues 428–443 in the numbering of Ratner et al. (87) or 421–436 in the Los Alamos database numbering, KQIINMWQEVGKAMYA], we found that two of the substitutions made at one position [residue 436 in the numbering of Ratner et al. (87)], replacing the Glu with Ala or Gln, produced peptides that were active at stimulating helper T cells specific for T1 at concentrations several logs lower than concentrations required for unmodified T1 itself (78). In contrast, the substitution of Asp for Glu did not affect antigenic potency. Since Ala is smaller than Glu and uncharged, and Gln is the same size and uncharged, whereas Asp is smaller but retains the negative charge, we concluded that the essential change is removal of the negative charge. We showed that the substituted peptides with increased antigenic potency had a higher affinity for binding to the class II MHC molecule, I-E^k, that presented the peptide (78). Therefore, we reasoned that if a peptide had higher affinity for the class II MHC molecule and stimulated existing helper T cells specific for the natural viral sequence at much lower concentrations, then this modified peptide might make a more potent vaccine in vivo that could still elicit T cells that reacted with the wild-type sequence (25,26,77,78).

To test this hypothesis, we first immunized mice expressing I-E^k with the Ala-substituted peptide T1–436A and compared the lymph node cells elicited with those from mice immunized with the wild-type T1 peptide. We measured T-cell proliferation in response to the wild type T1 peptide, since only T cells that reacted with the natural viral sequence were relevant from the point of view of a vaccine. We found that in mice immunized with an optimal dose of peptide (6 nmol), the response to T1 elicited by T1–436A was higher than that elicited by T1 itself (80). More importantly, at a 10-fold lower dose for immunization, T1 elicited almost no response, but T1–436A elicited a response to T1 that was still higher than that elicited by the 10-fold higher dose of T1 (80). Thus, we clearly had a more potent immunogen, at least for eliciting T-cell proliferation.

More important than T-cell proliferation was the ability to provide help for a CTL response. Thus, we incorporated the Glu-to-Ala substitution in the PCLUS3 helper portion of our peptide vaccine construct, since T1 is contained within the longer PCLUS3 helper sequence. We asked whether the modified second-generation vaccine construct, altered only in the portion binding the class II MHC molecules, would be more effective at eliciting CTL specific for the unaltered CTL epitope presented by a class I MHC molecule. Indeed, the improved peptide vaccine elicited 33-fold more lytic units than the original vaccine construct (80). To confirm that the improvement was indeed due to improved class II restricted T-cell help, and not just some nonspecific effect like greater stability of the peptide in vivo, we performed a genetic experiment in which two strains of mice were used, both expressing the same class I molecule presenting the CTL epitope but differing in the class II molecule available to present the helper epitope. Only the strain with the class II molecule that showed higher affinity for the Ala form than the Glu form produced a higher CTL response with the Ala-substituted peptide, whereas the strain with a class II molecule that did not distinguish these helper epitopes produced an identical response to both peptides. This experiment maps the improvement in the class I–restricted CTL response to a class II MHC molecule and thus confirms the mechanism of action of the epitope enhancement (80). This study leads to two conclusions: 1) it shows that class II MHC–restricted T-cell help is critical to optimization of a class I MHC–restricted CTL response, consistent with the earlier results we had observed in studying the need for covalently linked epitopes; 2) it provides proof of principle that epitope enhancement can be utilized to produce a more potent vaccine for induction of CTL (80).

Enhancement of CTL Epitopes

To extend the epitope enhancement approach to peptides presented by class I MHC molecules to CTL, and in particular to extend it to human MHC molecules, we applied the approach to a peptide of the hepatitis C virus (HCV) core protein that we had identified as presented by HLA-A2.1, the most common human class I molecule, to CTL from HCV-infected patients (88–91). Comparing a large number of substituted peptides, we identified several that bound to HLA-A2.1 with higher affinity and, of these, a subset that were more potent at sensitizing target cells for lysis by human HCV-specific CTL (81). Since the goal was a more immunogenic vaccine in vivo and we could not immunize humans, these peptides were then used to immunize HLA-A2.1 transgenic mice as a surrogate. The CTL response of HLA-A2.1 transgenic mice has been shown to be predictive of the response of humans (89,92,93), since the limitations in peptide binding to the MHC molecule generally outweigh any rare limitations in the T-cell repertoire of either species. One peptide, with an Ala substituted at position 8, was found to be more immunogenic in the HLA-A2.1-transgenic mice, and the CTL elicited were actually more active against the wild-type HCV sequence than the CTL raised against the wild-type peptide (81). Thus, we had made an enhanced peptide vaccine for HCV.

An alternative type of epitope enhancement was also first observed in the case of a CTL epitope from HIV-1. We found that the P18 epitope from the V3 loop of HIV-1 gp120 was a dominant CTL epitope in H-2^d mice in both the IIIB and MN strains, but the two strains did not cross-react (95,96). Moreover, we mapped the key epitopic residue that distinguished these two homologous peptides to the TCR as residue 325 in the Ratner (87) numbering, which is a Val in the IIIB strain and a Tyr in the MN strain (95,96). Interchanging the residues at just this single position completely reversed the specificity for lysis by the IIIB- and MN-specific CTL (95). Further, we found that the IIIB-specific CTL saw peptides with any aliphatic amino acid at that position, such as Val, Leu, or Ile, whereas the MN-specific CTL saw peptides with any aromatic amino acid at that position, including Tyr, Phe, Trp, His, and even Pro, which is a nonaromatic ring structure (79). When we then made chimeric peptides in which the sequence derived from MN but the Tyr residue at that position was replaced with an aliphatic residue, the resulting chimeric peptides were found to elicit broadly cross-reactive CTL, recognizing peptides with aliphatic, aromatic, or even polar Lys or Gln at that position (79). Thus, the sequence modification to make the chimeric peptide created an enhanced epitope, not by increasing the affinity for the MHC molecule, but by eliciting much more broadly cross-reactive CTL. Such a vaccine may be valuable in cases such as the V3 loop which is highly variable. Thus, this alternative type of epitope enhancement complements the modifications that increase antigenic potency.

ROLE OF CTL AVIDITY IN CLEARING VIRUS INFECTION

Although the affinity of antibodies has long been known to play an important role in their efficacy, it was not known whether the affinity of the TCR of CTL played a role in the efficacy of viral clearance. We addressed this question by raising CTL lines of differing avidity for the same peptide-MHC complex, by immunizing BALB/c mice with a recombinant vaccinia virus expressing HIV-1 IIIB gp160, vPE16 (97), and then stimulating the spleen cells with syngeneic presenting cells pulsed with a wide range of concentrations of the immunodominant peptide from gp160 IIIB, P18-I10 (RGPGRAFVTI) (35,49,98,99). After repetiitive stimulation with spleen cells pulsed with exquisitely low concentrations of peptide (down to 0.001–0.0001 μM), very high-avidity CTL grew out, whereas stimulation with spleen cells pulsed with very high concentrations of peptide (50–100 μM) selectively grew out only low-avidity CTL (100). At intermediate concentrations, cells of intermediate avidity grew out. The avidity was assessed functionally by the concentration of peptide pulsed onto target cells that was required to get an equivalent level of lysis. The same rank order of avidities (but not the identical concentrations) was found if the response being measured was interferon-γ production or proliferation. Thus, the CTL of both high and low avidity were phenotypically Tc1 in their cytokine profile. Furthermore, the difference in apparent avidity was not attributable to differences in the level of surface TCR, CD8, or several adhesion molecules tested (100). Therefore, we believe that the predominant molecular mechanism to account for the difference in functional avidity is a difference in the intrinsic affinity of the TCR, but which can be determined only by cloning the TCR genes, expressing a recombinant TCR, and measuring the affinity directly.

We then asked whether there was a difference in the ability of the high- and low-avidity CTL to kill virus-infected target cells expressing gp160 endogenously. High-, intermediate-, and low-avidity CTL killed cells infected with vPE16 recombinant vaccinia (97) expressing gp160 IIIB to a considerable, albeit not identical level (100). Therefore, one might have predicted that they would all be effective in clearing virus in vivo. To test this hypothesis, we adoptively transferred the CTL lines into SCID mice, which have no T or B cells of their own, and determined the effect on viral load after challenge with vPE16, which has a predilection for replication in the ovary. The viral load was reduced about 1000-fold by the high-avidity CTL, but hardly at all by the low-avidity CTL, and this result was reproducible with several independently derived high- and low-avidity CTL lines (100). When the CTL lines were titrated, we could not achieve a number of low-avidity CTL that gave a reduction in viral load in vivo equivalent to that produced by the high-avidity CTL, but as we reduced the number of high-avidity CTL, it looked as though they were at least 10-fold as potent on a per cell basis as the low-avidity CTL (94). Furthermore, the difference in reduction in viral load was not simply due to a delay in clearance by the low-avidity lines, as measurement of viral load at later times (6 days vs. 3 days) showed similar differences. We conclude that high-avidity CTL are much more effective at clearing virus, that in vitro ability to kill infected cells is not always a good predictor of efficacy in vivo, and that the quality of the CTL is therefore as important as the quantity of CTL in controlling viral infection (27,100).

The differential efficacy of high- vs. low-avidity CTL has now been confirmed with several other viruses, such as LCMV (101,102). Moreover, we predicted that it might apply to tumor rejection as well, and several labs have demonstrated that high-avidity CTL are more effective at killing human tumors (103) or causing clinical remissions in animal tumor models (104).

We hypothesized that, at least in the case of viruses, one mechanism explaining the difference in efficacy in vivo, despite the ability of both high- and low-avidity CTL to kill infected cells in vitro, might be related to the kinetics of viral infection. Early in virus infection of a cell, when very little viral protein has been synthesized, there may be only enough processed viral peptides presented on MHC molecules to allow recognition by high-avidity CTL. Later in viral infection, when more viral protein has been made, low-avidity CTL may also be able to kill the infected cells, but by then viral progeny have been made and it is too late to have as great an impact on viral replication as if the cells had been killed early in the infectious process. To test this hypothesis, we infected cells with vPE16 and measured their susceptibility to lysis by high- and low-avidity CTL at time points ranging from 2 to 24 hours of infection. As predicted, lysis by high-avidity CTL could be detected as early as 2 and 4 hours after infection, whereas killing by low-avidity CTL could not be detected until at least 8 hours of infection (94). This result strongly supports our working hypothesis.

We also wondered why high concentrations of antigen resulted in only low-avidity CTL and not also high-avidity CTL. We hypothesized that the high densities of peptide-MHC complexes might actually tolerize or delete the high-avidity CTL. To test this question, we measured proliferation of the CTL over a wide range of peptide concentration used to pulse the stimulator cells and found that, indeed, high densities of peptide-MHC led to a decrease in proliferation of high-avidity CTL (105). This effect turned out to be an apoptotic deletion of the cells, initiated by supraoptimal antigen stimulation through the TCR and associated CD8 molecules, but requiring also TNF-α production and a signal through the TNF-receptor II (105,106). Thus, high-avidity CTL were more susceptible to deletion by high densities of antigen, and this could be a mechanism for peripheral tolerance induction as well as clonal exhaustion (107), in which chronic high viral loads lead to loss of virus-specific CTL (108). Furthermore, since many tumor antigens are either autoantigens or present at high levels, it is possible that this mechanism may lead to deletion of the high-avidity CTL that are the most effective CTL for controlling tumor growth.

INCORPORATION OF CYTOKINES TO ENHANCE AND STEER IMMUNE RESPONSES TO VACCINES

Conventional adjuvants not only enhance immune responses, but also can bias the type of response produced (109–112). To accomplish both enhancement and steering toward desired response, phenotypes in a more rational and selective way, we explored the use of cytokines incorporated in the adjuvant with the vaccine antigen. In our earlier studies of MHC-lined Ir genes controlling immune responses to myoglobin and the malaria circumsporozoite protein, we found that incorporation of IL-2 into the incomplete Freund's adjuvant with the antigen could elicit antibody responses in genetic low-responder strains of mice that were close to the levels produced by genetic high-responder strains (113). The cytokine functional activity of IL-2 was necessary for this effect, because a variant of the recombinant human IL-2 used that had a single point mutation abrogating the cytokine activity eliminated the enhancement of the antibody response (114). Thus, the effect was not just a carrier effect of a foreign (human) protein. Furthermore, multiple daily doses of IL-2 given parenterally, IV., at the time of the immunization and for several days thereafter had no effect on the antibody response, whereas a single dose incorporated with the antigen in the emulsion adjuvant had a profound effect. The potential advantages of the latter method, besides simplicity and ease of administration, is that the cytokine is present in depot form for slow release at the same site as the antigen, and thus both may go to the same draining lymph nodes over a prolonged period of time. Such depot administration also potentially avoids some of the side effects that may accompany repeated parenteral administration.

To steer the immune response to peptide or other vaccines toward particular types of responses such as Th1, Th2, CTL, or particular antibody isotypes, we therefore explored an extension of this approach, namely use of other cytokines in incomplete Freund's adjuvant with our synthetic peptide HIV vaccine constructs, PCLUS3–18MN and PCLUS6.1–18MN. A comprehensive matrix comparison was carried out of eight different cytokines and their effect on seven different immune responses (115). The matrix was made further multidimensional by use of two different vaccine peptides and studies in two genetically distinct mouse strains, BALB/c, which has a predisposition toward Th2 responses, and B10 congenics, which have a tendency toward Th1 response. Although the resulting matrix was obviously complex, certain general conclusions could be drawn. First, GM-CSF was the most broadly effective enhancer of almost all the types of immune responses studies, without altering the balance between Th1 and Th2 responses. Presumably, its effect was on antigen-presenting cells, and we have recently confirmed this mechanism (150). Other cytokines had a more selective effect. IL-12, IL-2, and interferon-γ all increased the Th1 cytokine responses and the switch to IgG2a antibody isotype. GM-CSF enhanced neutralizing antibody titers in all strains, whereas IL-12 enhanced neutralizing antibodies primarily in B10 congenics and IL-4 did so primarily in BALB/c. The only cytokine besides GM-CSF that substantially enhanced the CTL response was IL-12. Others have also manipulated the immune response to vaccines using individual cytokines as adjuvants (116–121) and to DNA vaccines with plasmids encoding cytokines (122), although such a broad matrix was not compared nor were possible synergies examined.

Since we supposed that the mechanism of IL-12, presumably acting on the CTL precursor or influencing the helper cytokine profile, was different from the mechanism of GM-CSF, acting on the presenting cell, we hypothesized that the two might be synergistic. Indeed, we found that the combination of GM-CSF and IL-12 incorporated in the adjuvant was synergistic compared to either cytokine alone in enhancing the CTL response (115). Similar synergy was subsequently reported between these cytokines administered as genes in a DNA vaccine (123). A clinical trial of GM-CSF and IL-12 with a peptide HIV-1 vaccine is currently being developed in collaboration with the groups of Dr. Robert Yarchoan and Dr. Gene Shearer (NCI). We further asked whether TNF-α, which does not by itself enhance the CTL response, would synergize with IL-12 in enhancing the CTL response, and found that indeed it did (115). Moreover, this combination of IL-12 and TNF-α was the most potent inducer of interferon-γ response, inducing markedly more interferon than either cytokine alone (115).

We therefore asked whether all three cytokines, GM-CSF, IL-12, and TNF-α, would show triple synergy for enhancing the CTL and interferon-γ responses and also for improving the protective response against viral challenge. Indeed, we found such triple synergy (150). Under conditions in which the response was suboptimal, such as a single immunization, the triple combination of cytokines induced the strongest CTL response. When the immunized mice were challenged with a recombinant vaccinia virus expressing HIV-1 gp160 as a surrogate virus (97) since mice cannot be infected with HIV-1, only the mice immunized with the peptide vaccine combined with the triple combination of cytokines consistently showed complete protection, although the double combination of IL-12 and TNF often showed a marked level of protection as well, consistent with its ability to induce high interferon-γ levels, which are known to contribute to protection against vaccinia (124). Indeed, we showed that the protection was mediated more by CD4+ cells than CD8+ cells in this case, although adoptively transferred CD8+ CTL could also protect, and that the protection required interferon-γ (150).

Current studies have been designed to explore the mechanisms of this synergy. As mentioned above, we confirmed our hypothesis that GM-CSF enhances antigen-presenting cell function (150). The mechanism of action of TNF-α was less apparent. We hypothesized that this, or the combination of TNF-α and IL-12, might enhance the level of IL-12 receptor and thus synergize compared to IL-12 alone. There is no antibody available to measure IL-12 receptors on cell surfaces, so the receptor levels are usually inferred from mRNA levels. Using this approach in an anti-CD3–driven system in which the effect of these cytokines on the T-cell can be measured directly, we have recently shown that TNF-α plus IL-12 can increase levels of IL-12 receptor expression (151). Our results suggest both an instructive role for TNF-α/IL-12 in Th1 differentiation by regulating IL-12R expression at the single cell level, and selection, favoring a Th1 response at the population level, by upregulating IFN-γ production. Other groups have also found that cyto-kines introduced into peptide, protein, DNA, or cellular vaccines can enhance immune responses (119,122,123,125,126). Thus, the use of cytokines as an integral part of engineered vaccines may allow a level of immunogenicity and an ability to manipulate the type of response achieved that has not been possible with conventional adjuvants and vaccine constructs.

IMPORTANCE OF MUCOSAL CTL IN PROTECTION AGAINST MUCOSAL VIRAL TRANSMISSION

Induction of Mucosal CTL with a Peptide Vaccine and with a Recombinant Attenuated Vaccinia Virus Vaccine

The primary route of natural HIV transmission is through mucosa in either the genital or the gastrointestinal tract (28). For a vaccine to prevent such transmission, mucosal immunity may be as important as, or more important than, systemic immunity. Yet the majority of HIV vaccine research has focused on systemic immunity. We sought to ask whether an engineered vaccine that we had been developing for systemic use would also induce mucosal immunity, and if so, how critical mucosal CTL might be in preventing mucosal transmission of a virus.

To test first whether a synthetic peptide vaccine administered mucosally could elicit CTL in mucosal sites, such as Peyer's patches and lamina propria of the intestine, as well as in systemic sites, we immunized BALB/c mice with the PCLUS3–18 vaccine construct, mixed with (but not attached to) cholera toxin (CT) as a mucosal adjuvant, via several mucosal routes, and compared the CTL elicited in the gastrointestinal Peyer's patches and lamina propria as well as in the spleen with those of mice immunized subcutaneously (SC) with the peptide vaccine in incomplete Freund's adjuvant (127). The mice immunized SC made a substantial CTL response in the spleen but no detectable response in the mucosal sites. In contrast, mice immunized intrarectally, intragastrically, or intranasally with the peptide and CT demonstrated a CTL response in both the mucosal sites and the spleen (127). However, the intrarectal route was by far the most effective in eliciting CTL not only in the mucosal sites, but also in the spleen, where the levels approximated those achieved with the SC immunization. Since the mucosal sites monitored were in the gastrointestinal tract, it was possible that the greater efficacy of intrarectal immunization was biased by the proximity of the mucosal sites monitored. However, the far greater CTL response in the spleen induced by intrarectal rather than intragastric or intranasal immunization suggested that the intrarectal route was more effective in eliciting a broader immune response, not just a local one, and that the rank order represented more than just sampling bias. Even 6 months after the start of a 3-week course of four immunizations with peptide and CT, without further boosting thereafter, the level of CTL precursors in both the mucosal sites and the spleen was about as high as it was only 2 weeks after the last dose (127). Thus, CTL memory was surprisingly long-lived, given that the peptide was administered into the lumen of the gut, where it should be susceptible to proteases, without the benefit of any protective emulsion or other depot formulation. We concluded that the most effective mucosal route for our future studies was the intrarectal one.

We also made note of the striking asymmetry between the mucosal and systemic immunizations, in that all three mucosal routes of immunization induced CTL in the spleen as well as in mucosal sites, whereas the SC immunization induced only splenic but not mucosal CTL (127). This suggests that trafficking between mucosal and systemic compartments is not symmetrical, but that CTL precursors migrate more effectively from mucosal inductive sites (such as the Peyer's patches) to the systemic circulation than in the other direction. Studies are underway to study homing and homing receptors to understand the mechanisms of this asymmetry. The mucosal immunizations were performed atraumatically with a very soft, flexible, human umbilical vein catheter, and there is usually no evidence of bleeding or trauma, so we do not believe that the mucosal immunization induces systemic immunity due to movement of antigen, rather than of cells, although this possibility cannot be definitively excluded. However, evidence against leakage of antigen into the bloodstream as a mechanism for the induction of systemic CTL by mucosal immunization comes from experiments in which intentional inoculation of HIV peptide vaccine intravenously did not induce splenic CTL (I. M. Belyakov and J. A. Berzofsky, unpublished observations). Furthermore, in the case of vaccinia immunization by these routes, evidence described later suggests that the asymmetry observed there cannot be due primarily to movement of the virus rather than the immune cells elicited. Thus, it is likely that the asymmetry relates to the migration pattern of cells, not antigen. This asymmetry was found to have several practical implications and applications noted below.

The induction of CTL by intrarectal administration of synthetic peptide vaccine and cholera toxin was found to be dependent both on IL-12, as shown by treating the mice before and after each immunization with 0.5 mg of anti-IL-12 antibody, and on interferon-γ, as shown by use of interferon-γ knockout BALB/c mice (127). However, we could not determine whether both act directly on CTL induction or one acts through the other. Because IL-12 is important for inducing production of interferon-γ and for differentiation of Th1 cells that make this cytokine (128), and interferon-γ is necessary to upregulate the receptor for IL-12 and thus the response to this cytokine (129), each is necessary for the other. The problem becomes a classic chicken-egg circular one, and we can only conclude that both are necessary.

We also examined mucosal immunization with recombinant vaccinia virus vector vaccines, expressing the HIV-1 envelope protein containing the homologous immunodominant CTL epitope (P18 in the V3 loop) as the synthetic peptide vaccine. However, these vectors were made with the envelope protein from the dual-tropic primary isolate strain 89.6, which is more homologous to the MN strain than the IIIB strain of HIV. We found that the homologous sequence in strain 89.6 was also immunodominant in BALB/c mice, and that this peptide (IGPGRAFYAR), presented by H-2D^d, cross-reacted with that of the MN strain (IGPGRAFYTT), in that CTL raised against either reacted almost equally with both (46). We compared this envelope protein delivered in an attenuated virus, modified vaccinia Ankara (MVA), which is replication incompetent in mammalian cells (130–133), with a conventional replication-competent recombinant vaccinia virus based on the WR strain expressing the same envelope protein. Given by the intrarectal route, the MVA-89.6 was at least as effective at eliciting CTL as the conventional WR-89.6, both in the mucosal sites and in the spleen (46), despite the inability of the former virus to produce progeny virus and thus expand beyond the size of the initial inoculum. Because the MVA is nonlytic, it may stay in the local mucosal cells for a longer period without lysing them, continuing to produce recombinant gp160 in the infected cells, whereas the replication competent WR strain may produce more virus, but much of the progeny may seed the bloodstream and not stay at the mucosal site. In any case, this greater efficacy is consistent with the observations of others examining antibody responses induced by such viruses (131,134–136). When given intraperitoneally, these viruses elicited only splenic, but not mucosal CTL. Thus, the same asymmetry between mucosal and systemic compartments was seen for recombinant vaccinia immunization as for peptide immunization: systemic immunization yielded only systemic immunity, whereas mucosal immunization induced both mucosal and systemic immunity.

Demonstration of the Necessity of CTL in the Mucosal Site to Resist Mucosal Transmission

We asked whether mucosal immunization with the synthetic peptide vaccine could protect against transmission of a virus through the mucosal route. Since mice cannot be infected with HIV-1 itself, as a surrogate virus we used vPE16, a recombinant vaccinia virus expressing the HIV-1 envelope protein from the IIIB strain (97). It may be important that this virus does not incorporate the gp160 into the viral particle, but expresses it only in the infected cells (137). Thus, unlike HIV-1 itself, the surrogate virus used should not be susceptible to neutralizing antibodies against gp160. This difference simplified our examination of protection and its mechanism, since we could study the role of CTL without the complicating factor of neutralizing antibodies.

We challenged mice with vPE16 intrarectally and 6 days later measured titers of virus in the ovaries, where this virus preferentially replicates. Mice immunized intrarectally with peptide four times weekly, when challenged intrarectally with vPE 16 2 weeks later, showed a 10,000-fold reduction in viral pfu compared to unimmunized mice, and this protection was specific for HIV-1 gp160, in that mice challenged similarly with a control vaccinia recombinant expressing only β-galactosidase, vSC8, were not protected at all (127,138). Furthermore, this resistance to mucosal transmission lasted at least 6 months (138). The long-lived protection, in the absence of a depot form of antigen, when synthetic peptide antigen administered into the lumen of the colon should not be expected to have a long half-life, suggested the possibility that immune memory was sustained in this case without a continuous presence of antigen (139,140). Beyond the presence of memory CTL precursors, the protection in this assay, in which virus is measured 6 days after challenge, suggests that either the CTL remain in a state able to perform effector functions for 6 months or more or that the memory CTL can be rapidly reactivated by infection.

Although the virus does not incorporate gp160 into the virus particle, and thus should not be susceptible to neutralization by antibodies to gp160, the presence of protection and of CTL does not prove cause and effect. The specificity for gp160 suggests that the action is on the infected cell, where the gp160 is produced. However, antibodies could also contribute through complement-mediated effects or antibody-dependent cellular cytotoxicity (ADCC), and CD4+ T cells might also play a role, for example, through cytokine secretion. To test the dependence of protection on CD8+ cells, we depleted the mice of CD8+ cells in vivo by treatment with a monoclonal anti-CD8 antibody. Whether the antibody was given before and during the immunization process or only before the time of challenge, in either case the protection against mucosal transmission was completely abrogated (138). Thus, the resistance to mucosal transmission of virus was completely dependent on CD8+ cells. From this information we cannot conclude that the protective mechanism involves lysis of infected cells by CTL or the action of a cytokine produced by these cells, as it is known that interferon-γ plays an important role in protection against vaccinia (124). However, regardless of the mechanism used by these cells, we can conclude that it is carried out by CD8+ cells.

However, because the intrarectal immunization with peptide vaccine induced CTL in the spleen as well as in the mucosal sites, and because the virus titer was measured primarily in the ovaries, where it was greatest, it remained possible that the protection was mediated by systemic CTL acting, for example, directly in the ovary, and that mucosal CTL were not necessary. To test this question, we took advantage of the asymmetry noted earlier. Because mice immunized SC had levels of CTL in the spleen at least as high as those induced by intrarectal immunization, if the splenic CTL were sufficient to protect, one would expect the mice immunized SC should also be protected against mucosal transmission of the virus. However, if CTL in the Peyer's patches and/or lamina propria were necessary, then only the intrarectally immunized mice would be expected to be protected. To test this hypothesis, we compared mice immunized SC or intrarectally and found that only the intrarectally immunized mice showed any protection at all against the mucosal challenge with virus (138). We conclude that systemic CTL are not sufficient to protect, and that CTL must be present in the mucosa at the site of challenge to protect against mucosal transmission of virus and, therefore, that the virus inoculum is being limited at the mucosal barrier by eliminating the first set of infected cells locally, before the virus can spread systemically.

Several ancillary pieces of data support this interpretation. First, intrarectal immunization did not protect against virus administered intraperitoneally, only mucosally, whereas if the protection were occurring at a systemic site such as the ovary itself, then one would expect it to be independent of the challenge route. Second, the CTL generated in the spleen by intrarectal immunization did not appear quantitatively or qualitatively different from those generated by SC immunization. For example, there was no apparent difference in avidity (138) that might account for a difference in efficacy as an alternative interpretation. Third, the resistance to mucosal challenge was evident in the ovary even 2 days after challenge, when the virus had little time to replicate after reaching the ovary and so was more representative of virus that had just arrived from the initial mucosal site (138). Fourth, when virus titers were measured in the gastrointestinal tract, although they were much lower than those in the ovary, a reduction was seen from around 15,000 to <100 pfu. Therefore, clearance of virus was occurring at the mucosal site. All of this evidence, taken together strongly supports the interpretation that CTL must be present in the mucosa to protect against mucosal transmission and that they do so by eliminating the cells initially infected at the first site of exposure and so reduce the inoculum of progeny virus that gets beyond the mucosal site to become a systemic infection. Put another way, we believe that the CTL must make their stand at the mucosal barrier and that if the virus once gets beyond this mucosal barrier to produce a viremia, it is much harder to control.

This conclusion is important for vaccine development, since it implies that one cannot depend on systemic CTL to protect against mucosal transmission of a virus. If the major route of transmission is mucosal, a vaccine, to be successful, must elicit not only strong mucosal antibody responses (141), but also CTL locally in the mucosa, which is at risk for exposure to the virus. The most effective way to elicit such local mucosal immunity seems, at this point, to be by mucosal immunization, whether with a peptide or with a recombinant viral vector, such as the MVA recombinant expressing HIV-1 envelope discussed above.

Enhancement of the Mucosal CTL Response and Protection by Use of Cytokines as Mucosal Adjuvants in the Vaccine

Given that induction of CTL in the mucosa was so important for protection, we sought a way to enhance this immunity. We took advantage of our observation that the mucosal CTL response was dependent on endogenous IL-12, since we could block its induction by treatment of the mice with anti-IL-12 given before and after each immunization (127). Further, we reasoned that if we could block the response completely with the limited amount of antibody we could administer (0.5 mg before and after each dose of vaccine), perhaps endogenous production of IL-12 was limiting. Therefore, we hypothesized that delivery of additional exogenous IL-12 with the vaccine might increase the CTL response and the protection.

To test this hypothesis, we compared administration of IL-12 intraperitoneally at the time of intrarectal immunization with peptide with administration of IL-12 intrarectally together with the peptide and CT. In this case, the IL-12 was partially protected by mixing with DOTAP, a cationic lipofection agent used to introduce DNA into cells. As a control, saline mixed with DOTAP was administered intrarectally along with the peptide. The mice given IL-12 intrarectally with the peptide vaccine showed a significant increase in CTL activity, whereas those given the IL-12 intraperitoneally did not (138,142). Thus, the IL-12 must exert a local effect. Furthermore, when the mice were challenged intrarectally with vPE16, the mice immunized intrarectally with peptide vaccine and IL-12 showed a 6-log reduction in virus titer compared with the 4-log reduction seen in mice immunized with peptide and DOTAP without IL-12 (138). Thus, protection as well as CTL activity was enhanced by IL-12 as an adjuvant.

Given our earlier observation that GM-CSF synergized with IL-12 in enhancing a CTL response to peptide when all were emulsified together in incomplete Freund's adjuvant for systemic immunization (115), as described above, we asked whether GM-CSF would synergize with IL-12 for mucosal immunization. By immunizing the mice only twice instead of four times to be better able to detect synergy, we found that indeed the combination of GM-CSF and IL-12 with the peptide was substantially more effective at inducing CTL than peptide alone or in combination with either of the cytokines singly (143).

We also wanted to determine whether CT was necessary, since it is too toxic for human use. Although immunization with the peptide vaccine intrarectally without any adjuvant also induced CTL, the level was lower than that induced when CT was added (127). As a less toxic substitute, we examined mutant *E. coli*–labile toxin (LT), developed by John D. Clements at Tulane University (144). LT has been used as a mucosal adjuvant similar to CT but is somewhat less toxic. The mutation used prevents cleavage to the active form of the toxin but leaves the enzymatic active site intact, and the net result is to retain adjuvant function while eliminating most of the toxicity (144). When mutant LT (mLT) was compared with CT as a mucosal adjuvant for induction of mucosal and splenic CTL by immunization with peptide intrarectally, we found that the mLT induced levels of CTL that were at least as high as, and usually higher than, those induced using CT as adjuvant (143). Indeed, the level of CTL induction was usually more like that induced by CT plus IL-12. Furthermore, additional IL-12 did not induce further improvement in the response when mLT was used, in contrast to CT. Because CT has been shown to inhibit the induction of endogenous IL-12 (145), we propose that the CTL response is more dependent on exogenous IL-12 when CT is used as adjuvant and that probably mLT does not similarly inhibit endogenous IL-12 production (143). Similar apparently IL-12–independent induction of CTL using LT as a mucosal adjuvant was recently reported by Simmons et al. (146). Thus, mLT may be not only a safer adjuvant, but also a more effective one. We are therefore currently using mLT as an adjuvant in a trial to translate these results into mucosal immunization of rhesus macaques against SIV. In the initial study, comparing intrarectal and subcutaneous immunization of Mamu-A*01-positive rhesus macaques with the same HIV/SIV peptide vaccine, followed by intrarectal challenge with pathogenic SHIV-ku, we found that the mucosal immunization was more effective at reducing plasma viral set point than the subcutaneous immunization. Importantly, the intrarectally immunized animals also had a lower viral load in the gut mucosa, and higher levels of ex vivo CTL in this site, suggesting that the greater efficacy of the mucosal immunization in reducing viral load was due to more effective induction of CTL in the gut, resulting in greater clearance of virus from this major reservoir that was seeding the bloodstream (152). These results strongly emphasize that, to be effective, an HIV vaccine will probably have to elicit CTL in the gut mucosa as well as any other sites of transmission.

USE OF MUCOSAL IMMUNIZATION TO CIRCUMVENT THE BARRIER OF PREEXISTING POXVIRUS IMMUNITY FOR VACCINIA VECTOR VACCINES

The finding of asymmetry between the mucosal and systemic compartments after mucosal versus systemic immunization with either a peptide vaccine or a recombinant vaccinia virus vaccine led us to consider a new approach to an old problem. Since the advent of attenuated recombinant vaccinia virus vectors such as MVA and NYVAC, allowing for adequate safety of such vaccines, a remaining drawback to recombinant vaccinia vector vaccines is their poorer immunogenicity in individuals with prior poxvirus immunity. Since most individuals born before 1970 were immunized against smallpox with a vaccinia vaccine, it has been harder to vaccinate this sizable portion of the population (147), and similar resistance to induction of antibodies by recombinant vaccinia vaccines has been observed in mice with prior vaccinia immunity (148). It occurred to us that if systemic immunization leaves the mucosal immune system naive, it may still be possible to immunize such individuals via a mucosal route. Furthermore, since we found that mucosal immunization with recombinant vaccinia viral vaccines induces systemic as well as mucosal immunity (46), this would be a way of achieving systemic immunity to a recombinant protein expressed by the vaccinia vector in individuals already immune to vaccinia itself.

We tested this hypothesis by immunizing mice with a control vaccinia virus, vSC8, expressing only β-galactosidase, via the subcutaneous route. Four weeks later, when we attempted to immunize these vaccinia-immune mice subcutaneously with either MVA89.6 or vPE16, two vaccinia vectors expressing different variants of the HIV-1 envelope protein, we were unable to elicit any CTL response, whereas control animals without prior vaccinia immunity made a strong CTL response (149). This extended the problem of preexisting poxvirus immunity, previously studied primarily for antibody responses, to CTL responses. To see if the mucosal route of immunization would circumvent this problem, we immunized the mice that had previously received vSC8 subcutaneously, and control animals, with MVA89.6 or vPE16 intrarectally. The mice with prior vaccinia immunity showed almost as high a CTL response in the spleen as the vaccinia-naive mice (149). This result confirmed our hypothesis. The intranasal route also was capable of circumventing prior vaccinia immunity, but not as well as the intrarectal route, and the same results were found for the antibody response to gp160. In addition, the mucosal route was more effective for boosting a response in mice. We conclude that the asymmetry of the mucosal and systemic compartments can be used to advantage to allow the effective use of recombinant vaccinia vector vaccines in cases of prior poxvirus immunity. This approach may provide a solution to one of the last remaining problems in the widespread use of this family of otherwise very potent vaccine vectors.

This result also allowed us to address the question of whether the systemic immunity induced by mucosal immunization is due to movement of immune cells or vaccine from the mucosal to the systemic compartment. Since intentional immunization with the recombinant vaccinia systemically did not induce systemic immunity in the previously vaccinia-immune mice, the induction of systemic CTL immunity by mucosal immunization with recombinant vaccinia cannot be due simply to the leakage of the recombinant vaccinia into the systemic system. Rather, at least in this case, it must be the migration of immune cells from the mucosal to the systemic compartment that results in mucosal immunity. These results also emphasize and confirm the striking asymmetry between systemic and mucosal compartments after immunization by different routes and demonstrate the practical significance of this asymmetry.

CONCLUSIONS

To overcome some of the limitations of natural viruses that cause chronic infections, such as HIV and HCV, in inducing responses adequate to clear the infection, engineered vaccines can use a wide armamentarium of approaches. The magnitude of the response can be increased by sequence modifications resulting in epitope enhancement as well as by the appropriate use of cytokine adjuvants. Broadening the immune response to include less dominant epitopes can also be accomplished by epitope enhancement applied to subdominant epitopes and by cytokine adjuvants. Cytokine adjuvants can also steer the immune response toward desirable response phenotypes that may be more protective, such as Th1 and CTL rather than Th2. We have seen that the avidity of the CTL response may be critical in clearance of viral infection, and methods are needed to selectively induce high-avidity CTL. Engineered vaccines can alter the balance between helpful and harmful immune responses by selective use of epitopes. Mucosal immunization can target the immune response to the site of transmission, and we have seen that this local CTL immunity may be critical to protection against mucosal transmission. Finally, prophylactic immunization with a vaccine can potentially establish an immune response that can clear the virus before the establishment of latent infection or the diversification of the virus. Thus, the approaches described here may serve as building blocks to develop engineered vaccines that could potentially succeed in cases in which vaccines that simply mimic natural infection may not.

REFERENCES

1. Levy JA. Pathogenesis of human immunodeficiency virus infection. Microbiol Rev 1993; 57:183–289.
2. Haynes BF, Pantaleo G, Fauci AS. Toward an understanding of the correlates of protective immunity to HIV infection. Science 1996; 271:324–328.
3. Goudsmit J, Back NKT, Nara PL. Genomic diversity and antigenic variation of HIV-1: links between pathogenesis, epidemiology and vaccine development. FASEB J 1991; 5:2427–2436.
4. Rowland-Jones S, Tan R, McMichael A. Role of cellular immunity in protection against HIV infection. Adv Immunol 1997; 65:277–346.
5. Cease KB, Berzofsky JA. Towards a vaccine for AIDS: the emergence of immunobiology-based vaccine development. Annu Rev Immunol 1994; 12:923–989.
6. Yang OO, Walker BD. CD8+ cells in human immunodeficiency virus type I pathogenesis: cytolytic and noncytolytic inhibition of viral replication. Adv Immunol 1997; 66:273–311.
7. Goulder PJR, Rowland-Jones SL, McMichael AJ, Walker BD. Anti-HIV cellular immunity: recent advances towards vaccine design. AIDS 1999; 13:S121-S136.
8. Parren PWHI, Moore JP, Burton DR, Sattentau QJ. The neutralizing antibody response to HIV-1: viral evasion and escape from humoral immunity. AIDS 1999; 13:S137-S162.
9. Daniel MD, Kirchhoff F, Czajak SC, Sehgal PK, Desrosiers RC. Protective effects of a live attenuated SIV vaccine with a deletion in the *nef* gene. Science 1992; 258:1938–1941.
10. Desrosiers RC. HIV with multiple gene deletions as a live attenuated vaccine for AIDS. AIDS Res Hum Retroviruses 1992; 8:411–421.
11. Ruprecht RM. Live attenuated AIDS viruses as vaccines: promise or peril. Immunol Rev 1999; 170:135–149.
12. Clerici M, Giorgi JV, Chou C-C, Gudeman VK, Zack JA, Gupta P, Ho H-N, Nishanian PG, Berzofsky JA, Shearer GM. Cell mediated immune response to human immunodeficiency virus type I (HIV-1) in seronegative homosexual men with recent sexual exposure to HIV-1. J Infect Dis 1992; 165:1012–1019.
13. Rowland-Jones S, Sutton J, Ariyoshi K, Dong T, Gotch F, McAdam S, Whitby D, Sabally S, Gallimore A, Corrah T, Takiguchi M, Schultz T,

McMichael A, Whittle H. HIV-specific cytotoxic T-cells in HIV-exposed but uninfected Gambian women. Nat Med 1995; 1:59–64.

14. Harrer E, Harrer T, Barbosa P, Feinberg M, Johnson RP, Buchbinder S, Walker BD. Recognition of the highly conserved YMDD region in the human immunodeficiency virus type 1 reverse transcriptase by HLA-A2-restricted cytotoxic T lymphocytes from an asymptomatic long-term non-progressor. J Infect Dis 1996; 173:476–479.
15. Pinto LA, Sullivan J, Berzofsky JA, Clerici M, Kessler HA, Landay AL, Shearer GM. *Env*-specific cytotoxic T lymphocyte responses in HIV sero-negative health care workers occupationally exposed to HIV-contaminated body fluids. J Clin Invest 1995; 96:867–876.
16. Clerici M, Shearer GM. A $T_H1 \rightarrow T_H2$ switch is a critical step in the etiology of HIV infection . Immunol Today 1993; 14:107–111.
17. Salk J, Bretscher PA, Salk PL, Clerici M, Shearer GM. A strategy for prophylactic vaccination against HIV. Science 1993; 260:1270–1272.
18. Clerici M, Berzofsky JA. Cellular immunity and cytokines in HIV infection . AIDS 1994; 8 (suppl 1):S175-S182.
19. Clerici M, Shearer GM. The Th1-Th2 hypothesis of HIV infection: new insights. Immunol Today 1994; 15:575–581.
20. Letvin NL, Schmitz JE, Jordan HL, Seth A, Hirsch VM, Reimann KA, Kuroda MJ. Cytotoxic T lymphocytes specific for the simian immunodeficiency virus. Immunol Rev 1999; 170:127–134.
21. Robinson WE, Jr., Kawamura T, Lake D, Masuho Y, Mitchell WM, Hersh EM. Antibodies to the primary immunodominant domain of human immunodeficiency virus type 1 (HIV-1) glycoprotein gp41 enhance HIV-1 infection in vitro. J Virol 1990; 64:5301–5305.
22. Takeda A, Robinson JE, Ho DD, Debouck C, Haigwood NL, Ennis FA. Distinction of human immunodeficiency virus type 1 neutralization and infection enhancement by human monoclonal antibodies to glycoprotein 120. J Clin Invest 1992; 89:1952–1957.
23. Golding H, Robey FA, Gates FT, III, Linder W, Beining PR, Hoffman T, Golding B. Identification of homologous regions in human immunodeficiency virus I gp41 and human MHC class II β 1 domain I. Monoclonal antibodies against the gp41-derived peptide and patients' sera react with native HLA class II antigens, suggesting a role for autoimmunity in the pathogenesis of acquired immune deficiency syndrome. J Exp Med 1988; 167:914–923.
24. Golding H, Shearer GM, Hillman K, Lucas p, Manischewitz J, Zajac RA, Clerici M, Gress RE, Boswell NR, Golding B. Common epitope in human immunodeficiency virus (HIV) 1-GP41 and HLA class II elicits immunosuppressive autoantibodies capable of contributing to immune dysfunction in HIV 1-infected individuals. J Clin Invest 1989; 83:1430–1435.

25. Berzofsky JA. Epitope selection and design of synthetic vaccines: molecular approaches to enhancing immunogenicity and crossreactivity of engineered vaccines. Ann N Y Acad Sci 1993; 690:256–264.
26. Berzofsky JA, Berkower IJ. Novel approaches to peptide and engineered protein vaccines for HIV using defined epitopes: advances in 1994–95. AIDS 1995; 9 (suppl A):S143-S157.
27. Berzofsky JA, Ahlers JD, Derby MA, Pendleton CD, Arichi T, Belyakov IM. Approaches to improve engineered vaccines for human immunodeficiency virus (HIV) and other viruses that cause chronic infections. Immunol Rev 1999; 170:151–172.
28. Lehner T, Bergmeier L, Wang Y, Tao L, Mitchell E. A rational basis for mucosal vaccination against HIV infection. Immunol Rev 1999; 170:183–196.
29. Palker TJ, Clark ME, Langlois AJ, Matthews TJ, Weinhold KJ, Randall RR, Bolognesi DP, Haynes BF. Type-specific neutralization of the human immunodeficiency virus with antibodies to env-encoded synthetic peptides. Proc Natl Acad Sci USA 1988; 85:1932–1936.
30. Rusche JR, Javaherian K, McDanal C, Petro J, Lynn DL, Grimaila R, Langlois A, Gallo RC, Arthur LO, Fischinger PJ, Bolognesi DP, Putney SD, Matthews TJ. Antibodies that inhibit fusion of HIV infected cells bind a 24 amino acid sequence of the viral envelope, gp120. Proc Natl Acad Sci USA 1988; 85:3198–3202.
31. Goudsmit J, Debouck C, Meloen RH, Smit L, Bakker M, Asher DM, Wolff AV, Gibbs CJ,Jr., Gajdusek DC. Human immunodeficiency virus type 1 neutralization epitope with conserved architecture elicits early type-specific antibodies in experimentally infected chimpanzees. Proc Natl Acad Sci USA 1988; 85:4478–4482.
32. Cease KB, Margalit H, Cornette JL, Putney SD, Robey WG, Ouyang C, Streicher HZ, Fischinger PJ, Gallo RC, DeLisi C, Berzofsky JA. Helper T-cell antigenic site identification in the AIDS virus gp120 envelope protein and induction of immunity in mice to the native protein using a 16-residue synthetic peptide. Proc Natl Acad Sci USA 1987; 84:4249–4253.
33. Berzofsky JA, Bensussan A, Cease KB, Bourge JF, Cheynier R, Lurhuma Z, Salaün J-J, Gallo RC, Shearer GM, Zagury D. Antigenic peptides recognized by T lymphocytes from AIDS viral envelope-immune humans. Nature 1988; 334:706–708.
34. Hale PM, Cease KB, Houghten RA, Ouyang C, Putney S, Javaherian K, Margalit H, Cornette JL, Spouge JL, DeLisi C, Berzofsky JA. T-cell multideterminant regions in the human immunodeficiency virus envelope: toward overcoming the problem of major histocompatibility complex restriction. Int Immunol 1989; 1:409–415.
35. Takahashi H, Cohen J, Hosmalin A, Cease KB, Houghten R, Cornette J,

DeLisi C, Moss B, Germain RN, Berzofsky JA. An immunodominant epitope of the HIV gp160 envelope glycoprotein recognized by class I MHC molecule-restricted murine cytotoxic T lymphocytes. Proc Natl Acad Sci USA 1988; 85:3105–3109.

36. Clerici M, Stocks NI, Zajac RA, Boswell RN, Bernstein DC, Mann DL, Shearer GM, Berzofsky JA. Interleukin-2 production used to detect antigenic peptide recognition by T-helper lymphocytes from asymptomatic HIV seropositive individuals. Nature 1989; 339:383–385.
37. Hosmalin A, Clerici M, Houghten R, Pendleton CD, Flexner C, Lucey DR, Moss B, Germain RN, Shearer GM, Berzofsky JA. An epitope in HIV-1 reverse transcriptase recognized by both mouse and human CTL. Proc Natl Acad Sci USA 1990; 87:2344–2348.
38. Berzofsky JA, Pendleton CD, Clerici M, Ahlers J, Lucey DR, Putney SD, Shearer GM. Construction of peptides encompassing multideterminant clusters of HIV envelope to induce in vitro T-cell responses in mice and humans of multiple MHC types. J Clin Invest 1991; 88:876–884.
39. Clerici M, Lucey DR, Zajac RA, Boswell RN, Gebel HM, Takahashi H, Berzofsky J, Shearer GM. Detection of cytotoxic T lymphocytes specific for synthetic peptides of gp160 in HIV-seropositive individuals. J Immunol 1991; 146:2214–2219.
40. Berzofsky JA. Development of artificial vaccines against HIV using defined epitopes. FASEB J 1991; 5:2412–2418.
41. Oscherwitz J, Gotch FM, Cease KB, Berzofsky JA. New insights and approaches regarding B- and T-cell epitopes in HIV vaccine design. AIDS 1999; 13:S163–S174.
42. Walker BD, Plata F. Cytotoxic T lymphocytes against HIV. AIDS 1990; 4:177–184.
43. McMichael AJ, Walker BD. Cytotoxic T lymphocyte epitopes: implications for HIV vaccines. AIDS 1994; 8(suppl 1):S155–S173.
44. Plata F, Autran B, Martins LP, Wain-Hobson S, Raphaël M, Mayaud C, Denis M, Guillon J-M, Debré P. AIDS virus-specific cytotoxic T lymphocytes in lung disorders. Nature 1987; 328:348–351.
45. Hadida F, Haas G, Zimmermann N, Hosmalin A, Spohn R, Samri A, Jung G, Debre P, Autran B. CTLs from lymphoid organs recognize an optimal HLA-A2-restricted and HLA-B52-restricted nonapeptide and several epitopes in the C-terminal region of HIV-1 Nef. J Immunol 1995; 154:4174–4186.
46. Belyakov IM, Wyatt LS, Ahlers JD, Earl P, Pendleton CD, Kelsall BL, Strober W, Moss B, Berzofsky JA. Induction of mucosal CTL response by intrarectal immunization with a replication-deficient recombinant vaccinia virus expressing HIV 89.6 envelope protein. J Virol 1998; 72:8264–8272.

47. Gulukota K, DeLisi C. HLA allele selection for designing peptide vaccines. Genet Anal 1996; 13:81–86.
48. Javaherian K, Langlois AJ, McDanal C, Ross KL, Eckler LI, Jellis CL, Profy AT, Rusche JR, Bolognesi DP, Putney SD, Matthews TJ. Principal neutralizing domain of the human immunodeficiency virus type 1 envelope protein. Proc Natl Acad Sci USA 1989; 86:6768–6772.
49. Shirai M, Pendleton CD, Berzofsky JA. Broad recognition of cytotoxic T-cell epitopes from the HIV-1 envelope protein with multiple class I histocompatibility molecules. J Immunol 1992; 148:1657–1667.
50. Bergmann CC, Tong L, Cua RV, Sensintaffar JL, Stohlman SA. Cytotoxic T-cell repertoire selection: a single amino acid determines alternative class I restriction. J Immunol 1994; 152:5603–5612.
51. Nehete PN, Casement KS, Arlinghaus RB, Sastry KJ. Studies on in vivo induction of HIV-1 envelope-specific cytotoxic T lymphocytes by synthetic peptides from the V3 loop region of HIV-1 IIIB gp 120. Cell Immunol 1995; 160:217–223.
52. Achour A, Picard O, Mbika J-P, Willer A, Snart R, Bizzini B, Carelli C, Burny A, Zagury D. Envelope protein and p18(IIIB) peptide recognized by cytotoxic T lymphocytes from humans immunized with human immunodeficiency virus envelope. Vaccine 1993; 11:699–701.
53. Achour A, Lemhammedi S, Picard O, M'Bika JP, Zagury JF, Moukrim Z, Willer A, Beix F, Burny A, Zagury D. Cytotoxic T lymphocytes specific for HIV-1 gp160 antigen and synthetic P18III_B peptide in an HLA-A11-immunized individual. AIDS Res Hum Retroviruses 1994; 10:19–25.
54. Alexander-Miller MA, Parker KC, Tsukui T, Pendleton CD, Coligan JE, Berzofsky JA. Molecular analysis of presentation by HLA-A2.1 of a promiscuously binding V3 loop peptide from the HIV-1 envelope protein to human CTL. Int Immunol 1996; 8:641–649.
55. LaRosa GJ, Davide JP, Weinhold K, Waterbury JA, Profy AT, Lewis JA, Langlois AJ, Dreesman GR, Boswell RN, Shadduck P, Holley LH, Karplus M, Bolognesi DP, Matthews TJ, Emini EA, Putney SD. Conserved sequence and structural elements in the HIV-1 principal neutralizing determinant. Science 1990; 249:932–935.
56. Javaherian K, Langlois AJ, LaRosa GJ, Profy AT, Bolognesi DP, Herlihy WC, Putney SD, Matthews TJ. Broadly neutralizing antibodies elicited by the hypervariable neutralizing determinant of HIV-1. Science 1990; 250: 1590–1593.
57. Mitchison NA. The carrier effect in the secondary response to hapten-protein conjugates. II. Cellular cooperation. Eur J Immunol 1971; 1:18.
58. Shirai M, Pendleton CD, Ahlers J, Takeshita T, Newman M, Berzofsky JA. Helper-CTL determinant linkage required for priming of anti-HIV

CD8$^+$ CTL in vivo with peptide vaccine constructs. J Immunol 1994; 152: 549–556.

59. Shirai M, Chen M, Arichi T, Nishioka M, Newman M, Nakazawa T, Feinstone SM, Berzofsky JA. Use of intrinsic and extrinsic helper epitopes for in vivo induction of anti-hepatitis C virus cytotoxic T lymphocytes (CTL) with CTL epitope peptide vaccines. J Infect Dis 1996; 173:24–31.
60. Widmann C, Romero P, Maryanski JL, Corradin G, Valmori D. T helper epitopes enhance the cytotoxic response of mice immunized with MHC class I-restricted malaria peptides. J Immunol Methods 1992; 155:95–99.
61. Lasarte JJ, Sarobe P, Gullón A, Prieto J, Borrás-Cuesta F. Induction of cytotoxic T lymphocytes in mice against the principal neutralizing domain of HIV-1 by immunization with an engineered T-cytotoxic-T-helper synthetic peptide construct. Cell Immunol 1992; 141:211–218.
62. Guerder S, Matzinger P. A fail-safe mechanism for maintaining self-tolerance. J Exp Med 1992; 176:553–564.
63. Ridge JP, Di Rosa F, Matzinger P. A conditioned dendritic cell can be a temporal bridge between a CD4+ T-helper and a T-killer cell. Nature 1998; 393:474–478.
64. Schoenberger SP, Toes REM, van der Voort EIH, Offringa R, Melief CJM. T-cell help for cytotoxic T lymphocytes is mediated by CD40-CD40L interactions. Nature 1998; 393:480–483.
65. Bennett SRM, Carbone FR, Karamalis F, Flavell RA, Miller JFAP, Heath WR. Help for cytotoxic-T-cell responses is mediated by CD40 signalling. Nature 1998; 393:478–480.
66. Ahlers JD, Pendleton CD, Dunlop N, Minassian A, Nara PL, Berzofsky JA. Construction of an HIV-1 peptide vaccine containing a multideterminant helper peptide linked to a V3 loop peptide 18 inducing strong neutralizing antibody responses in mice of multiple MHC haplotypes after two immunizations. J Immunol 1993; 150:5647–5665.
67. Palker TJ, Matthews TJ, Langlois A, Tanner ME, Martin ME, Scearce RM, Kim JE, Berzofsky JA, Bolognesi DP, Haynes BF. Polyvalent human immunodeficiency virus synthetic immunogen comprised of envelope gp120 T helper cell sites and B cell neutralization epitopes. J Immunol 1989; 142:3612–3619.
68. Hart MK, Palker TJ, Matthews TJ, Langlois AJ, Lerche NW, Martin ME, Scearce RM, McDanal C, Bolognesi DP, Haynes BF. Synthetic peptides containing T and B cell epitopes from human immunodeficiency virus envelope gp120 induce anti-HIV proliferative responses and high titers of neutralizing antibodies in rhesus monkeys. J Immunol 1990; 145:2677–2685.
69. Hart MK, Weinhold KJ, Scearce RM, Washburn EM, Clark CA, Palker TJ, Haynes BF. Priming of anti-human immunodeficiency virus (HIV)

CD8+ cytotoxic T cells *in vivo* by carrier-free HIV synthetic peptides. Proc Natl Acad Sci USA 1991; 88:9448–9452.

70. Haynes BF, Torres JV, Langlois AJ, Bolognesi DP, Gardner MB, Palker TJ, Scearce RM, Jones DM, Moody MA, McDanal C, Matthews TJ. Induction of HIVMN neutralizing antibodies in primates using a prime-boost regimen of hybrid synthetic gp120 envelope peptides. J Immunol 1993; 151:1646–1653.
71. Yasutomi Y, Palker TJ, Gardner MB, Haynes BF, Letvin NL. Synthetic peptide in mineral oil adjuvant elicits simian immunodeficiency virus-specific CD8+ cytotoxic T lymphocytes in Rhesus monkeys. J Immunol 1993; 151:5096–5105.
72. Haynes BF, Moody MA, Heinley CS, Korber B, Millard WA, Scearce RM. HIV type 1 V3 region primer-induced antibody suppression is overcome by administration of C4-V3 peptides as a polyvalent immunogen. AIDS Res Hum Retroviruses 1995; 11:211–221.
73. Ahlers JD, Dunlop N, Pendleton CD, Newman M, Nara PL, Berzofsky JA. Candidate HIV type1 multideterminant cluster peptide-P18MN vaccine constructs elicit type 1 helper T cells, cytotoxic T cells, and neutralizing antibody, all using the same adjuvant immunization. AIDS Res Hum Retroviruses 1996; 12:259–272.
74. Humphrey RW, Pinto LA, Fowke K, Merced-Galindez F, Ahlers JD, Little R, Dunlop N, Pendleton CD, Kohler D, Nara P, Shcarer GM, Berzofsky JA, Yarchoan R. A phase I protocol for the evaluation of the safety and immunogenicity of vaccination with synthetic HIV envelope peptides in patients with early HIV: a preliminary report [abstract]. J Human Virol 1997; 1:181.
75. Pinto LA, Berzofsky JA, Fowke KR, Littles RF, Merced-Galindez F, Humphreys R, Ahlers J, Dunlop N, Cohen RB, Steinberg SM, Nara P, Shearer GM, Yarchoan R. HIV-specific immunity following immunization with HIV synthetic envelope peptides in asymptomatic HIV-infected patients. AIDS 1999; 13:2003–2012.
76. Bartlett JA, Wasserman SS, Hicks CB, Dodge RT, Weinhold KJ, Tacket CO, Ketter N, Wittek AE, Palker TJ, Haynes BF, Datri 010 Study Group . Safety and immunogenicity of an HLA-based HIV envelope polyvalent synthetic peptide immunogen. AIDS 1998; 12:1291–1300.
77. Berzofsky JA. Designing peptide vaccines to broaden recognition and enhance potency. Ann NY Acad Sci 1995; 754:161–168.
78. Boehncke W-H, Takeshita T, Pendleton CD, Sadegh-Nasseri S, Racioppi L, Houghten RA, Berzofsky JA, Germain RN. The importance of dominant negative effects of amino acids side chain substitution in peptide-MHC molecule interactions and T-cell recognition. J Immunol 1993; 150: 331–341.

79. Takahashi H, Nakagawa Y, Pendleton CD, Houghten RA, Yokomuro K, Germain RN, Berzofsky JA. Induction of broadly cross-reactive cytotoxic T cells recognizing an HIV-1 envelope determinant. Science 1992; 255: 333–336.
80. Ahlers JD, Takeshita T, Pendleton CD, Berzofsky JA. Enhanced immunogenicity of HIV-1 vaccine construct by modification of the native peptide sequence. Proc Natl Acad Sci USA 1997; 94:10856–10861.
81. Sarobe P, Pendleton CD, Akatsuka T, Lau D, Engelhard VH, Feinstone SM, Berzofsky JA. Enhanced in vitro potency and in vivo immunogenicity of a CTL epitope from hepatitis C virus core protein following amino acid replacement at secondary HLA-A2.1 binding positions. J Clin Invest 1998; 102:1239–1248.
82. Pogue RR, Eron J, Frelinger JA, Matsui M. Amino-terminal alteration of the HLA-A*0201-restricted human immunodeficiency virus pol peptide increases complex stability and *in vitro* immunogenicity. Proc Natl Acad Sci USA 1995; 92:8166–8170.
83. Parkhurst MR, Salgaller ML, Southwood S, Robbins PF, Sette A, Rosenberg SA, Kawakami Y. Improved induction of melanoma-reactive CTL with peptides from the melanoma antigen gp100 modified at HLA-A*0201-binding residues. J Immunol 1996; 157:2539–2548.
84. Rosenberg SA, Yang JC, Schwartzentruber DJ, Hwu P, Marincola FM, Topalian SL, Restifo NP, Dudley ME, Schwartz SL, Spiess PJ, Wunderlich JR, Parkhurst MR, Kawakami Y, Seipp CA, Einhorn JH, White DE. Immunologic and therapeutic evaluation of a synthetic peptide vaccine for the treatment of patients with metastatic melanoma. Nature Medicine 1998; 4:321–327.
85. Rammensee H-G, Friede T, Stevanovíc S. MHC ligands and peptide motifs: first listing. Immunogenetics 1995; 41:178–228.
86. Ruppert J, Sidney J, Celis E, Kubo RT, Grey HM, Sette A. Prominent role of secondary anchor residues in peptide binding to HLA-A2.1 molecules. Cell 1993; 74:929–937.
87. Ratner L, Haseltine W, Patarca R, Livak KJ, Starcich B, Josephs SF, Doran ER, Rafalski JA, Whitehorn EA, Baumeister K, Ivanoff L, Petteway SR, Jr., Pearson ML, Lautenberger JA, Papas TS, Ghrayeb J, Chang NT, Gallo RC, Wong-Staal F. Complete nucleotide sequence of the AIDS virus HTLV-III. Nature 1985; 313:277–284.
88. Shirai M, Okada H, Nishioka M, Akatsuka T, Wychowski C, Houghten R, Pendleton CD, Feinstone SM, Berzofsky JA. An epitope in hepatitis C virus core region recognized by cytotoxic T cells in mice and humans. J Virol 1994; 68:3334–3342.
89. Shirai M, Arichi T, Nishioka M, Nomura T, Ikeda K, Kawanishi K, Engelhard VH, Feinstone SM, Berzofsky JA. CTL responses of HLA-A2.1-

transgenic mice specific for hepatitis C viral peptides predict epitopes for CTL of humans carrying HLA-A2.1.J Immunol 1995; 154:2733–2742.
90. Battegay M, Fikes J, Di Bisceglie AM, Wentworth PA, Sette A, Celis E, Ching W-M, Grakoui A, Rice CM, Kurokohchi K, Berzofsky JA, Hoofnagle JH, Feinstone SM, Akatsuka T. Patients with chronic hepatitis C have circulating cytotoxic T cells which recognize hepatitis C virus-encoded peptides binding to HLA-A2.1 molecules. J Virol 1995; 69:2462–2470.
91. Cerny A, McHutchison JG, Pasquinelli C, Brown ME, Brothers MA, Grabscheid B, Fowler P, Houghton M, Chisari FV. Cytotoxic T lymphocyte response to hepatitis C virus-derived peptides containing the HLA A2.1 binding motif. J Clin Invest 1995; 95:521–530.
92. Man S, Newberg MH, Crotzer VL, Luckey CJ, Williams NS, Chen Y, Huczko EL, Ridge JP, Engelhard VH. Definition of a human T cell epitope from influenza A non-structural protein 1 using HLA-A2.1 transgenic mice. Int Immunol 1995; 7:597–605.
93. Vitiello A, Marchesini D, Furze J, Sherman LA, Chesnut RW. Analysis of the HLA-restricted influenza-specific cytotoxic T lymphocyte response in transgenic mice carrying a chimeric human-mouse class I major histocompatibility complex. J Exp Med 1991; 173:1007–1015.
94. Derby MA, Alexander-Miller MA, Tse R, Berzofsky JA. High avidity CTL exploit two complementary mechanisms to provide better protection against viral infection than low avidity CTL. J Immunol 2001; 166:1690–1697.
95. Takahashi H, Merli S, Putney SD, Houghten R, Moss B, Germain RN, Berzofsky JA. A single amino acid interchange yields reciprocal CTL specificities for HIV gp160. Science 1989; 246:118–121.
96. Takahashi H, Houghten R, Putney SD, Margulies DH, Moss B, Germain RN, Berzofsky JA. Structural requirements for class-I MHC molecule-mediated antigen presentation and cytotoxic T-cell recognition of an immunodominant determinant of the HIV envelope protein. J Exp Med 1989; 170:2023–2035.
97. Earl PL, Hugin AW, Moss B. Removal of cryptic poxvirus transcription termination signals from the human immunodeficiency virus type 1 envelope gene enhances expression and immunogenicity of a recombinant vaccinia virus. J Virol 1990; 64:2448–2451.
98. Kozlowski S, Corr M, Takeshita T, Boyd LF, Pendleton CD, Germain RN, Berzofsky JA, Margulies DH. Serum angiotensin-1 converting enzyme activity processes an HIV 1 gp160 peptide for presentation by MHC class I molecules. J Exp Med 1992; 175:1417–1422.
99. Takeshita T, Takahashi H, Kozlowski S, Ahlers JD, Pendleton CD, Moore RL, Nakagawa Y, Yokomuro K, Fox BS, Margulies DH, Berzofsky JA.

Molecular analysis of the same HIV peptide functionally binding to both a class I and a class II MHC molecule. J Immunol 1995; 154:1973–1986.
100. Alexander-Miller MA, Leggatt GR, Berzofsky JA. Selective expansion of high or low avidity cytotoxic T lymphocytes and efficacy for adoptive immunotherapy. Proc Natl Acad Sci USA 1996; 93:4102–4107.
101. Gallimore A, Dumrese T, Hengartner H, Zinkernagel RM, Rammensee HG. Protective immunity does not correlate with the hierarchy of virus-specific cytotoxic T-cell responses to naturally processed peptides. J Exp Med 1998; 187:1647–1657.
102. Herrath MGV, Coon B, Oldstone MBA. Low-affinity cytoxic T-lymphocytes require IFN-γ to clean an acute viral infection. Virology 1997; 229: 349–359.
103. Yee C, Savage PA, Lee PP, Davis MM, Greenberg PD. Isolation of high avidity melanoma-reactive CTL from heterogeneous populations using peptide-MHC tetramers. J Immunol 1999; 162:2227–2234.
104. Zeh III HJ, Perry-Lalley D, Dudley ME, Rosenberg SA, Yang JC. High avidity CTLs for two self-antigens demonstrate superior in vitro and in vivo antitumor efficacy. J Immunol 1999; 162:989–994.
105. Alexander-Miller MA, Leggatt GR, Sarin A, Berzofsky JA. Role of antigen, CD8, and Cytotoxic T lymphocyte avidity in high dose antigen induction of apoptosis of effector CTL. J Exp Med 1996; 184:485–492.
106. Alexander-Miller MA, Derby MA, Sarin A, Henkart PA, Berzofsky JA. Supra-optimal peptide/MHC causes a decrease in Bcl-2 and allows TNF-α receptor II-mediated apoptosis of CTL. J Exp Med 1998; 188(8):1391–1399.
107. Moskophidis D, Lechner F, Pircher H, Zinkernagel RM. Virus persistence in acutely infected immunocompetent mice by exhaustion of antiviral cytotoxic effector T cells. Nature 1993; 362:758–761.
108. Gallimore A, Glithero A, Godkin A, Tissot AC, Pluckthun A, Elliott T, Hengartner H, Zinkernagel R. Induction and exhaustion of lymphocytic choriomeningitis virus-specific cytotoxic T lymphocytes visualized using soluble tetrameric major histocompatibility complex class I-peptide complexes. J Exp Med 1998; 187:1383–1393.
109. Warren HS, Vogel FR, Chedid LA. Current status of immunological adjuvants. Ann Rev Immunol 1986; 4:369–388.
110. Levi M, Rudén U, Birx D, Loomis L, Redfield R, Lövgren K, Åkerblom L, Sandström E, Wahren B. The effects of adjuvants and multiple antigen peptides on humoral and cellular immune responses to gp160 of HIV-1. J AIDS 1993; 6:855–864.
111. Xu-Amano J, Kiyono H, Jackson RJ, Staats HF, Fujihashi K, Burrows PD, Elson CO, Pillai S, McGhee JR. Helper T-cell subsets for immuno-

globulin A responses: oral immunization with tetanus toxoid and cholera toxin as adjuvant selectively induces Th2 cells in mucosa associated tissues. J Exp Med 1993; 178:1309–1320.
112. Alving CR, Detrick B, Richards RL, Lewis MG, Shafferman A, Eddy GA. Novel adjuvant strategies for experimental malaria and AIDS vaccines. Ann N Y Acad Sci 1993; 690:265–275.
113. Kawamura H, Rosenberg SA, Berzofsky JA. Immunization with antigen and interleukin-2 in vivo overcomes Ir genetic low responsiveness. J Exp Med 1985; 162:381–386.
114. Good MF, Pombo D, Lunde MN, Maloy WL, Halenbeck R, Koths K, Miller LH, Berzofsky JA. Recombinant human interleukin-2 (IL-2) overcomes genetic nonresponsiveness to malaria sporozoite peptides.Correlation of effect with biological activity of IL-2. J Immunol 1988; 141:972–977.
115. Ahlers JD, Dunlop N, Alling DW, Nara PL, Berzofsky JA. Cytokine-in-adjuvant steering of the immune response phenotype to HIV-1 vaccine constructs: GM-CSF and TNFα synergize with IL-12 to enhance induction of CTL. J Immunol 1997; 158:3947–3958.
116. Tagliabue A, Boraschi D. Cytokines as vaccine adjuvants: interleukin 1 and its synthetic peptide 163–171. Vaccine 1993; 11:594–595.
117. Afonso LCC, Scharton TM, Vieira LQ, Wysocka M, Trinchieri G, Scott P. The adjuvant effect of interleukin-12 in a vaccine against *Leishmania major*. Science 1994; 263:235–237.
118. Bliss J, Van Cleave V, Murray K, Wiencis A, Ketchum M, Maylor R, Haire T, Resmini C, Abbas AK, Wolf SF. IL-12, as an adjuvant, promotes a T helper 1 cell, but does not suppress a T helper 2 cell recall response. J Immunol 1996; 156:887–894.
119. Disis ML, Bernhard H, Shiota FM, Hand SL, Gralow JR, Huseby ES, Gillis S, Cheever MA. Granulocyte-macrophage colony-stimulating factor: An effective adjuvant for protein and peptide-based vaccines. Blood 1996; 88:202–210.
120. Rao JB, Chamberlain RS, Bronte V, Carroll MW, Irvine KR, Moss B, Rosenberg SA, Restifo NP. IL-12 is an effective adjuvant to recombinant vaccinia virus-based tumor vaccines: enhancement by simultaneous B7–1 expression. J Immunol 1996; 156:3357–3365.
121. Arulanandam BP, O'Toole M, Metzger DW. Intranasal interleukin-12 is a powerful adjuvant for protective mucosal immunity. J Infect Dis 1999; 180:940–949.
122. Xiang Z, Ertl HCJ. Manipulation of the immune response to a plasmid-encoded viral antigen by coinoculation with plasmids expressing cytokines. Immunity 1995; 2:129–135.

123. Iwasaki A, Stiernholm BJN, Chan AK, Berinstein NL, Barber BH. Enhanced CTL responses mediated by plasmid DNA immunogens encoding costimulatory molecules and cytokines. J Immunol 1997; 158:4591–4601.
124. Harris N, Buller RM, Karupiah G. Gamma interferon-induced, nitric oxide-mediated inhibition of vaccinia virus replication. J Virol 1995; 69: 910–915.
125. Dranoff G, Jaffee E, Lazenby A, Golumbek P, Levitsky H, Brose K, Jackson V, Hamada H, Pardoll D, Mulligan RC. Vaccination with irradiated tumor cells engineered to secrete murine granulocyte-macrophage colony-stimulating factor stimulates potent, specific, and long-lasting anti-tumor immunity. Proc Natl Acad Sci USA 1993; 90:3539–3543.
126. Sin J-I, Kim JJ, Ugen KE, Ciccarelli RB, Higgins TJ, Weiner DB. Enhancement of protective humoral (Th2) and cell-mediated (Th1) immune responses against herpes simplex virus-2 through co-delivery of granulocyte-macrophage colony-stimulating factor expression cassettes. Eur J Immunol 1998; 28:3530–3540.
127. Belyakov IM, Derby MA, Ahlers JD, Kelsall BL, Earl P, Moss B, Strober W, Berzofsky JA. Mucosal immunization with HIV-1 peptide vaccine induces mucosal and systemic cytotoxic T lymphocytes and protective immunity in mice against intrarectal recombinant HIV-vaccinia challenge. Proc Natl Acad Sci USA 1998; 95:1709–1714.
128. Trinchieri G. Interleukin-12: a proinflammatory cytokine with immunoregulatory functions that bridge innate resistance and antigen-specific adaptive immunity. Annu Rev Immunol 1995; 13:251–276.
129. Szabo SJ, Dighe AS, Gubler U, Murphy KM. Regulation of the Interleukin (IL)-12R β2 subunit experession in developing T helper 1 (Th1) and Th2 cells. J Exp Med 1997; 185:817–824.
130. Mayr A, Hochstein-Mintzel V, Stickl H. Abstammung, eigenschaften and verwendung des attenuierten vaccinia-stammes MVA. Infection 1975; 3: 6–14.
131. Sutter G, Wyatt LS, Foley PL, Bennink JR, Moss B. A recombinant vector derived from the host range-restricted and highly attenuated MVA strain of vaccinia virus stimulates protective immunity in mice to influenza virus. Vaccine 1994; 12:1032–1040.
132. Meyer H, Sutter G, Mayr A. Mapping of deletions in the genome of the highly attenuated vaccinia virus MVA and their influence on virulence. J Gen Virol 1991; 72:1031–1038.
133. Carroll MW, Moss B. Host range and cytopathogenicity of the highly attenuated MVA strain of vaccinia virus: propagation and generation of recombinant viruses in a nonhuman mammalian cell line. Virology 1997; 238:198–211.
134. Wyatt LS, Shors ST, Murphy BR, Moss B. Development of a replication-

deficient recombinant vaccinia virus vaccine effective against parainfluenza virus 3 infection in an animal model. Vaccine 1996; 14:1451–1458.
135. Bender BS, Rowe CA, Taylor SF, Wyatt LS, Moss B, Small PAJr. Oral immunization with a replication-deficient recombinant vaccinia virus protects mice against influenza. J Virol 1996; 70:6418–6424.
136. Hanke T, Blanchard TJ, Schneider J, Ogg GS, Tan R, Becker M, Gilbert SC, Hill AV, Smith GL, McMichael A. Immunogenicities of intravenous and intramuscular administrations of modified vaccinia virus Ankara-based multi-CTL epitope vaccine for human immunodeficiency virus type 1 in mice. J Gen Virol 1998; 79:83-90.
137. Katz E, Wolffe EJ, Moss B. The cytoplasmic and transmembrane domains of the vaccinia virus B5R protein target a chimeric human immunodeficiency virus type 1 glycoprotein to the outer envelope of nascent vaccinia virions. J Virol 1997; 71:3178–3187.
138. Belyakov IM, Ahlers JD, Brandwein BY, Earl P, Kelsall BL, Moss B, Strober W, Berzofsky JA. The Importance of local mucosal HIV-specific $CD8^+$ cytotoxic T lymphocytes for resistance to mucosal-viral transmission in mice and enhancement of resistance by local administration of IL-12. J Clin Invest 1998; 102(12):2072–2081.
139. Ahmed R, Gray D. Immunological memory and protective immunity: understanding their relation. Science 1996; 272:54–60.
140. Kündig TM, Bachmann MF, Oehen S, Hoffmann UW, Simard JJL, Kalberer CP, Pircher H, Ohashi PS, Hengartner H, Zinkernagel RM. On the role of antigen in maintaining cytotoxic T-cell memory. Proc Natl Acad Sci USA 1996; 93:9716–9723.
141. Czerkinsky C, Anjuere F, McGhee JR, George-Chandy A, Holmgren J, Kieny MP, Fujiyashi K, Mestecky JF, Pierrefite-Carle V, Rask C, Sun J-B. Mucosal immunity and tolerance: relavance to vaccine development. Immunol Rev 1999; 170:197–222.
142. Belyakov IM, Kelsall B, Strober W, Berzofsky JA. Use of rIL-12 for enhancing the mucosal cytotoxic T lymphocyte response to a peptide HIV vaccine. J Invest Med 1998; 46:216A.
143. Belyakov IM, Ahlers JD, Clements JD, Strober W, Berzofsky JA. Interplay of cytokines and adjuvants in the regulation of mucosal and systemic HIV-specific cytotoxic T lymphocytes. J Immunol 2000; 165:6454–6462.
144. Dickinson BL, Clements JD. Dissociation of *Escherichia coli* heat-labile enterotoxin adjuvanticity from ADP-ribosyltransferase activity. Infect Immun 1995; 63:1617–1623.
145. Braun MC, He J, Wu C-Y, Kelsall BL. Cholera toxin suppresses interleukin (IL)-12 production and IL-12 receptor B1 and B2 chain expression. J Exp Med 1999; 189:541–552.
146. Simmons CP, Mastroeni P, Fowler R, Ghaem-Maghami M, Lycke N,

Pizza M, Rappuoli R, Dougan G. MHC class I-restricted cytotoxic lymphocyte responses induced by enterotoxin-based mucosal adjuvants. J Immunol 1999; 163:6502–6510.

147. Cooney EL, Collier AC, Greenberg PD, Coombs RW, Zarling J, Arditti DE, Hoffman MC, Hu SL, Corey L. Safety of and immunological response to a recombinant vaccinia virus vaccine expressing HIV envelope glycoprotein. Lancet 1991; 337:567–572.
148. Rooney JF, Wohlenberg C, Cremer KJ, Moss B, Notkins AL. Immunization with a vaccinia virus recombinant expressing herpes simplex virus type 1 glycoprotein D: Long-term protection and effect of revaccination. J Virol 1988; 62(5):1530–1534.
149. Belyakov IM, Moss B, Strober W, Berzofsky JA. Mucosal vaccination overcomes the barrier to recombinant vaccinia immunization caused by preexisting poxvirus immunity. Proc Natl Acad Sci USA 1999; 96:4512–4517.
150. Ahlers JD, Belyakov IM, Matsui S, Berzofsky JA. Mechanisms of cytokine synergy essential for vaccine protection against viral challenge. Int Immunol 2001; 13:897–908.
151. Ahlers JD, Belyakov IM, Matsui S, Berzofsky JA. Signals delivered through TCR instruct IL-12R expression: IL-12 and TNFα synergize for IL-12R expression at low antigen dose. Int Immunol 2001. In press.
152. Belyakov IM, Hel Z, Kelsall B, Ahlers JD, Nacsa J, Watkins DI, Allen TM, Sette A, Altman J, Woodward R, Markham P, Clements JD, Kuznetsov VA, Franchini G, Strober W, Berzofsky JA. The importance of mucosal CTL vs systemic CTL in reducing viral load after intrarectal challenge of rhesus macaques with pathogenic SHIV [abstr]. Scand J Immunol 2001; 54(suppl 1):120.

7

DNA Vaccines for Immunodeficiency Viruses

Harriet L. Robinson

Emory Vaccine Center and
Yerkes Primate Research Center
Emory University
Atlanta Georgia

CHALLENGES FOR AN AIDS VACCINE

HIV-1, first recognized in 1983, now scourges the world as the fourth leading cause of death. Most HIV-1 infections strike sexually active young adults, depleting both developed and developing countries of innovators, breadwinners, and parents. Why has this emergent epidemic so devastated populations, and why, with the tools of modern biology, has it been so hard to develop a vaccine. Within 4 years of the ability to culture polio virus, the Salk vaccine was reaching the public. We have been able to grow HIV-1 and have known the complete sequence of its genome for 15 years, yet are still without a vaccine. What is it about this virus that so challenges our ability to imprint an immune system with a protective memory response?

Features of HIV-1 infections that defy vaccination include the high variability of its genome, an inherent resistance to antibodies, and the ability of the virus to establish latent infections. The variability of HIV-1 results from its polymerase, an RNA-directed DNA polymerase introducing one to two mutations per genome

(~10,000 bp) at each round of infection (1,2). These large numbers of mutations (no two viruses are the same) afford HIV-1 unrivaled opportunity for evading immune responses. A second feature of HIV-1 that confounds vaccination is the very poor ability of this virus to be blocked by neutralizing antibodies (3,4). This ''invisibility'' to neutralizing antibody is in large part due to very high levels of glycosylation of the envelope glycoprotein (Env) (25 glycosylation sites on the gp120 receptor binding subunit of Env) (5). These glycosyl groups, along with variable loops of amino acid sequences, shield conserved entry-mediating regions of Env from antibody (6). A third feature contributing to the difficulty of vaccination is the ability of HIV-1 to lie latent in infected cells (7). Proviral DNA, inserted and therefore immortalized in the chromosomal DNA of hosts, permits infections to lie latent, unavailable for clearance by antiretroviral drugs or immune responses.

DNA VACCINES

DNA-based vaccines use bacterial plasmids to express protein immunogens in vaccinated hosts (for reviews, see Refs. 8, 9). Recombinant DNA technology is used to clone cDNAs encoding immunogens of interest into eukaryotic expression plasmids. Vaccine plasmids are then amplified in bacteria, purified, and directly inoculated into the hosts being vaccinated. DNA can be inoculated by a saline-needle injection or by a gene gun device, which delivers DNA-coated gold beads into skin. The plasmid DNA is taken up by host cells, the vaccine protein is expressed, processed, and presented in the context of self-major histocompatibility class I and class II molecules, and an immune response against the DNA-encoded immunogen is generated.

DNA vaccines generate immune responses with ng levels of expressed protein (9). Initial skepticism about DNA vaccines was rooted in the belief that such low levels of expressed protein, approximately 1000 times lower than those in killed whole virus or protein vaccines, could not possibly raise immune responses. So why do DNA vaccines work? The answer probably lies in the high efficiencies of antigen presentation that are achieved by the direct transfection of professional antigen-presenting cells (10–14). Cross-priming of dendritic cells or macrophages has played different roles in different experimental models (12,14,15). Cross-priming occurs when a bone marrow–derived cell (such as a dendritic cell) presents peptides derived from proteins synthesized in another cell (16). And finally, an adjuvant activity of unmethylated CpG sequences in plasmid DNA appears to contribute to the efficiency of DNA vaccines (for reviews, see Refs. 17, 18).

INCREASING THE EFFICIENCY OF DNA VACCINES

Although DNA vaccines for most antigens work quite well in inbred strains of mice, their early use in nonhuman primates and humans has required both larger doses (up to 5 mg) and more boosters (three to four) than may be practical for mass vaccination (19–21). The early ''proof of concept'' experiments for HIV-1 DNAs in humans also have been disappointing in that trials have resulted in lower immune responses than are generally considered to be required for protective immunizations against HIV-1 (22,23). Thus, a major effort has been directed towards improving the efficiency of DNA-based immunizations for HIV-1. The most successful of these approaches are briefly presented below.

RNA and Codon-Optimized Genes

Markedly increased levels of HIV-1 gene expression have been achieved by using RNA-optimized and/or codon-optimized sequences (Table 1). These optimized sequences are sometimes referred to as ''humanized'' sequences. Optimizations initially focused on mutating inhibitory sequences that govern the transport of HIV-1 mRNAs to the cytoplasm (Table 1, study 1) (24). These mutations rendered the HIV-1 gag gene independent of Rev and greatly increased its expression. Second-generation optimizations of sequences focused on rendering codons the same as those in highly expressed human sequences as well as the removal of INS sequences (Table 1, studies 2 and 3) (25,26). Both forms of optimization changed HIV-1 genes from being AT-rich (~60% AT) to being GC-rich (~60% GC) and increased levels of expression in the absence of Rev by at least two orders of magnitude. The optimized sequences raised much higher antibody and T-cell responses in mice and nonhuman primates than nonoptimized sequences (27,28).

Formulations of DNA

Considerable efforts have focused on identifying and developing formulations of DNA that improve the efficiency of immunizations by both stabilizing the DNA against degradation and increasing the efficiency of the delivery of DNA into antigen-presenting cells. At present, two formulations, the use of alum and adsorbing DNA onto cationic biodegradable microparticles, are of particular interest (Table 2). Both of these formulations have had adjuvant effects of more than 10-fold (29,30). When these two approaches were combined by mixing DNA microparticles with alum, antibody titers were increased 250-fold (30). Both alum and the microparticles have proven safe for human use. Alum is an approved vaccine adjuvant for human use. The microparticles are composed of poly(lactide-co-glycolide) formulated with cetyltrimethylammonium bromide, both of which are currently used in humans.

Genetic Adjuvants

At least 18 different immunostimulatory molecules have been tested as genetic adjuvants for HIV-1 DNA vaccines (Table 3) (for review, see Ref. 31). Most have

Table 1 RNA-Optimized and Codon-Optimized HIV-1 Vaccine Inserts

Study	Modification	Expression/ immunogenicity	Comment	Ref.
1	Inactivation of multiple INS (AU-rich regions and AUUUA motifs) to achieve Rev-independent expression of Gag and PR	140-fold increase in Gag expression, expression slightly higher than achieved with Rev Tc raised in mice with mutated gag, the levels of these not as high as raised with a recombinant vaccinia virus expressing gag	Activity attributed to the stabilization of RNA All elements in a sequence must be optimized for high expression INS sequences act whether or not the sequence is translated and are independent of splicing	24,27
2	Optimization of codons to those for highly expressed human genes in Gag-PR Optimal consensus sequence for the initiation of translation, GCCACCAUGG Hepatitis B virus posttranscriptional regulatory element, PRE	300- to 1000-fold increase in Gag expression, 500–1000 ng of Gag produced in transient transfections in 293 cells In mice, Tc raised with 100 times less DNA, 30% of cells score in IFN-γ ICC for a Gag epitope following a single administration of 20 μg of DNA 4/4 rhesus had Tc after 2 or 3 1 mg doses of DNA delivered at 4-week intervals; 2 out of 4 macaques react with 2 or 3 peptide pools. Only 1/4 rhesus recieving unmodified Gag showed low and transient Tc	Inactivation of INS and codon optimization of protease led to lower levels of particle production than only inactivation of INS, hypothesized to reflect protease prematurely cleaving the Pr55 Gag precursor	25
3	Optimization of codons in Env for highly expressed human genes	Env expression became Rev-independent and increased from barely detectable to dominant bands on Western blots Gene gun immunizations in mice reveal earlier and higher antibody responses		26,28

Table 2 Formulations That Improve the Efficacy of DNA Immunizations

Formulation	Effect	Comment	Ref.
DNA plus alum	Up to 100-fold increases in antibody responses in mice 5- to 10-fold increases in antibody responses in nonhuman primates	Alum must be comprised of negatively charged aluminum salts that do not bind to DNA Alum did not affect levels of antigen expression in situ, but exerted effects post-expression Alum did not affect the Th1 bias of saline injections of DNA	29,44
DNA formulated on cationic polylactide-coglycolide microspheres	Up to 250-fold increases in antibody responses in mice 1 μg doses of formulated DNA raise equivalent levels of Tc as 2×10^7 pfu of recombinant vaccinia virus	The best increases currently obtained by a delivery vehicle Hypothesized to act by preventing degradation and delivering DNA to APC Small particles more effective than large ones	30

had fairly modest effects. This may be due in part to the expressed lymphokines, chemokines, or costimulatory molecules acting against an endogenous background of similar molecules. Consistent with this, we have found genetic adjuvants to have more pronounced effects in neonates than adults (T. Pertmer and H. L. Robinson, unpublished). In neonates, lower backgrounds of endogenous immunomodulatory molecules may afford introduced genetic adjuvants the opportunity for a greater impact on immune response.

The relatively small effects of genetic adjuvants on immune responses may also reflect more stringent temporal requirements for the expressed adjuvant than evaluated in initial experiments. A study comparing the temporal relationship between the delivery of IL-2 or GM-CSF–expressing DNA and a plasmid-expressing HIV-1 gp120 revealed increases in immune responses when cytokine DNA were delivered after but not at the time of the delivery of the DNA immunogen (32,33). Pre- or codelivery of the cytokine DNA resulted in augmentation of nonspecific proliferative responses and decreases in the specific response (32).

Table 3 Genetic Adjuvants and HIV-1 DNA Immunizations[a]

Immunomodulator expressed by genetic adjuvant	HIV-1 DNA immunogen	Outcome	Comment	Ref.
IL-1α	Env Gag-pol	Increased antibody 2- to 5-fold		45
IL-2	Env Gag	Increase antibody and CD8 responses when IL-2–Ig DNA administered two days after Gag or Env-DNA	IL-2 must be used as an IL-2–Ig fusion Adjuvant effect seen in different strains of mice as well as macaques	20,32 45 45
		In another study, simultaneous administration of IL-2 DNA increased antibody responses 2- to 5-fold and had marginal effects on Tc responses	IL-2–Ig DNA more effective than IL-2–Ig protein	46
		In a third study, co-delivered IL-2 increased antibody responses in 2 rhesus		
IL-4	Env	Simultaneous administration reduced antibody responses 10-fold		32
		Other studies report enhancement of antibody 5- to 10-fold in mice		45
		A 3rd study reports enhanced antibody in rhesus macaques		46
IL-5	Env Gag-pol	Simultaneous administration increased antibody 5- to 10-fold		45
IL-10	Env Gag-pol	Simultaneous administration increased antibody by 5- to 10-fold Increased Th1-biased immunity		45
IL-12	Env	Simultaneous administration reduced antibody but enhanced Tc	IL-12 DNA caused splenomegaly in mice Levels of IFN-γ in serum increased	47
IL-15	Env Gag-pol	Simultaneous administration increased antibody responses 2- to 5-fold, increased Tc responses		45

IL-18	Env Gag-pol	Simultaneous administration increased antibody responses 2- to 5-fold, marginal effects on Tc responses		45
IFN-γ	Env Gag-pol	Simultaneous administration had no effect on antibody in rhesus macaques		46
G-CSF	Env Gag-pol	Simultaneous administration had no effect		48
GM-CSF	Env Gag-pol Vif Nef	Two studies find that administration at two days after Env DNA enhanced antibody responses Another study found enhanced antibody and proliferative responses for codelivered GM-CSF DNA	Simultaneous administration found to reduce antibody repsonses in mice, other studies report enhanced antibody responses	33,47,48
M-CSF	Env Gag-pol	Simultaneous administration enhanced Tc	Associated with cd11c+ cells at the site of injection and antigen-specific induction of mip-1β	48
TNF-α	Env Gag-pol	Simultaneous administration increased antibody by 2- to 5-fold, increased Tc responses		45
TNF-β	Env Gag-pol	No clear effect on antibody or Tc responses		45
RANTES	Env Gag-pol	Simultaneous administration increased Tc	Studies done in mice as well as two HIV-1–infected chimpanzees, possible increase in the stimulation index in the chimpanzees after the 2nd of 3 immunizations	49
MIP-1a	Env Gag-pol	Simultaneous administration increased stimulation index but not Tc		49
CD80 (B7.1)	Env Gag-pol	Simultaneous administration did not affect immune responses		50
CD86 (B7.2)	Env Gag-pol	Simultaneous administration increased Tc, did not affect antibody		50

[a] Unless otherwise stated, studies were done in mice.
Tc, Cytotoxic T cells.

In contrast, delivery at 2 days postimmunization augmented the specific immune response that had just been primed. In these studies, all effects were less than 10-fold, and delivery of DNAs expressing IL-2, IL-4, or GM-CSF at the same time as the delivery of the vaccine DNA uniformly resulted in reduced (not enhanced) responses. Delivery of IL-2 as an IL-2–Ig fusion was more effective than IL-2 alone (32). This was hypothesized to reflect 1) a longer serum half-life of the IL-2 as an IL-2–Ig fusion protein, 2) the divalent avidity of the IL-2 in the Ig-fusion protein, and 3) the ability of the Ig-fusion proteins to augment signaling via initiating receptor clustering (32). Recently, studies with DNA-expressing and L-2–Ig fusion have been extended into macaques. In rhesus, the IL-2–Ig plasmid was more effective than multiple deliveries of IL-2–Ig protein at enhancing both the peak and memory levels of specific CD8 responses (20). Augmentation of immune responses was about 10-fold, achieving memory levels of p11c-m-epitope–specific CD8 cells of 0.2–0.3%.

HETEROLOGOUS PRIME/BOOST PROTOCOLS: PRINCIPLES FROM RODENT MODELS

The basic principles for boosting DNA primes with other immunogens have been worked on in rodent models (Table 4). These studies reveal that DNA priming should precede immunization with the heterologous immunogen. Not unexpectedly, heterologous prime/boost studies reveal protein boosters both increasing antibody responses and in certain instances impacting the avidity maturation of the antibody responses (34). Recombinant viral boosters increase both antibody and cell-mediated immune responses (35,36). The protocols in Table 4 are but a few of the myriad of potential heterologous prime/boost protocols. By the correct use of vectors one should be able to bias immune responses towards type one or type 2 T-cell help (37) or raise mucosal as well as systemic immune responses. Indeed, in mice DNA priming followed by intranasal delivery of an adenoviral vector raised vaginal IgA (38) (Table 4).

Among the currently tested heterologous prime/boost protocols, of particular note are the boosts for T-cell responses that occur when recombinant poxviruses are used to boost DNA-primed responses (Table 4; Fig. 1). Among the tested poxvirus vectors, modified vaccinia Ankara (MVA) has been more effective than NYVAC (New York Department of Health vaccinia virus) or fowl pox. The strong boosting of DNA-primed CD8 responses by poxvirus boosters is likely to reflect memory cells induced by the DNA being very effectively boosted by the recombinant poxvirus infection. For DNA-raised responses, submicrogram levels of antigen raise low peaks of both effector and memory cells (typically $<1\%$ of total CD8 cells) (20,39; H. L. Robinson, unpublished findings). These low levels of memory cells are boosted both by the larger amount

Table 4 Heterologous Prime/Boost Protocols: Principles from Rodent Models

Prime	Boost	Outcome	Comment	Ref.
DNA	Protein	Increased antibody responses	Antibody to the HIV-1 Env undergoes avidity maturation following the protein booster but does not acquire cross-neutralizing activity for primary isolates	34
DNA	Recombinant poxviruses	Increased antibody responses 5- to 100-fold increases in CD8 cells	DNA has to be first MVA superior to NYVAC i.d. or i.v. injections best for boosters	35,51–54
DNA	Recombinant poxvirus Followed by protein	Increased antibody responses, specific for homologous Env	Best antibody responses seen with the protein boosters Cell-mediated responses not studied	55
DNA	Adenovirus	Increased antibody responses	Intranasal boosters with adenovirus raise vaginal IgA Cell-mediated responses not studied	38

of antigen and the proinflammatory cytokines expressed by poxvirus-infected cells.

PRECLINICAL EXPERIENCE WITH DNA PRIMING AND PROTEIN OR POXVIRUS BOOSTERS FOR AN AIDS VACCINE

Early studies using DNA priming and protein or recombinant poxvirus boosters to raise protective immunity in macaques have had a number of provocative re-

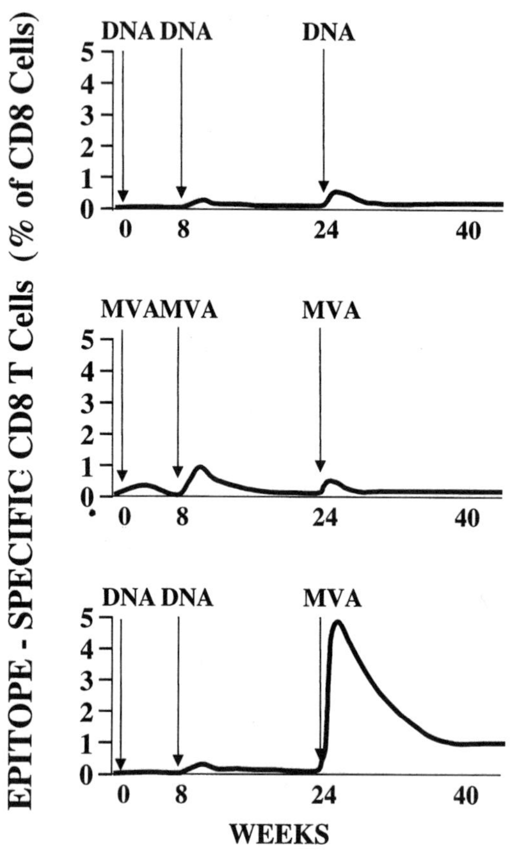

Figure 1 Temporal CD8 cell responses following DNA priming and recombinant MVA boosters. Data are hypothetical, but based on results from laboratories using DNA, MVA, or DNA + MVA immunizations.

sults (Table 5). One of four protein booster immunizations has provided sterilizing immunity (Table 5, experiment 1). One of three poxvirus boosters has resulted in containment of a reasonably virulent challenge (Table 5, experiment 6). Given the caveat that experiments were run in different models and with different immunogen, some generalizations/hypotheses can be formulated.

Hypothesis 1

Protein boosters of DNA primes protect if, and only if, they raise neutralizing antibody for the challenge virus. The success of DNA priming and protein boost-

Table 5 Preclinical DNA Prime and Protein or Poxvirus Boosters in AIDS Models

Exp/boost	DNA	Booster	Challenge	Success	Comment	Ref.
1/prt	IIIb Env-rev expressing DNA, multiple inoculations	100 μg of IIIb gp160 in QS21, one booster	Rhesus macaques, SHIV-IIIb challenge at 2 weeks postboost, challenge delivered i.v.	Sterilizing protection	High titers of neutralizing antibody and Tc on the day of challenge Protection against a homologous challenge	56
2/prt	IIIb Env-, Gag-, Tat-, Rev-, and Nef-expressing DNAs 10 μg of DNA delivered by gene gun at 0, 1, 3, and 5 months	50 μg of p24Gag, gp160, Tat, Rev, and Nef in Ribi adjuvant at 5 and 7 months	Cynomologus macaques, SHIV-IIIb challenge at 4 weeks post the final booster, challenge delivered i.v.	Immunizations failed to protect Immunizations induced B- and T-cell responses Low levels of neutralizing antibody on the day of challenge	Absence or neutralizing antibody on the day of challenge likely to correlate with failure Gene gun deliveries of DNA followed by protein immunizations likely to have primed less protective Th2-biased responses (see 4, 6, 7)	57
3/prt	5 SHIV-IIIb DNAs representing all viral genes delivered at 0, 1, 24 weeks 500 μg each for a total of 2.5 mg delivered i.d. 4 μg of each for a total of 20 μg delivered by gene gun	100 μg of IIIb gp160 in incomplete Freunds adjuvant, two boosters at 44 and 66 weeks	Rhesus macaques, SHIV-IIIb challenge at 2 weeks post the final booster, followed 43 weeks later by rechallenge with SHIV-IIIb, followed 19 weeks later by rechallenge with SHIV89.6p, all challenges delivered i.v.	Animals with good titers of neutralizing antibody on the day of challenge protected against the 1st challenge; only i.d. primed animals protected against subsequent challenges	Requirement for neutralizing antibody for protection against 1st challenge Cell-mediated responses appeared to contribute to protection in i.d. DNA-primed but not gene gun DNA–primed animals Following two deliveries of protein, titers of neutralizing antibody were highest for animals immunized with only protein, suggesting that DNA priming had blunted the protein booster	19

Table 5 Continued

Exp/boost	DNA	Booster	Challenge	Success	Comment	Ref.
4/prt	Multiple SIVmne clone 8 DNAs comprising the entire genome except the LTRs delivered i.m. and i.d. at 0 and 8 weeks 3 mg of plasmid DNA	25 μg of gp160 plus 250 μg gag-pol particles delivered in MF-59 adjuvant at weeks 16 and 36	Pig tail macaques, uncloned SIVmne at 2 weeks post the final booster, challenge delivered i.r.	Four DNA immunizations reduced viral loads at set point more effectively than the DNA plus protein boosters Macaques with Th-1 biased immune responses contained the challenge more effectively than macaques with Th2-biased responses	Another example of the requirement for neutralizing antibody for protein boosters to be effective Better protection in macaques with Th1 biased cell-mediated immunity, consistent with interpretation of exp 6.	58
5/pox	dpol-DNA (expresses HIV-1 viruslike particle), delivered by gene gun at 0 and 8 weeks 4 μg of DNA	2 fowlpox vectors (expressing gag-pol and env), 2×10^8 pfu by scarification 3 fowlpox immunizations at 16, 24, and 32 weeks	Pig tail macaques, 10^5 $TCID_{50}$ of HIV-1 LAI delivered i.v. at 38 weeks	Specific CTL precursors boosted 5- to 20-fold by the poxvirus Infection not detected in 3 out of 4 macaques, contained in the 4th macaque	A highly avirulent challenge model: in control animals, HIV-1 infections had peak titers of plasma viral RNA of less than 400	59
6/pox	5 SHIV immunizations at IIIb DNAs representing all viral genes delivered at 0, 1, 24 weeks 500 μg each for a total of 2.5 mg delivered i.d. 4 μg or each for a total of 20 μg delivered by gene gun	3 fowlpox vectors expressing SHIV-IIIb, Gag-pol, Env, and Nef., 5×10^8 of each administered i.m. 2 fowlpox immunizations at 44 and 66 weeks	Rhesus macaques, SHIV-IIIb challenge at 68 weeks, followed 43 weeks later by rechallenge with SHIV-IIIb, followed 19 weeks later by rechallenge with SHIV89.6p, all challenges delivered i.v.	i.d. but not g.g.-primed animals contained SHIV-IIIb infections below detection by RT-PCR i.d. primed animals also contained SHIV-89.6P challenge with reductions in viral load by 10^5 to $>10^7$-fold (below detection)	Containment did not require the presence of neutralizing antibody Ability to contain infections persisted over the 62-week period of challenges Containment of the 2nd and 3rd challenges likely contributed to by prior challenges boosting immunity	

				"Contained" SHIV-IIIb infection that had not been scored by PCR transmitted to a naive macaque by transfusion of 10 mL of blood	The difference in protective efficacy of i.d. and gene gun deliveries of DNA hyposthesized to reflect i.d. deliveries raising Th1-biased responses and gene gun deliveries raising Th2-biased responses (for precedent in mouse models, see Ref. 37	
7/pox	String of epitopes containing the SIV-Gag p11c-m epitope, delivered by gene gun at 0 and 8 weeks 8 μg DNA	MVA expressing the same string of epitopes, 5×10^8 pfu Three MVA immunizations at weeks 17, 22, and 44	Rhesus macaques, uncloned SIVmac251, intrarectal challenge at 45 weeks	2/3 infected 7/8 controls infected	High levels of p11c-m specific CD8 cells (1–6%) on the day of challenge did not protect, no escape mutants for the p11c-m epitope detected at 16 weeks postchallenge Poor protection likely to correlate with the string of epitopes not containing a SIV helper epitope and the potential TH2-bias of gene gun DNA priming	39

Pox, recombinant vaccinia or fowlpox vectors; Tc, cytotoxic T cells; Th1, T-helper type 1; Th2; T-helper type 2.

ing has been limited by the requirement for neutralizing antibody on the day of challenge (see experiments 1 and 3). Thus, for protein boosters to be effective in a human vaccine, they will need to raise persisting titers of cross-neutralizing antibody for patient isolates. At present, the ability to raise such neutralizing antibody in primate models has not been realized.

Hypothesis 2

DNA priming and recombinant poxvirus boosters raise high titers of CD8 T cells in primates. Experiments 5 and 7 in Table 5 clearly demonstrate the potential for DNA priming followed by poxvirus boosters to raise high-titer CD8 cell responses in primate models. These responses are particularly important for AIDS vaccines as they recognize epitopes in sequences that are highly conserved among immunodeficiency viruses. Conservation within clade B varies from 80% for the least variable protein (p24) to just over 40% for the most variable protein (gp120) (40). Thus, if a clade B vaccine is used in an area in which clade B viruses are endemic, the majority of the vaccine-raised CD8 epitopes will be matched to the clade B challenge infections.

Hypothesis 3

Th1 are superior to Th2 cellular immune responses at containing immunodeficiency virus infections. Although highly hypothetical, the data in Table 5 suggest that Th1-biased cellular immune responses will be important for cell-mediated control of immunodeficiency virus infections. This is suggested by findings in experiments 4 and 6, in which protection correlated with immunizations that were either demonstrated or hypothesized to raise Th1-biased immune responses. In experiment 4, protein-boosted macaques were less well protected than animals that received only DNA. This correlated with the protein-boosted macaques tending to have Th2-biased responses. In experiment 6, a saline injection of DNA was more effective than a gene gun delivery of DNA at priming protective immunity ($p = 0.01$). This difference in efficacy did not manifest itself in prechallenge assays for Tc or antibody and would not have been realized in the absence of the challenge. In murine models, saline injections of DNA tend to bias immune responses towards type 1 help, whereas gene gun deliveries of DNA tend to bias immune responses towards type 2 T-cell help (37). The raising of Th1 cells by saline injections of DNA has also been demonstrated in macaques (41).

Hypothesis 4

Challenge infections can be contained but not eliminated by cell-mediated immune responses. One of the hopes for cell-mediated immunity had been that it could clear as well as limit challenge infections. This hope became less realistic when a transfusion study demonstrated that a challenge virus that had not been detected by RT-PCR could be transmitted to a naive macaque by transfusion of blood (Table 5, experiment 6) (19). The transmitted virus had been used to challenge the transmitting monkey 70 and 27 weeks prior to the transmission and had never been detected by real-time polymerase chain reaction (PCR) for plasma viral RNA. This result demonstrates that CD8 cells may not clear infections. It also suggests that as yet poorly understood ''suppressive'' activities of CD8 cells may contribute to the ability of immunodeficiency virus infections to remain latent (42) (for review, see Ref. 43).

OUTLOOK

Although the current approaches to improving DNA vaccines (Tables 1–4) are sobering in their limited and sometimes disappointing findings (Table 5), the platform that these studies provide for future vaccine development should not be underestimated. Phase 1/2 clinical trials are currently being initiated by Merck with a highly expressed codon-optimized Gag gene that raises good levels of CD8 cells in macaques. Volunteers in this trial will receive DNA by intramuscular (i.m.) injection. Teams led by Andrew McMichael of Oxford University and myself at Emory University, Bernard Moss at the National Institutes of Allergy and Infectious Diseases, and Janet McNicholl at the Centers for Disease Control are actively preparing for phase 1/2 clinical trials using DNA priming followed by MVA boosters. The Oxford group plans to use a codon-optimized Gag gene plus a string of CD8 epitopes for priming and boosting immunogens, while we are preparing immunogens encoding viral-like particles. The results of these trials will be crucially important for determining whether the success of the second generation of DNA approaches in nonhuman primate models will translate into human models.

Meanwhile, as these key trials are undertaken, basic science must continue on the optimization of DNA vectors (Table 1), the optimization of DNA formulations (Table 2), the optimizations of adjuvants (Table 3), and improved understanding of heterologous prime/boost protocols (Table 4). Only with a concerted research effort will the background knowledge be available to take results from the second-generation trials forward to an effective AIDS vaccine.

ACKNOWLEDGMENT

This work was supported in part by Public Health Service Grants P01-AI-43045 and RR00165.

REFERENCES

1. Preston BD, Poiesz BJ, Loeb LA. Fidelity of HIV-1 reverse transcriptase. Science 1988; 242(4882):1168–1171.

2. Roberts JD, Bebenek K, Kunkel TA. The accuracy of reverse transcriptase from HIV-1. Science 1988; 242(4882):1171–1173.
3. Moore JP, Ho DD. HIV-1 neutralization: the consequences of viral adaptation to growth on transformed T cells. AIDS 1995; 9(suppl A):S117–136.
4. Burton DR, Moore JP. Why do we not have an HIV vaccine and how can we make one? Nat Med 1998; 4(5 suppl):495–498.
5. Leonard CK, Spellman MW, Riddle L, Harris RJ, Thomas JN, Gregory TJ. Assignment of intrachain disulfide bonds and characterization of potential glycosylation sites of the type 1 recombinant human immunodeficiency virus envelope glycoprotein (gp120) expressed in Chinese hamster ovary cells. J Biol Chem 1990; 265(18):10373–10382.
6. Kwong PD, Wyatt R, Robinson J, Sweet RW, Sodroski J, Hendrickson WA. Structure of an HIV gp120 envelope glycoprotein in complex with the CD4 receptor and a neutralizing human antibody [comments]. Nature 1998; 393(6686):648–659.
7. Finzi D, Silliciano RF. Viral dynamics in HIV-1 infection. Cell 1998; 93(5): 665–671.
8. Donnelly JJ, Ulmer JB, Shiver JW, Liu MA. DNA vaccines. Annu Rev Immunol 1997; 15:617–648.
9. Robinson HL, Pertmer TM. DNA Vaccines for viral infections: basic studies and applications. In: Maramorosch K, Murphy FA, Shatkin AJ, eds. Advances in Virus Research. Vol 55. San Diego: Academic Press, 2000: 1–74.
10. Condon C, Watkins SC, Celluzzi CM, Thompson K, Falo LD Jr. DNA-based immunization by in vivo transfection of dendritic cells. Nat Med 1996; 2(10):1122–1128.
11. Casares S, Inaba K, Brumeanu TD, Steinman RM, Bona CA. Antigen presentation by dendritic cells after immunization with DNA encoding a major histocompatibility complex class II-restricted viral epitope. J Exp Med 1997; 186(9):1481–1486.
12. Porgador A, Irvine KR, Iwasaki A, Barber BH, Restifo NP, Germain RN. Predominant role for directly transfected dendritic cells in antigen presentation to CD8+ T cells after gene gun immunization. J Exp Med 1998; 188(6):1075–1082.
13. Banchereau J, Steinman RM. Dendritic cells and the control of immunity. Nature 1998; 392(6673):245–252.
14. Akbari O, Panjwani N, Garcia S, Tascon R, Lowrie D, Stockinger B. DNA vaccination: transfection and activation of dendritic cells as key events for immunity. J Exp Med 1999; 189(1):169–178.
15. Corr M, von Damm A, Lee DJ, Tighe H. In vivo priming by DNA injection occurs predominantly by antigen transfer. J Immunol 1999; 163(9):4721–4727.

16. Carbone FR, Bevan MJ. Class I-restricted processing and presentation of exogenous cell-associated antigen in vivo. J Exp Med 1990; 171(2):377–387.
17. Krieg AM, Yi AK, Schorr J, Davis HL. The role of CpG dinucleotides in DNA vaccines. Trends Microbiol 1998; 6(1):23–27.
18. Pisetsky DS. Immune activation by bacterial DNA: a new genetic code. Immunity 1996; 5(4):303–310.
19. Robinson HL, Montefiori DC, Johnson RP, Manson KH, Kalish ML, Lifson JD, et al. Neutralizing antibody-independent containment of immunodeficiency virus challenges by DNA priming and recombinant pox virus booster immunization. Nat Med 1999; 5(5):526–534.
20. Barouch DH, Craiu A, Kuroda MJ, Schmitz JE, Zheng XX, Santra S, et al. Augmentation of immune responses to HIV-1 and simian immunodeficiency virus DNA vaccines by IL-2/Ig plasmid administration in rhesus monkeys. Proc Natl Acad Sci USA 2000; 97:4192–4197.
21. Wang R, Doolan DL, Le TP, Hedstrom RC, Coonan KM, Charoenvit Y, et al. Induction of antigen-specific cytotoxic T lymphocytes in humans by a malaria DNA vaccine. Science 1998; 282(5388):476–480.
22. MacGregor RR, Boyer JD, Ugen KE, Lacy KE, Gluckman SJ, Bagarazzi ML, et al. First human trial of a DNA-based vaccine for treatment of human immunodeficiency virus type 1 infection: safety and host response. J Infect Dis 1998; 178(1):92–100.
23. Boyer JD, Cohen AD, Vogt S, Schumann K, Nath B, Ahn L, et al. Vaccination of seronegative volunteers with a human immunodeficiency virus type 1 env/rev DNA vaccine induces antigen-specific proliferation and lymphocyte production of beta-chemokines. J Infect Dis 2000; 181(2):476–483.
24. Schneider R, Campbell M, Nasioulas G, Felber BK, Pavlakis GN. Inactivation of the human immunodeficiency virus type 1 inhibitory elements allows Rev-independent expression of Gag and Gag/protease and particle formation. J Virol 1997; 71(7):4892–4903.
25. zur Megede J, Chen MC, Doe B, Schaefer M, Greer CE, Selby M, et al. Increased expression and immunogenicity of sequence-modified human immunodeficiency virus type 1 gag gene. J Virol 2000; 74(6):2628–2635.
26. Haas J, Park EC, Seed B. Codon usage limitation in the expression of HIV-1 envelope glycoprotein. Curr Biol 1996; 6(3):315–324.
27. Qiu JT, Song R, Dettenhofer M, Tian C, August T, Felber BK, et al. Evaluation of novel human immunodeficiency virus type 1 Gag DNA vaccines for protein expression in mammalian cells and induction of immune responses. J Virol 1999; 73(11):9145–9152.
28. Vinner L, Nielsen HV, Bryder K, Corbet S, Nielsen C, Fomsgaard A. Gene gun DNA vaccination with Rev-independent synthetic HIV-1 gp160 envelope gene using mammalian codons. Vaccine 1999; 17(17):2166–2175.

29. Ulmer JB, DeWitt CM, Chastain M, Friedman A, Donnelly JJ, McClements WL, et al. Enhancement of DNA vaccine potency using conventional aluminum adjuvants. Vaccine 1999; 18(1–2):18–28.
30. Singh M, Briones M, Ott G, O'Hagan D. Cationic microparticles: a potent delivery system for DNA vaccines. Proc Natl Acad Sci USA 2000; 97(2): 811–816.
31. Cohen AD, Boyer JD, Weiner DB. Modulating the immune response to genetic immunization. FASEB J 1998; 12(15):1611–1626.
32. Barouch DH, Santra S, Steenbeke TD, Zheng XX, Perry HC, Davies ME, et al. Augmentation and suppression of immune responses to an HIV-1 DNA vaccine by plasmid cytokine/Ig administration. J Immunol 1998; 161(4):1875–1882.
33. Kusakabe K, Xin KQ, Katoh H, Sumino K, Hagiwara E, Kawamoto S, et al. The timing of GM-CSF expression plasmid administration influences the Th1/Th2 response induced by an HIV-1-specific DNA vaccine. J Immunol 2000; 164(6):3102–3111.
34. Richmond JF, Lu S, Santoro JC, Weng J, Hu SL, Montefiori DC, et al. Studies of the neutralizing activity and avidity of anti-human immunodeficiency virus type 1 Env antibody elicited by DNA priming and protein boosting. J Virol 1998; 72(11):9092–9100.
35. Richmond JF, Mustafa F, Lu S, Santoro JC, Weng J, O'Connell M, et al. Screening of HIV-1 Env glycoproteins for the ability to raise neutralizing antibody using DNA immunization and recombinant vaccinia virus boosting. Virology 1997; 230(2):265–274.
36. Schneider J, Gilbert SC, Hannan CM, Degano P, Sheu EG, Plebanski M, et al. Induction of CD8+ T cells using heterologous prime-boost immunisation strategies. Immunol Rev 1999; 170:29–38.
37. Feltquate DM, Heaney S, Webster RG, Robinson HL. Different T helper cell types and antibody isotypes generated by saline and gene gun DNA immunization. J Immunol 1997; 158(5):2278–2284.
38. Xiang ZQ, Pasquini S, Ertl HC. Induction of genital immunity by DNA priming and intranasal booster immunization with a replication-defective adenoviral recombinant. J Immunol 1999; 162(11):6716–6723.
39. Hanke T, Samuel RV, Blanchard TJ, Neumann VC, Allen TM, Boyson JE, et al. Effective induction of simian immunodeficiency virus-specific cytotoxic T lymphocytes in macaques by using a multiepitope gene and DNA prime-modified vaccinia virus Ankara boost vaccination regimen. J Virol 1999; 73(9):7524–7532.
40. Korber B, Foley B, Gaschen B, Kuiken C. Epidemiological and immunological implications of the global variability of HIV-1. In: Pantaleo G, Walker B, eds. Retroviral Immunology. Totowa, NJ: The Humana Press, 2001:1–32.

41. Lekutis C, Letvin NL. HIV-1 envelope-specific CD4+ T helper cells from simian/human immunodeficiency virus-infected rhesus monkeys recognize epitopes restricted by MHC class II DRB1*0406 and DRB*W201 molecules. J Immunol 1997; 159(4):2049–2057.
42. Walker CM, Moody DJ, Stites DP, Levy JA. CD8+ lymphocytes can control HIV infection in vitro by suppressing virus replication. Science 1986; 234(4783):1563–1566.
43. Levy JA, Mackewicz CE, Barker E. Controlling HIV pathogenesis: the role of the noncytotoxic anti-HIV response of CD8+ T cells. Immunol Today 1996; 17(5):217–224.
44. Wang S, Liu X, Fisher K, Smith JG, Chen F, Tobery TW, et al. Enhanced type I immune response to a hepatitis B DNA vaccine by formulation with calcium- or aluminum phosphate. Vaccine 2000; 18(13):1227–1235.
45. Kim JJ, Trivedi NN, Nottingham LK, Morrison L, Tsai A, Hu Y, et al. Modulation of amplitude and direction of in vivo immune responses by co-administration of cytokine gene expression cassettes with DNA immunogens. Eur J Immunol 1998; 28(3):1089–1103.
46. Kim JJ, Yang JS, VanCott TC, Lee DJ, Manson KH, Wyand MS, et al. Modulation of antigen-specific humoral responses in rhesus macaques by using cytokine cDNAs as DNA vaccine adjuvants. J Virol 2000; 74(7): 3427–3429.
47. Kim JJ, Ayyavoo V, Bagarazzi ML, Chattergoon MA, Dang K, Wang B, et al. In vivo engineering of a cellular immune response by coadministration of IL-12 expression vector with a DNA immunogen. J Immunol 1997; 158(2):816–826.
48. Kim JJ, Yang JS, Lee DJ, Wilson DM, Nottingham LK, Morrison L, et al. Macrophage colony-stimulating factor can modulate immune responses and attract dendritic cells in vivo. Hum Gene Ther 2000; 11(2):305–321.
49. Boyer JD, Kim J, Ugen K, Cohen AD, Ahn L, Schumann K, et al. HIV-1 DNA vaccines and chemokines. Vaccine 1999; 17(suppl 2):S53–64.
50. Kim JJ, Bagarazzi ML, Trivedi N, Hu Y, Kazahaya K, Wilson DM, et al. Engineering of in vivo immune responses to DNA immunization via codelivery of costimulatory molecule genes. Nat Biotechnol 1997; 15(7): 641–646.
51. Schneider J, Gilbert SC, Blanchard TJ, Hanke T, Robson KJ, Hannan CM, et al. Enhanced immunogenicity for CD8+ T cell induction and complete protective efficacy of malaria DNA vaccination by boosting with modified vaccinia virus Ankara. Nat Med 1998; 4(4):397–402.
52. Sedegah M, Jones TR, Kaur M, Hedstrom R, Hobart P, Tine JA, et al. Boosting with recombinant vaccinia increases immunogenicity and protective efficacy of malaria DNA vaccine. Proc Natl Acad Sci USA 1998; 95(13):7648–7653.

53. Hanke T, Blanchard TJ, Schneider J, Hannan CM, Becker M, Gilbert SC, et al. Enhancement of MHC class I-restricted peptide-specific T cell induction by a DNA prime/MVA boost vaccination regime. Vaccine 1998; 16(5): 439–445.
54. Irvine KR, Chamberlain RS, Shulman EP, Surman DR, Rosenberg SA, Restifo NP. Enhancing efficacy of recombinant anticancer vaccines with prime/boost regimens that use two different vectors. J Natl Cancer Inst 1997; 5:89.
55. Caver TE, Lockey TD, Srinivas RV, Webster RG, Hurwitz JL. A novel vaccine regimen utilizing DNA, vaccinia virus and protein immunizations for HIV-1 envelope presentation. Vaccine 1999; 17(11–12):1567–1572.
56. Letvin NL, Montefiori DC, Yasutomi Y, Perry HC, Davies ME, Lekutis C, et al. Potent, protective anti-HIV immune responses generated by bimodal HIV envelope DNA plus protein vaccination. Proc Natl Acad Sci USA 1997; 94(17):9378–9383.
57. Putkonen P, Quesada-Rolander M, Leandersson AC, Schwartz S, Thorstensson R, Okuda K, et al. Immune responses but no protection against SHIV by gene-gun delivery of HIV-1 DNA followed by recombinant subunit protein boosts. Virology 1998; 250(2):293–301.
58. Haigwood NL, Pierce CC, Robertson MN, Watson AJ, Montefiori DC, Rabin M, et al. Protection from pathogenic SIV challenge using multigenic DNA vaccines. Immunol Lett 1999; 66(1–3):183–188.
59. Kent SJ, Zhao A, Best SJ, Chandler JD, Boyle DB, Ramshaw IA. Enhanced T-cell immunogenicity and protective efficacy of a human immunodeficiency virus type 1 vaccine regimen consisting of consecutive priming with DNA and boosting with recombinant fowlpox virus. J Virol 1998; 72(12): 10180–10188.

8

Replication-Deficient, Pseudotyped HIV-1 Vectors as HIV Vaccines

June Kan-Mitchell

Karmanos Cancer Institute
Wayne State University School of Medicine
Detroit, Michigan

Flossie Wong-Staal

Center for AIDS Research
University of California, San Diego
La Jolla, California

INTRODUCTION

The AIDS epidemic continues to spread through the human population, now opening new fronts in Asia. The development of a safe and efficacious vaccine for either prophylaxis or treatment is the best hope for the control of this epidemic. Several vaccine strategies are under investigation, including recombinant poxviruses encoding viral proteins or epitopes, DNA vaccines, whole attenuated or inactivated viruses, and combinations of the above (see elsewhere in this book). However, developing an effective vaccine against HIV-1 has proven to be difficult, even with the benefit of the expertise derived from successful vaccines against viruses such as smallpox and polio. Although acute HIV-1 infection is frequently associated with a vigorous immune response, which includes neutralizing antibodies and helper and cytotoxic T cells (1,2), this response invariably fails to eradicate the virus. Most of those infected will progress to AIDS and ultimately death. Similarly, most vaccines would elicit a transient immune response that fails to completely prevent infection or persistently suppress viral replication. The most effective vaccine tested in the rhesus macaque model is a live, attenuated SIV deleted in several nonessential genes including nef (3). However, the safety concerns for such a vaccine for people are formidable, and in fact there is evidence that such attenuated viruses have been able to induce AIDS in some experimental animals (4). Our rationale, therefore, is to further attenuate the virus such that it is conditionally infectious (i.e., upon pseudotyping with a heterologous viral envelope protein) for only one round. This is achieved by removing the envelope and accessory genes from an infectious HIV provirus and generating viral particles by pseudotyping with a heterologous viral envelope protein, e.g., the glycoprotein from vesicular stomatitis virus (VSV-G). By this means, we are essentially delivering HIV proteins (Gag, Env, Tat, and Rev) in an HIV-based gene delivery vector. The use of lentiviral vectors to express viral antigens as vaccines can be extended to other infectious agents as well.

LENTIVIRAL VECTORS

Retroviral vectors derived from murine onco-retroviruses have been more commonly used for gene delivery. They have a large cloning capacity, close to 10 kb, integrate their cargo into the chromosomes of target cells, which is a prerequisite for long-term expression, and do not transfer virus-derived DNA sequences, avoiding the induction of virus-specific immunity. However, retroviral vectors are incapable of infecting cells that do not divide within a few hours or transduction of most adult, postmitotic cells. The last 3 years have witnessed dramatic progress in the development of lentiviral vectors, including those derived from HIV-1 and HIV-2, which are capable of delivering transgenes into nondividing and terminally differentiated cells. Lentiviruses, a subfamily of retroviruses, can replicate in nonmitotic cells because of the ability of their preintegration complex to traverse the intact membrane of the nucleus in the target cells. For HIV-1, this process appears to be facilitated by several viral proteins: the integrase protein, the matrix protein from Gag, and the accessory protein Vpr. Both integrase and matrix protein contain signal sequences for nuclear localization. In contrast, Vpr appears to bind directly to the nuclear pore complex. While the roles of these elements in viral replication are not completely understood, several independent mechanisms may be at play because removal of one or the other genes does not prevent infection of the nondividing cells. In fact, because of the complexity and redundancy of the HIV genome, it was possible to dissociate the genes essential for single round transduction/infection from those that encode for virulence and pathogenicity.

Lentiviruses have proven extremely efficient at providing long-term gene expression in cells in culture including weakly activated T lymphocytes, terminally differentiated macrophages (5), hematopoietic stem/progenitor cells (6,7), and functionally mature fully differentiated dendritic cells (8). HIV-based vectors can mediate efficient in vivo delivery and the long-term expression of transgenes in tissues. Animal studies showed that HIV-1 vectors efficiently infect terminally differentiated neural cells in the central nervous system and that marker gene expression was stable for months (9,10). HIV vectors also infect retinal (11), hepatic, and muscle cells (12). Because these vectors can efficiently transduce human CD34+ hematopoietic stem cells in the absence of cytokine stimulation, these cells were capable of engrafting and differentiating into multiple hematopoietic cell lineages in the diabetic/severe combined immunodeficient (NOD/SCID) mice (13). Although the HIV-1 vector systems have been the most extensively studied, other lentiviral vectors have been produced, including the human immunodeficiency virus type 2 (HIV-2) and simian immunodeficiency virus (SIV) vectors (6,14). It is also possible to generate chimeric vector systems consisting of HIV-1 and HIV-2 (5) or HIV-1 and SIV components (15). In addition, lentiviral vectors from nonprimates, including felines and equines, are also being developed. These appear to have the same general properties as their HIV counterpart (6,16,17).

A major advantage of using lentiviral vectors as vaccines is their ability to transduce professional antigen-presenting cells (APCs), particularly dendritic cells (DCs), such that intact or large fragments of selected viral proteins will be processed and presented on both class I and class II MHC molecules to stimulate cytotoxic and helper T lymphocytes (CTL and Th) simultaneously. This obviates the need to customize vectors for patients based on their HLA allotypes, since the dendritic cells will process and present these viral antigens in the context of all major and minor HLA loci. In this manner, prior knowledge and specific inclusion of the relevant epitopes, particularly the less characterized Th epitopes, is not required. A prophylactic vaccine against HIV may also have to induce both humoral and cell-mediated immune responses to achieve protection (18). Increasing understanding of what constitutes relevant HIV-specific T-cell responses and the exact role DCs play in eliciting them will permit modifications to optimize the current HIV vectors as vaccines.

DENDRITIC CELLS

Dendritic cells are the most potent stimulators of CD4+ Th and CD8+ CTLs in the immune system and have been referred to as ''nature's adjuvant.'' Their central role in eliciting effective antiviral immunity is well accepted. These unique antigen-presenting cells have specialized mechanisms whereby an antigen encountered in the peripheral tissues such as skin and mucosa are brought to T cells in the lymph nodes and mucosal-associated lymphoid tissues to elicit a successful antigen-specific T-cell immune responses (19).

DCs have been tested for use therapeutically (20). A clinical trial of HIV-antigen pulsed DCs showed that three of three patients with CD4+ T cells > $400/mm^3$ had an increase in HIV-specific immune responses after HIV gp160-pulsed DC infusions (21). Our approach is to design highly attenuated, replication-deficient HIV-based vectors that allow only one round of infection of DCs. The virus load is directly controlled by the immunizing dose and can be designed not to reach a pathogenic threshold causing disease.

HIV-based vectors may also be used in ex vivo transduction of DCs followed by reinfusion into autologous patients. This procedure should be even safer and may be conceivable as a therapeutic vaccine, although somewhat impractical as a preventive vaccine. Strategies to increase safety may include removal of all nonessential HIV accessory genes and extensive testing of replication-competent retrovirus (RCR). It should be noted that there is no evidence to date for RCRs after in vitro or in vivo applications of even the early lentiviral systems (22). Based on clinical trials in cancer, the number of DCs transferred is relatively small, in the range of 10^9–10^{10}. Because a transduction efficiency of up to 50–80% is routinely attainable (8), a high-output packaging cell line is not needed to initiate these studies.

The principal population of DCs in the tissues, exemplified by Langerhans cells in epithelial and mucosal surfaces, is considered to be immature DCs that are specialized for antigen capture by phagocytosis or pinocytosis. These cells express chemokine receptors, including CCR5, which facilitate their recruitment to sites of inflammation where chemokine ligands MIP-1α, MIP-1β, MIP-3α, and RANTES are being produced (23). Immature DCs are therefore optimally situated at the surface epithelia to encounter virus that breaches the mucosa during the earliest stages of infection. They are likely to be the first cells targeted by HIV during transmission. Once loaded with the virus, DCs differentiate or "mature" with alterations of their surface profiles to facilitate migration to lymph nodes via the lymphatic vessels. There is also upregulation of adhesion, CD40, and costimulatory molecules and production of large quantities of IL-12, features important for their subsequent function in the lymph nodes to attract and trigger a potent immune response. The inherent migratory capacity of DCs therefore ensures the rapid spread of the HIV to their next targets, the T-cell areas in the lymphatic system (24).

In vitro studies examining skin- and blood-derived DCs revealed that immature and mature DCs have different capacity to capture and support the replication of HIV. Freshly isolated LCs infected by macrophage-tropic (R5) HIV-1 transmitted infection to T-cell blasts, while those infected by a CXCR4-using T-cell–tropic (X4) isolate did not (25), unless the LCs were further cultured to express CXCR4 (26). Immature monocyte-derived DCs can be productively infected with R5 HIV, while monocytes and mature DCs are difficult to infect (27). Only early RU5 transcripts were formed by monocytes and mature DCs, while immature DCs complete reverse transcription showing strong LTR-gag signals (28). Factors in addition to surface receptors may be at play, since functional CCR5 and CXCR4 are expressed by mature DCs (29). However, the virus in mature DCs is triggered by CD40-CD40L interactions with T cells to set up a vigorous and productive infection transmitting both M-tropic and T-tropic virus to the latter. Thus, it appears that one mechanism by which HIV establishes a primary infection is facilitated by infection of immature DCs. The virus replicates at a low level until the now mature DCs arrive at the T-cell areas of lymphoid tissues. There the natural attractions and interactions between mature DCs and T cells release the block to the virus life cycle in the DCs, allowing HIV particles to be made rapidly.

The identification of a novel DC surface molecule, DC-SIGN, provides a new pathway by which HIV establishes an infection (30). This molecule, expressed by immature DCs, also has a strong affinity for HIV gp120 (31), thereby entrapping viral particles in the periphery and transmitting them to secondary lymphoid tissues. There DC-SIGN mediates a transient clustering between DCs and T cells, allowing a DC to screen thousands of T cells to find the few that express a compatible TCR. DC-SIGN, a type I C-type lectin, is the first member to be characterized by an increasing number of receptors that may perform dual functions as scavenger receptors as well as costimulatory molecules in DC–T-cell interactions (32). Various cellular processes in the DCs regulate the capture of antigens and eventual presentation of their epitopes to elicit an optimal immune response. For example, the timing of antigen loading onto class II molecules and transport of these antigenic complexes to the cell surface are dependent on the state of maturation of the DCs (33). It is therefore important to consider the possibility that expression of viral promoters as well as the transgenes may have profound effects on cellular processes critical to the DCs' ability to function effectively.

Despite the inadvertent role DCs may play in establishing and promoting an HIV infection, they are clearly capable of eliciting vigorous HIV-specific CTLs in a proportion of patients that seemed much larger than for other viruses (34). Many lines of evidence support the premise that the CTL response is capable of controlling HIV replication, and this will not be discussed here.

TRANSDUCTION WITH PSEUDOTYPED LENTIVIRAL VECTORS

We and others have transduced cells of the monocyte-macrophage-DC series with pseudotyped lentiviral vectors (8,28,36). We found immature DCs to be efficiently transduced by VSV-G pseudotyped nonreplicating HIV vectors deficient in nef or all four accessory genes. There were no significant alterations on the surface CD markers that are typical of DCs. Furthermore, the phagocytic potential of immature DCs as well as their ability to differentiate into mature DCs capable of stimulating allogeneic T-cell proliferation were not affected. HIV-specific CTL from nonprogressor patients were stimulated to proliferate by transduced DCs from the patients themselves or from HLA-A locus–matched donors (unpublished data). Most importantly, transduced DCs were capable of priming naive CD8+ T cells from seronegative donors, stimulating the proliferation and expansion of HIV-specific CTL (8). In fact, an oligoclonal expansion of limited Vβ gene products was observed in these T-cell cultures (unpublished data). HIV vectors efficiently targeted other antigen-presenting cells or their progenitors, including macrophages (5) or primitive hematopoietic progenitor cells (6). Transduced CD34+ cells continued to differentiate in vitro into different subsets of progeny cells, including those with normal DC morphology and phenotypes (7). The introduction of transgenes into antigen-presenting cells should lead to more effective antigen presentation, particularly for MHC class I–restricted epitopes. The protein products of the transgenes are synthesized endogenously and presented via the customary class I presentation pathway, which is more efficient than presenting foreign antigens by cross-presentation.

CONCLUSION

Future studies are necessary to address many of the remaining questions. For example, we showed that differentiation of monocytes from healthy donors into macrophages or DCs were not affected after transduction with our pseudotyped ΔEnv HIV-1 (Fig. 1). Negatively selected fresh monocytes were transduced and then cultured in the presence of GM-CSF or GM-CSF + IL-4 to generate macrophages and DCs, respectively. In vitro differentiation to these cell types was not affected with respect to cell morphology or the expression of the CD surface markers HLA-DR, CD80, CD86, and ICAM-1. These results will be further verified in the humanized SCID mouse model. It appears that lentiviral vectors show some promise for use as vaccines directly in humans, without resorting to ex vivo custom transductions of fully differentiated DCs, a technically elaborate and costly procedure. This is an important practical consideration if such vaccines are to be made available to developing countries.

Despite the remarkable progress in terms of antiretroviral drug therapy against HIV in the past 5 years, HAART does not always fully suppress viral replication and is successful only approximately 50% of the time in the general patient population. A possible adjuvant therapy might be gene-based immunotherapy that has a completely different mechanism of action and, therefore, may act synergistically with HAART to improve outcome. It is therefore important

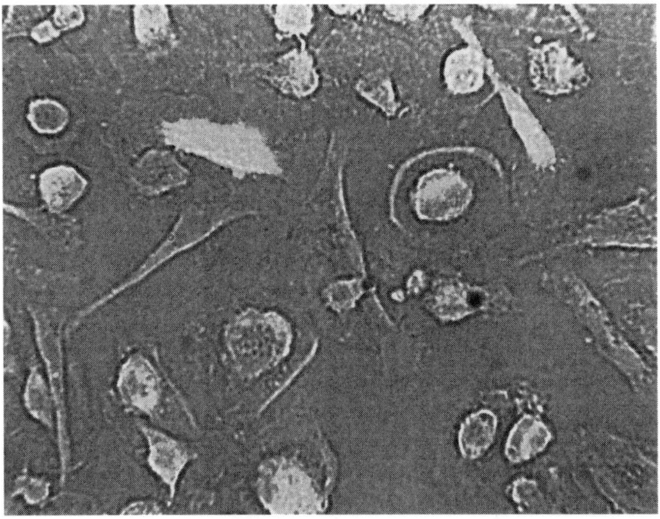

(A)

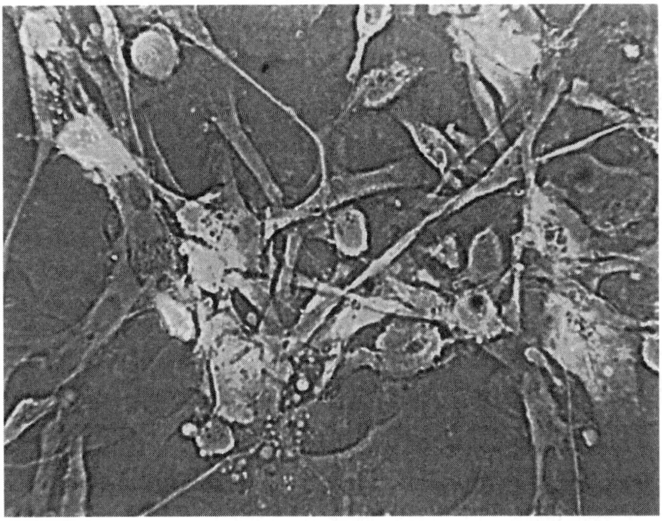

(B)

Figure 1 Monocytes transduced by the ΔEnv HIV-1 GFP vector differentiated to (A) macrophages and (B) immature DCs after culture for 15 days in the presence of appropriate cytokines. Cells were fixed in 4% paraformaldehyde in PBS, mounted in Gel-Mount (Biomedia) and examined under fluorescent microscopy.

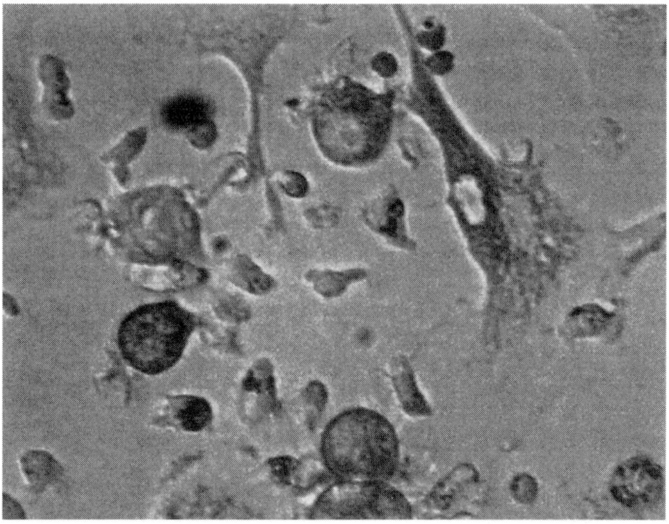

(A)

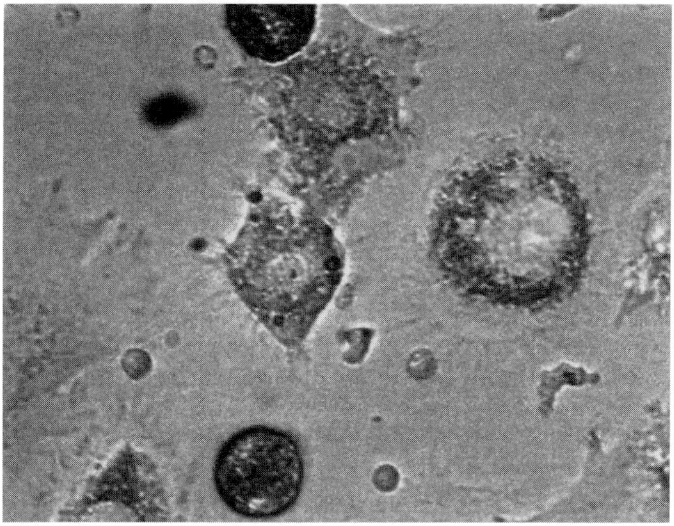

(B)

Figure 2 Immature DCs from nonprogressor patient before (A) and after (B) transduction by the ΔEnv HIV-1 GFP vector and cultured for an additional 5 days. Photographs were obtained with a 32× objective by fluorescent phase contrast microscopy.

to evaluate whether DCs from HIV-positive patients are functionally competent and whether there may be differences among groups of patients with different clinical status. Such information will help to design appropriate immunogens for each group of patients. We observed that blood monocytes from asymptomatic HIV-1–positive patients appeared to be uninfected and fully capable of inducing allogeneic T-cell proliferation (37). In contrast, DCs from two of two nonprogressor/slow-progressor patients were more sensitive to the deleterious effects of transduction, and the transduced DCs expressed significantly lower levels of the green fluorescent reporter protein than comparable DCs from healthy donors (Fig. 2). This suggests that the DCs from infected patients were less efficient at expressing the transgenes. Since it was previously shown that maturation of DCs or their differentiation from precursor monocytes could affect the ability of this series of cells to transcribe and express HIV-1 genes (28), our observation suggests that the monocytes may be immunologically altered by chronic infection. A parallel in the HIV-specific cytotoxic T-cell response is only beginning to become appreciated (38). Tetramers and intracellular staining were used to reveal functional heterogeneity among antigen-specific CD8+ T cells ex vivo. In this manner it was shown that HIV-specific T cells from patients are impaired in terms of maturation and cytotoxic activity (38). Additional studies on the ex vivo effect of lentiviral vectors and their transgenes on the biology of DCs from HIV patients are the first steps in continuing development of this novel gene-based therapeutic vaccine approach. Clinical trials, of course, will be the final arbiters of the effectiveness of transduced DCs as immunogens in vivo.

HIV or other lentiviral vectors represent a distinct and promising approach to the development of HIV vaccines. It is most likely that the current first-generation vectors will be optimized by inclusion of other transgene sequences. In particular, to activate DCs, CpG motifs (39,40) or chemokine and/or cytokine genes can be added to the constructs. A recent innovative strategy is to express mycobacterial antigens as fusion proteins with a destabilizing ubiquitin molecule, which produces a stronger Th1-type immunity and significant resistance to a tuberculous challenge (41). Conceivably, lentiviral vectors may eventually be used to deliver promising polyepitopic vaccines such as that undergoing clinical testing.

REFERENCES

1. Brander C, Walker BD. T lymphocyte responses in HIV-1 infection: implications for vaccine development. Curr Opin Immunol 1999; 11:451–459.
2. Parren PW, Moore JP, Burton DR, Sattentau QJ. The neutralizing antibody response to HIV-1: viral evasion and escape from humoral immunity. AIDS 1999; 13:S131–162.
3. Wyand MS, Manson KH, Garcia-Moll M, Montefiori D, Desrosiers RC.

Vaccine protection by a triple deletion mutant of simian immunodeficiency virus. J Virol 1996; 70:3724–3733.
4. Baba TW, Liska V, Khimani AH, Ray NB, Dailey PJ, Penninck D, Bronson R, Greene MF, McClure HM, Martin LN, Ruprecht RM. Live attenuated, multiply deleted simian immunodeficiency virus causes AIDS in infant and adult macaques. Nat Med 1999; 5:194–203.
5. Corbeau P, Kraus G, Wong-Staal F. Transduction of human macrophages using a stable HIV-1/HIV-2-derived gene delivery system. Gene Ther 1998; 5:99–104.
6. Poeschla EM, Looney DJ. CXCR4 is required by a nonprimate lentivirus: heterologous expression of feline immunodeficiency virus in human, rodent, and feline cells. J Virol 1998; 72:6858–6866.
7. Li X, Gervaix A, Kang D, Law P, Spector SA, Ho AD, Wong-Staal F. Gene therapy targeting cord blood-derived CD34+ cells from HIV-exposed infants: preclinical studies. Gene Ther 1998; 5:233–239.
8. Gruber A, Kan-Mitchell J, Kuhen KL, Mukai T, Wong-Staal F. Dendritic cells transduced by multiply deleted HIV-1 vectors exhibit normal phenotypes and functions and elicit an HIV-specific cytotoxic T-lymphocyte response in vitro. Blood 2000; 96:1327–1333.
9. Naldini L, Blomer U, Gage FH, Trono D, Verma IM. Efficient transfer, integration, and sustained long-term expression of the transgene in adult rat brains injected with a lentiviral vector. Proc Natl Acad Sci USA 1996; 93:11382–11388.
10. Blomer U, Naldini L, Kafri T, Trono D, Verma IM, Gage FH. Highly efficient and sustained gene transfer in adult neurons with a lentivirus vector. J Virol 1997; 71:6641–6649.
11. Miyoshi H, Takahashi M, Gage FH, Verma IM. Stable and efficient gene transfer into the retina using an HIV-based lentiviral vector. Proc Natl Acad Sci USA 1997; 94:10319–10323.
12. Kafri T, Blomer U, Peterson DA, Gage FH., Verma IM. Sustained expression of genes delivered directly into liver and muscle by lentiviral vectors. Nat Genet 1997; 17:314–317.
13. Miyoshi H, Smith KA, Mosier DE, Verma IM, Torbett BE. Transduction of human CD34+ cells that mediate long-term engraftment of NOD/SCID mice by HIV vectors. Science 1999; 283:682–686.
14. Rizvi TA, Panganiban AT. Simian immunodeficiency virus RNA is efficiently encapsidated by human immunodeficiency virus type 1 particles. J Virol 1993; 67:2681–2688.
15. White SM, Renda M, Nam NY, Klimatcheva E, Zhu Y, Fisk J, Halterman M, Rimel BJ, Federoff H, Pandya S, Rosenblatt JD, Planelles V. Lentivirus vectors using human and simian immunodeficiency virus elements. J Virol 1999; 73:2832–2840.

16. Johnston JC, Gasmi M, Lim LE, Elder JH, Yee JK, Jolly DJ, Campbell KP, Davidson BL, Sauter SL. Minimum requirements for efficient transduction of dividing and nondividing cells by feline immunodeficiency virus vectors. J Virol 1999; 73:4991–5000.
17. Buchschacher GL Jr, Wong-Staal F. Development of lentiviral vectors for gene therapy for human diseases. Blood 2000; 95:2499–2504.
18. Salk J, Bretscher PA, Salk PL, Clerici M, Shearer GM. A strategy for prophylactic vaccination against HIV. Science1993; 260:1270–1272.
19. Banchereau J, Steinman RM. Dendritic cells and the control of immunity. Nature 1998; 392:245–252.
20. Timmerman JM, Levy R. Dendritic cell vaccines for cancer immunotherapy. Annu Rev Med 1999; 50:507–529.
21. Kundu SK, Engleman E, Benike C, Shapero MH, Dupuis M, van Schooten WC, Eibl M, Merigan TC. A pilot clinical trial of HIV antigen-pulsed allogeneic and autologous dendritic cell therapy in HIV-infected patients. AIDS Res Hum Retrovir 1998; 14:551–560.
22. Amado RG, Chen IS. Lentiviral vectors—the promise of gene therapy within reach? Science 1999; 285:674–676.
23. Dieu MC, Vanbervliet B, Vicari A, Bridon JM, Oldham E, Ait-Yahia S, Briere F, Zlotnik A, Lebecque S, Caux C. Selective recruitment of immature and mature dendritic cells by distinct chemokines expressed in different anatomic sites. J Exp Med 1998; 188:373–386.
24. Rowland-Jones SL. HIV: the deadly passenger in dendritic cells. Curr Biol 1999; 9:R248–250.
25. Reece JC, Handley AJ, Anstee EJ, Morrison WA, Crowe SM., Cameron PU. HIV-1 selection by epidermal dendritic cells during transmission across human skin. J Exp Med 1998; 187:1623–1631.
26. Zaitseva M, Blauvelt A, Lee S, Lapham CK, Klaus-Kovtun V, Mostowski H, Manischewitz J, Golding H. Expression and function of CCR5 and CXCR4 on human Langerhans cells and macrophages: implications for HIV primary infection. Nat Med 1997; 3:1369–1375.
27. Granelli-Piperno A, Delgado E, Finkel V, Paxton W, Steinman RM. Immature dendritic cells selectively replicate macrophagetropic (M-tropic) human immunodeficiency virus type 1, while mature cells efficiently transmit both M- and T-tropic virus to T cells. J Virol 1998; 72:2733–2737.
28. Granelli-Piperno A, Zhong L, Haslett P, Jacobson J, Steinman RM. Dendritic cells, infected with vesicular stomatitis virus-pseudotyped HIV-1, present viral antigens to CD4(+) and CD8(+) T cells from HIV-1-infected individuals. J Immunol 2000; 165:6620–6626.
29. Delgado E, Finkel V, Baggiolini M, Mackay CR, Steinman RM, Granelli-Piperno A. Mature dendritic cells respond to SDF-1, but not to several beta-chemokines. Immunobiology 1998; 198:490–500.

30. Geijtenbeek TB., Kwon DS., Torensma R, van Vliet SJ, van Duijnhoven GC, Middel J, Cornelissen, I.L., Nottet HS., KewalRamani, V.N., Littman DR, Figdor CG, van Kooyk Y. DC-SIGN, a dendritic cell-specific HIV-1-binding protein that enhances trans-infection of T cells. Cell 2000; 100: 587–597.
31. Curtis BM, Scharnowske S, Watson AJ. Sequence and expression of a membrane-associated C-type lectin that exhibits CD4-independent binding of human immunodeficiency virus envelope glycoprotein gp120. PNAS 1992; 89:8356–8360.
32. Hartgers FC, Figdor CG, Adema GJ. Towards a molecular understanding of dendritic cell immunobiology. Immunol Today 2000; 21:542–545.
33. Steinman RM. DC-SIGN: a guide to some mysteries of dendritic cells. Cell 2000; 100:491–494.
34. McMichael AJ, Ogg G, Wilson J, Callan M, Hambleton S, Appay V, Kelleher T, Rowland-Jones S. Memory CD8+ T cells in HIV infection. Philos Trans R Soc Lond B Biol Sci 2000; 29:363–367.
35. Sewell AK, Price DA, Oxenius A, Kelleher AD, Phillips RE. Cytotoxic T lymphocyte responses to human immunodeficiency virus: control and escape. Stem Cells 2000; 8:230–244.
36. Schroers R, Sinha I, Segall H, Schmidt-Wolf IG, Rooney CM, Brenner MK, Sutton RE, Chen SY. Transduction of human PBMC-derived dendritic cells and macrophages by an HIV-1-based lentiviral vector system. Mol Ther 2000; 1:171–179.
37. Sapp M, Engelmayer J, Larsson M, Granelli-Piperno A, Steinman. R, Bhardwaj N. Dendritic cells generated from blood monocytes of HIV-1 patients are not infected and act as competent antigen presenting cells eliciting potent T-cell responses. Immunol Lett 1999; 66:121–128.
38. Appay V, Nixon DF, Donahoe SM, Gillespie GM, Dong T, King A, Ogg GS, Spiegel HM, Conlon C, Spina CA, Havlir DV, Richman DD, Waters A, Easterbrook P, McMichael AJ, Rowland-Jones, SL. HIV-specific CD8(+) T cells produce antiviral cytokines but are impaired in cytolytic function. J Exp Med 2000; 192:63–75.
39. Hartmann G, Weiner GJ, Krieg AM. CpG DNA: a potent signal for growth, activation, and maturation of human dendritic cells. Proc Natl Acad Sci 1999; 96:9305–9310.
40. Jakob T, Walker PS, Krieg AM, von Stebut E, Udey MC, Vogel JC. Bacterial DNA and CpG-containing oligodeoxynucleotides activate cutaneous dendritic cells and induce IL-12 production: implications for the augmentation of Th1 responses. Int Arch Allergy Immunol 1999; 118:457–461.
41. Delogu G, Howard A, Collins FM, Morris SL. DNA vaccination against tuberculosis: expression of a ubiquitin-conjugated tuberculosis protein enhances antimycobacterial immunity. Infect Immun 2000; 68:3097–3102.

9

Development of Mucosal DNA Vaccines Against HIV-1 Using Live Attenuated *Salmonella typhi* as a Vaccine-Delivery System

George K. Lewis, M. Tarek Shata, and David M. Hone

Institute of Human Virology
University of Maryland Biotechnology Institute
Baltimore, Maryland

INTRODUCTION

This chapter summarizes the development of a mucosal DNA vaccine against HIV-1. This vaccine is based on an emerging strategy, which uses live attenuated *Salmonella typhi* as a vaccine-delivery system. The discovery that intracellular bacteria can "transfect" host cells with plasmids encoding eukaryotic expression cassettes, allowing the expression of vaccine genes by the host cell rather than the bacterium, has opened up a new avenue for the development of affordable mucosal vaccines against HIV-1. This phenomenon has been described for three bacterial genera, *Shigella* (1), *Salmonella* (2–4), and *Listeria* (5), which replicate in the cytoplasm of eukaryotic cells. All of these organisms infect via mucosal surfaces and are strong candidates for bacterial mucosal vaccine-delivery systems. The relative merits of each genus as vector vaccines are discussed in detail elsewhere (6–8). Because of the availability of an increasingly large series of strains that are well tolerated in human volunteers (reviewed in Refs. 9 and 10), it is likely that attenuated *Salmonella typhi* will be the first of these organisms to be evaluated as a delivery vehicle for DNA vaccines in humans. For this reason, this chapter focuses on attenuated *S. typhi* as a mucosal delivery system for DNA vaccines against HIV-1.

DESIRABLE PROPERTIES OF AN EFFECTIVE MUCOSAL VACCINE AGAINST HIV-1

The ultimate goal of any effort that aims to develop a vaccine against HIV-1 is to come up with an immunogen and a formulation that induces protective immunity and that will be affordable for worldwide use. Reaching this goal is handicapped by three obstacles. First, the vaccine must induce protective immunity against HIV-1. This can be determined conclusively only by large-scale efficacy trials in human volunteers who are at high risk for infection with HIV-1. In our view, it is unlikely over the next few years that such trials will identify a protective vaccine. For this reason, there is an intensive effort underway to identify correlates of protective immunity against HIV-1. These studies are carried out primarily in animal models of vaccination and in clinical studies in which the progression to AIDS appears to be checked by host immunity to HIV-1. Currently, there is strong evidence that passive immunization of nonhuman primates with antibodies can protect against infection (11–18), including mucosal transmission (11,12) showing clearly that antibodies can afford protective immunity provided the correct antibodies are present in high concentration prior to infection. In addition, there is general agreement that CD8+ T-cell responses limit viremia during acute infection (19–23) and protect against infection (24–27). It is unclear whether this protection is afforded by CTL activity, the secretion of antiviral factors such as β-chemokines, or both. Without a clear-cut correlate of protective immunity in either an animal model or a clinical setting where infection is limited, most of the current vaccine strategies are aimed empirically toward the induction of strong humoral and cellular immunity.

Second, an effective vaccine against HIV-1 must elicit protective immunity at each portal through which HIV-1 enters the host. A successful vaccine must protect against mucosal and parenteral exposures to HIV-1. This poses a dilemma for vaccine candidates that are delivered parenterally. It is known that parenteral immunization with nonreplicating vaccines usually induce little or no mucosal immunity (28). It is also known that recall responses can be elicited in both the mucosal and systemic compartments after boosting in either compartment; however, this requires priming in the mucosal compartment (29). Priming in the systemic compartment only allows recall responses in the systemic compartment, and these only occur when the boost is given parenterally (29). The induction of mucosal immunity will be particularly important if it turns out that sterilizing immunity is required for protection against HIV-1. In this case, once HIV-1 gains a stronghold, the die is cast and an infected person almost always progresses to AIDS. Although there is debate as to whether an effective vaccine against HIV-1 must induce sterilizing immunity or whether it must simply limit viral load, our group is focusing on the development of vaccines that induce sterilizing immunity. This requires that our candidate vaccines elicit both mucosal and systemic immunity.

Third, because most new HIV-1 infections are occurring in developing nations, the practical consideration of affordability is of considerable importance. Most of the HIV-1 vaccines in clinical trials include a soluble envelope subunit protein immunogen in conjunction with one or another viral vector encoding this and other proteins of HIV-1. The high cost of producing quantities of highly purified recombinant proteins is likely to make such vaccines less affordable in developing nations.

The desirable features of an HIV-1 vaccine are summarized in Table 1. This table is organized to reflect the ''top-down'' strategy taken by most of the major HIV-1 vaccine programs. The initial focus has been to identify an immunogen that elicits strong humoral and cellular responses to HIV-1 in human volunteers, preferably after the demonstration of protective immunity using this immunogen in nonhuman primates. This approach is highly appropriate, but it does not take into account that problems such as affordability ultimately determine whether the vaccine is practical for use in developing nations. One need only consider the dearth of antiretroviral drugs available in developing countries to realize the impact of cost on the use of a vaccine in these countries. By focusing primarily on immunogenicity in the early phases of HIV-1 vaccine development, it is possible that a vaccine will be developed that is difficult to transport, difficult to administer, and difficult to pay for in much of the world. These considerations, in addition to potent immunogenicity, have prefigured our attempts to develop a vaccine against HIV-1. Our tack is a ''bottoms-up'' approach in the context of Table 1.

Our strategy is to exploit live attenuated intracellular bacteria, particularly

Table 1 Desirable AIDS Vaccine Properties

1. Should induce broadly protective immunity in all people
2. Should protect against mucosal and parenteral exposure to HIV-1
3. Should be well tolerated
4. Should be deliverable without needles
5. Should be affordable by all people
6. Should be transportable without maintenance of cold chain

S. typhi, as mucosal delivery systems for HIV-1 antigens. Vector vaccines based on *S. typhi* begin with the inherent properties of being well tolerated, affordable in developing countries, and transportable with a minimal cold chain. In addition, bacterial vector vaccines offer additional safety in that they can be cleared by antibiotic therapy if untoward reactions occur. This is not possible for current configurations of viral vector vaccines. Because of these considerations, and if combinations of vectors and immunogens can be found that elicit strong humoral and cellular responses against HIV-1, it is very likely that HIV-1 vaccines based on bacterial delivery systems will increase the access of developing countries to an HIV-1 vaccine. In the sections to follow, we will review the current status of the development of attenuated strains of *S. typhi* that can be used as live vector vaccines for HIV-1 antigens and complement this review with a discussion of current immunogens that can be delivered by these vectors.

ATTENUATED *S. TYPHI* AS A MUCOSAL ANTIGEN-DELIVERY SYSTEM IN HUMANS

In recent years, attenuated salmonellae have been pursued vigorously not only as typhoid vaccines but as mucosal vaccine-delivery systems for passenger immunogens from viral, bacterial, and metazoan pathogens (reviewed in Ref. 30). This interest is based on three attributes of *Salmonella* biology: 1) an easily manipulated genetic system, 2) the availability of attenuating mutations, and 3) the ability of *Salmonella* to infect monocytes or dendritic cells after entry via mucosal surfaces. In addition, the key genetic elements of *Salmonella* that are responsible for pathogenesis are becoming known at a rapid rate (reviewed in Refs. 31–36), and there is little doubt that this information will lead to better vectors for the delivery of vaccine antigens.

Attenuating Mutations of *Salmonella*

A number of attenuating mutations render *S. typhi* avirulent while preserving immunogenicity (for a complete list see the Appendix in Ref. 30). These include mutations in genes involved in lipopolysaccharide (LPS) biosynthesis (37–39), aromatic amino acid metabolism (40), purine biosynthesis (41–43), regulatory genes (44), and virulence factors (45–47). Among this list, the deletion of the genes involved in aromatic amino acid metabolism (i.e., the *aro* genes) stand out as favored attenuating mutations because the loci are on distal parts of the bacterial chromosome. This allows the creation of double *aro* deletion mutants by allelic exchange. These mutations have extremely low probabilities of reversion to wild type. Additionally, the use of homologous recombination to delete these genes obviates the need to use antibiotic resistance, plasmid sequences, or sequences from non-*typhi* strains of *Salmonella* to create and maintain the mutant genotype. These properties have led to the development and evaluation of a series of attenuated vectors based on parental *S. typhi* strain Ty2 (48–52).

The parental strain for these vectors, CVD 908, was created by deletion of the *AroC* and *AroD* genes in wild-type *S. typhi* strain Ty2 (48–50). CVD 908 has been evaluated in phase I and phase II studies as a typhoid vaccine (10,51–55) and in one phase I study to deliver the circumsporozoite protein of *Plasmodium falciparum* as a passenger immunogen (56). It is also under evaluation in AVEG-028, a phase I study using CVD 908 to express and deliver a truncated gp120 protein from HIV-1 as a passenger immunogen. The published phase I and phase II studies show CVD 908 to be well tolerated and immunogenic after inoculation of volunteers with a single oral dose of the vaccine; however, a transient, asymptomatic bacteremia is occasionally detected in the volunteers when blood was cultured on auxotrophic media. Although the bacteremia observed with *aro* mutants such as CVD 908 is asymptomatic and transient, it led to the addition of a third attenuating mutation to create CVD 908-*htrA*. The *htrA* locus encodes a *Salmonella* heat-shock protein, and deletion of this gene impairs the ability of *Salmonella* to survive in the host (57–59). In both phase I (52) and phase II (60) studies CVD 908-*htrA* has proven well tolerated and immunogenic at doses ranging from 5×10^7 colony forming units (cfu) to 5×10^9 cfu after a single oral inoculation. Most importantly, no vaccine bacteremias were observed and CVD 908-*htrA* retained immunogenicity. Thus, CVD 908-*htrA* appears both safe and immunogenic, making it a promising strain to be evaluated as a delivery system for DNA vaccines.

In addition to the mutations described above, the recent wealth of information emerging from studies of the molecular pathogenesis of *Salmonella* infections points the way toward ever more sophisticated attenuation strategies. For example, the identification of bacterial genes that control invasion encoded by the *inv* locus (reviewed in Refs. 31–36) offers promising new targets for the precise control of the *Salmonella* life cycle in vivo. Selected examples of how these genes control key steps in bacterial pathogenesis are described below.

Salmonella Infects Monocytes/Dendritic Cells After Entry via Mucosal Surfaces

Humans are the only natural host and reservoir of *S. typhi* (reviewed in Refs. 9 and 61), and the current picture of the pathogenesis of typhoid fever (or enteric fever) sets the stage for the exploitation of this organism as a mucosal vaccine-delivery system. This picture is presented in Figure 1. Typhoid is a systemic infection of the reticuloendothelial system of considerable severity. The appearance of disease requires approximately 1–3 weeks, with abdominal pain and fever being the classical signs of typhoid fever. These symptoms can be preceded by variable diarrhea, enterocolitis, chills, anorexia, weakness, and muscle pains. The

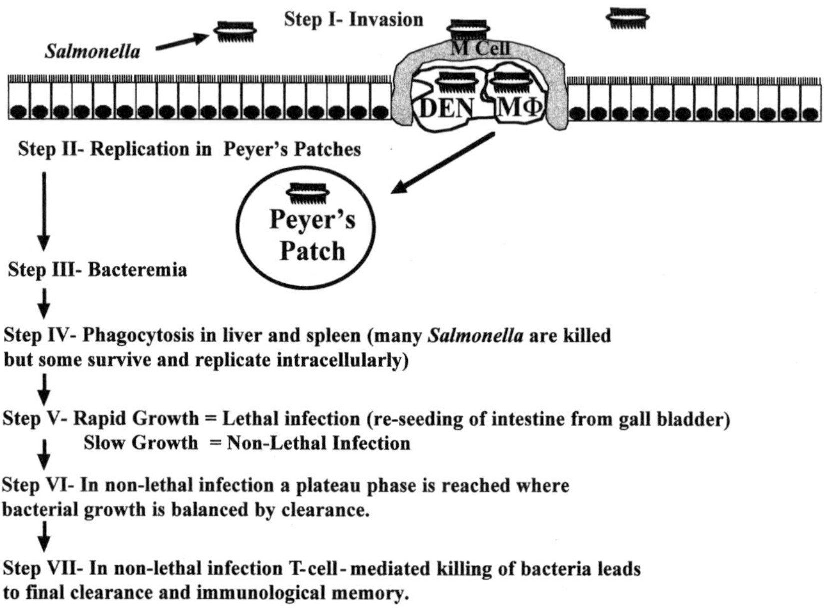

Figure 1 Depiction of the stages in the pathogenesis of enteric (typhoid-like) fevers. This information is synthesized from studies carried out in humans infected with *S. typhi* and in mice infected with *S. typhimurium.* DEN = Dendritic cells; MΦ = macrophages.

goal of the attenuating mutations described above is to obviate symptoms while preserving the ability of *S. typhi* to induce immune responses to itself and passenger antigens. This requires that the bacteria be allowed to enter the body and to elicit an immune response but not to disseminate and produce disease. The deepening understanding of the key steps in *Salmonella* pathogenesis at the molecular level makes this a real possibility over the next few years.

Since *S. typhi* is highly host adapted to humans, our picture of typhoid pathogenesis is a composite drawn from clinical studies in humans, vaccine studies in human volunteers, studies in chimpanzees, and studies carried out in a mouse typhoid (enteric fever) model using *Salmonella typhimurium*, which causes gastroenteritis in humans rather than enteric fever. In fact, most of what is known about the use of *Salmonella* as a mucosal delivery system for passenger antigens comes from studies that use *S. typhimurium* in mice (reviewed in Refs. 9 and 30). This is true also for studies of the mucosal cell types that are infected shortly after entry of *Salmonella* into the intestinal tract. With this caveat in mind, the following picture emerges of typhoid pathogenesis (Fig. 1).

After ingestion, *Salmonella* passes through the pylorus and enters the small intestine. The organisms bind to the surfaces of epithelial cells, including both enterocytes and M cells. M cells appear to be the major portal of entry for *Salmonella*, as they allow the bacteria to pass freely through the cytoplasm and exit through their basolateral surfaces to the underlying tissue space that is rich in dendritic cells, macrophages, and lymphocytes (Step I, Fig. 1). At this point, *Salmonella* appear to infect CD11c+ dendritic cells or macrophages that move deeper into the organized mucosal lymphoid tissues, including lymphoid follicles and Peyer's patches, which are the first sites to be colonized (62) (Step II, Fig. 1). This occurs within 3 hours of gastric inoculation of mice with *S. typhimurium* (63,64). Studies of ligated ileal loops in the mouse model have identified M cells as the primary portal of entry for *Salmonella* (63–66). Organized mucosal lymphoid tissues such as follicles and Peyer's patches are covered by M cells and enterocytes in an approximate 1:20 ratio (67–69). The M cells form tight junctions with the enterocytes and possess a unique lumenal surface with characteristic "microfolds." M cells have increased pinocytic activity as compared to enterocytes and allow safe conduct of macromolecules, viral particles, bacteria, and metazoan parasites to the underlying organized lymphoid tissue (reviewed in Refs. 70 and 71).

The entry of *Salmonella* into M cells is accompanied by the "ruffling" of the apical membrane and rearrangement of the cytoskeleton and death of the M cells, an apparently unique feature of this interaction (63,72). These events are controlled by *Salmonella* genes that map to one of two known pathogenicity islands, which control the entry of *Salmonella* into susceptible cells [*Salmonella* pathogenicity island 1 (SPI1) or survival in the cytoplasm of phagocytic cells (SPI2) (reviewed in Refs. 31–36)]. SP1 encodes a Type III secretion system that allows the delivery of bacterial proteins encoded by SP1 into the cytoplasm of the eukaryotic cell (31–36). These proteins are responsible for the cytoskeletal rearrangements necessary for entry of *Salmonella* into the susceptible cell.

Once past the M cell, virulent *Salmonella* infects cells of the underlying lymphoid follicles and Peyer's patches, which are the principal sites of initial *Salmonella* replication in vivo (62). It has been known for some time that *Salmonella* readily infects macrophages and that they are the primary targets of infection in the organized mucosal lymphoid tissue (reviewed in Ref. 61). Several recent studies suggest that *Salmonella* infect subepithelial CD11c+ dendritic cells as well (4,73–76). This is supported by a recent study demonstrating the co-localization of *Salmonella* with CD11c+ dendritic cells in the subepithelial dome of organized mucosal lymphoid tissue (73). Furthermore, recent studies showed that salmonellae infect CD11c+ dendritic cells in vitro, where they initiate proinflammatory cytokine synthesis (76) and the presentation of passenger antigens by both the class I and class II MHC pathways (74). The infection of dendritic cells by *Salmonella* is supported by a very recent study using a eukaryotic expression vector encoding green fluorescent protein (GFP) to identify target cells "transfected" by *Salmonella* carrying this plasmid clone (4). Thus, it appears that in addition to macrophages, *Salmonella* infect CD11c+ dendritic cells very early in infection.

It should be noted also that in addition to entry via M cells, there is an older literature suggesting that *Salmonella* can enter through enterocytes (77) and by destroying tight cell junctions between adjacent enterocytes (reviewed in Ref. 31). The importance of these pathways relative to the M cell is not established, and the current consensus favors the M cell as the primary portal of entry for *Salmonella*.

Despite this consensus, a new pathway for *Salmonella* entry has been described that appears to involve neither M cells nor enterocytes (31,78). *Salmonella typhimurium* in which SPI1 was functionally inactivated by mutagenesis of the *invA* gene does not enter via M cells or enterocytes, disrupt tight cell junctions, or replicate in Peyer's patches (31,78). Yet these organisms disseminate systemically producing a lethal infection. It was also found that dissemination was dependent upon the presence of CD18+ phagocytes and that IgG but not IgA anti-*Salmonella* antibodies were produced concomitantly (31,78). Thus, genes of SPI1 dictate not only the route of entry but also the quality of the immune response to this bacterium and the ability to establish a lethal infection. As more information emerges about the relationships among these variables, it is certain that new strategies will become available to exploit in the development of *Salmonella*-based delivery systems for many different candidate vaccines.

After these early steps, which occur in a matter of hours, infected monocytes/dendritic cells seed distal secondary lymphoid tissue via the blood producing a bacteremia (Step III, Fig. 1). These tissues include the mesenteric lymph nodes and subsequently the spleen and liver, where the *Salmonella* replicate in vacuoles within phagocytic cells (Step IV). Over time, the balance between the ability of the *Salmonella* to grow in these vacuoles and the ability of the phagocytes to kill the *Salmonella* determines the severity of symptoms and disease, which are associated with a secondary bacteremia that is accompanied by intestinal perforations and high fever. The genes encoded by SPI2 of *Salmonella* are likely to play key roles in determining this balance. The complexity of this process is underscored by the need for both antibody and class I plus class II MHC-restricted cell-mediated immunity to confer protective immunity against *Salmonella* in the mouse typhoid model (79).

Although the intermediate steps in typhoid pathogenesis are still incompletely characterized, it appears that certain attenuating mutations allow *Salmonella* to pass the M cell and to infect monocytes and dendritic cells, which then initiate both antibody- and T-cell–mediated responses. One key feature of the attenuated *Salmonella* strains studied by our group in both mice and humans is their ability to induce both mucosal and systemic immunity after oral inoculation

(30,53,54,80,81). This is consistent with the propensity of "antigen-loaded" dendritic cells to migrate to distal lymphoid tissues, where they initiate both humoral and cell-mediated immune responses (reviewed in Ref. 82). Currently, little is known about the precise mechanisms whereby passenger antigens are presented when they are delivered by *Salmonella* except that "cross-priming" appears to be involved between dendritic cells and apoptotic monocytes that are created by infection with *Salmonella* (83).

Delivery of Passenger Antigens by *Salmonella*

There is ample evidence that *S. typhi* can elicit both class I and class II MHC-restricted T-cell responses to passenger antigens (see the Appendix in Ref. 30 for review) in both the mucosal and systemic compartments. In this regard, it should be noted there are significant empirical differences among individual passenger antigens in their ability to induce these responses that are related to expression levels and antigen placement in the bacterium (81; reviewed in Ref. 7). In addition to cell-mediated responses, attenuated *Salmonella* also elicit both serum and mucosal antibody responses to passenger antigens (81). While it is very likely that the delivery of passenger antigens expressed by *Salmonella* will lead to new vaccines, there are two major problems in using this strategy to develop a vaccine against HIV-1. First, *Salmonella* cannot fold and glycosylate the HIV-1 Env protein, and we know that gp120 constructs expressed by *Salmonella* do not induce significant levels of neutralizing antibodies (81; unpublished data). Second, expression of HIV-1 proteins by *Salmonella* may "hyper-attenuate" the vector vaccine and reduce immunogenicity of these proteins. We have repeatedly found that the stable expression of even truncated gp120 is very difficult (81) due largely to the energetics of the protein-synthetic machinery of the bacterium to handle the expression of this protein. For this reason, we sought other means of expressing the HIV-1 antigens in order to exploit *Salmonella* as delivery system for a vaccine against HIV-1. This led to the use of *Salmonella* as a delivery vehicle for DNA vaccines.

Delivery of Passenger Antigens Encoded in DNA Vaccines by *Salmonella*

The ability of intracellular gram-negative bacteria to "transfect" infected cells with plasmids encoding eukaryotic expression systems was discovered independently by three groups (1,84,85), including ourselves (84). Although it is still early in the game, it appears that this is a robust method for the delivery of DNA vaccines. The first study to use intracellular bacteria to deliver a DNA vaccine reported that antigen-specific humoral and T-cell proliferative responses were elicited by *Shigella flexneri* carrying a DNA vaccine encoding β-galactosidase (LacZ) (86). A more extensive study reported the induction of antibody responses and both class I and class II MHC-restricted T-cell responses to LacZ after immunization with *S. typhimurium* carrying a eukaryotic expression plasmid encoding LacZ (2). Additionally, protection was induced against *Listeria monocytogenes* using this same system to deliver *Listeria* antigens (2). In similar studies, protective immunity was induced against tumor cells expressing LacZ when mice were immunized with attenuated *S. typhimurium* to deliver a eukaryotic expression plasmid encoding LacZ (4). This study also demonstrated dendritic cell expression of the transfected gene using the *Salmonella* to deliver a GFP gene on a eukaryotic expression plasmid (4). Most recently Fennelly and coworkers (3) provided detailed evidence for the induction of both antibodies and CTLs specific for measles virus proteins using *S. flexneri* to deliver a DNA vaccine encoding these proteins.

DEVELOPMENT OF A *SALMONELLA* HIV-1 DNA VACCINE

Our interest in the delivery of DNA vaccines by attenuated intracellular bacteria arose from our earlier studies using *Salmonella* to deliver gp120 of HIV-1. We initiated those studies approximately a decade ago at a time when it appeared possible that linear epitopes of gp120 might elicit meaningful neutralizing antibodies and when the first studies were appearing implicating a role for cellular immune responses in the control of HIV-1. We decided to express gp120 in attenuated *Salmonella* with the hope that such an immunogen would elicit neutralizing antibodies and cellular immune responses to this protein. It became apparent soon afterward that antibodies that neutralize HIV-1 with any degree of breadth typically recognize complex epitopes, and we showed that the gp120 expressed in *S. typhi* is misfolded and did not express such epitopes (87). After several iterations of construct refinement (88), we developed a truncated gp120 (tgp120) that consistently elicited both systemic and mucosal T-cell proliferative/cytokine responses and antibody responses after a single oral inoculation of mice using attenuated *S. typhimurium* (81). This led to the evaluation of our tgp120 construct in humans using attenuated *S. typhi* strain CVD 908 under the aegis of the NIAID AIDS Vaccine Evaluation Group protocol AVEG-028. Although AVEG-028 is still underway, two problems remained with our *S. typhimurium*–tgp120 system that required additional refinement.

First, even though this construct would elicit antibody, there was little chance that the tgp120 expressed by *Salmonella* would fold properly to create the discontinuous epitopes that elicit broadly neutralizing antibodies. Second, we obtained believable CD8+ CTL responses with this construct infrequently (about one experiment in 6). These problems became apparent as the first reports were appearing that described the induction of antibody responses and good CD8+ T-cell responses by DNA vaccines.

We postulated that intracellular gram-negative bacteria such as *Salmonella* and *Shigella*, which easily maintain the plasmids encoding eukaryotic expression vectors, might deliver such a vector to the cytoplasm in an infected cell in such a way that it would reach the nucleus and be expressed (Fig. 2). This turned out to be the case, as shown by the nearly simultaneous description of the phenomenon in late 1995 and early 1996 by Sizemore et al. (85), Courvalin et. al. (1), and ourselves (84). This phenomenon, which we call "bactofection," was extended by in vivo studies showing that immune responses could be elicited using *Shigella* delivering DNA vaccines encoding LacZ (3,85,86) or measles virus proteins (3), *S. typhimurium* delivering DNA vaccines encoding LacZ or *Listeria* antigens (2), or *S. typhi* delivering DNA vaccines encoding measles virus antigens (3). Our own studies using *Salmonella* to deliver DNA vaccines encoding HIV-1 Env proteins have required improvements in the DNA vaccine to obtain consistently strong CTL responses and are currently under submission for publication. They can be summarized as follows.

Our initial studies using *Salmonella* to deliver HIV-1 DNA vaccines employed an Env construct that requires the presence of the viral regulatory gene Rev in order for mRNA encoding Env to exit the nucleus. Similar Env constructs have been used for a number of years by others as naked DNA vaccines in which both humoral and cellular immune responses can be obtained against Env epitopes after inoculation of mice and primates with large doses of the naked DNA vaccine (89; reviewed in Ref. 90). In our hands, such constructs proved inadequate in that multiple large doses of the naked Env DNA vaccine were required

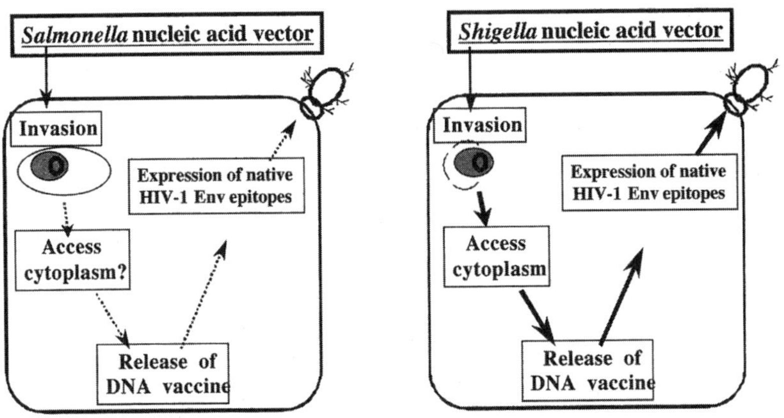

Figure 2 Depiction of "bactofection" by the intracellular bacteria *Salmonella* and *Shigella*.

to elicit such responses in mice (unpublished data). The difficulties of expressing Env in both human and rodent cells are now well known, and this problem severely hampered our use of *Salmonella* to deliver traditional (i.e., Rev-dependent) Env-based DNA vaccines in animal models. A solution to this dilemma emerged from the seminal studies from Brian Seed's group (91,92) that identified the importance of codon optimization for the *rev*-independent, high-level expression of HIV-1 *env* genes.

It was recognized that HIV-1 uses a highly unusual codon bias that is quite different from the optimal bias for human genes. Through a heroic synthesis of an entire *env* gene using an optimal human codon bias, it was shown that very high levels of *env* gene expression could be obtained leading to a 50- to 100-fold increase in the amount of Env protein synthesized in transfected cells (91,92). Most importantly, the expression of codon-optimized *env* genes was entirely independent of Rev (91,92). Seed's group quickly showed that codon-optimized Env DNA vaccines were much more immunogenic in mice than traditional Env DNA vaccines (92), which led to the development of a codon-optimized *env* gene for the R5 isolate HIV-$1_{\text{Ba-L}}$ (D. M. Hone et al., unpublished). Using attenuated *S. typhimurium* to deliver this codon-optimized DNA vaccine, we now obtain Env-specific CD8+ T-cell responses after a single oral inoculation with the bacteria that are comparable to those obtained by the same DNA vaccine delivered intramuscularly. An example of one such study is shown in Figure 3. In this experiment, BALB/cJ mice were immunized orally with a single dose of 5×10^9 attenuated *S. typhimurium* SL7207 carrying a codon-optimized DNA vaccine encoding a secreted form (gp140) of the HIV-1 envelope glycoprotein of HIV-$1_{\text{Ba-L}}$. As a negative control, the mice were immunized with SL7207 carrying an "empty" plasmid vector that we use to deliver DNA vaccines. Separate groups of BALB/cJ mice were immunized intramuscularly with 5 μg of endotoxin-free gp140 DNA vaccine or the empty expression vector in phosphate-buffered saline. One week later HIV-1–specific CD8+ T-cell responses were evaluated for an immunodominant CTL epitope in the V3 region of gp140 by IFN-γ ELISPOT assay. As shown in Figure 3, immunization with the DNA vaccine using either SL7207 as the delivery vehicle or naked plasmid DNA elicited specific CD8+ T-cell responses of comparable magnitude. No specific response was observed when the empty plasmid vector was used. This study shows that it is possible to generate CD8+ T-cell responses to HIV-1 DNA vaccines using attenuated *S. typhimurium* as the delivery vehicle. Furthermore, these responses approximate those obtained by intramuscular inoculation with the same HIV-1 DNA vaccine. We are currently identifying and optimizing the variables in this system that effect the immunogenicity of the DNA vaccine. These include the dose, the *Salmonella* strain used as the vector, the promoter used to drive the *env* gene, and the requirement for boosting with homologous and heterologous forms of the DNA vaccine.

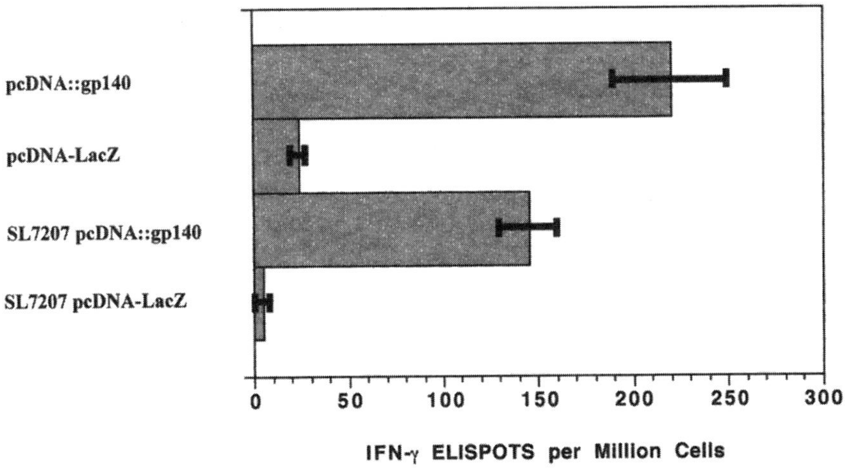

Figure 3 Induction of CD8+ T-cell responses by a codon-optimized gp140 DNA vaccine delivered by either a single oral inoculation with attenuated *S. typhimurium* strain SL7207 or a single intramuscular inoculation with 5 μg of the same DNA vaccine as naked DNA. Control DNA vaccines are pcDNA-LacZ, which is the same plasmid backbone used to deliver the pcDNA::gp140, except that the gp140-coding sequences were replaced by β-galactosidase–coding sequences.

In summary, it is now clear that attenuated intracellular bacteria, including *Salmonella*, can be used to deliver DNA vaccines after oral inoculation. The simplicity of this approach has the potential to overcome many of the problems of formulation, delivery, and cost that are likely to be significant impediments to the worldwide delivery of an effective vaccine against HIV-1. If the correct combination of protective immunogens can be found that can be delivered by attenuated *Salmonella*, these problems can be overcome, resulting in an affordable vaccine against HIV-1.

REFERENCES

1. Courvalin P, Goussard S, Grillot-Courvalin C. Gene transfer from bacteria to mammalian cells. C R Acad Sci III 1995; 318:1207–1212.
2. Darji, A, Guzman CA, Gerstel B, Wachholz P, Timmis KN, Wehland J, Chakraborty T, Weiss S. Oral somatic transgene vaccination using attenuated *S. typhimurium*. Cell 1997; 91:765–775.

3. Fennelly GJ, Khan SA, Abadi MA, Wild TF, Bloom BR. Mucosal DNA vaccine immunization against measles with a highly attenuated *Shigella flexneri* vector. J Immunol 1999; 162:1603–1610.
4. Paglia P, Medina E, Arioli I, Guzman CA, Colombo MP. Gene transfer in dendritic cells, induced by oral DNA vaccination with *Salmonella typhimurium*, results in protective immunity against a murine fibrosarcoma. Blood 1998; 92:3172–3176.
5. Cornell KA, Bouwer HG, Hinrichs DJ, Barry RA. Genetic immunization of mice against *Listeria monocytogenes* using plasmid DNA encoding listeriolysin O. J Immunol 1999; 163:322–329.
6. Darji A, zur Lage S, Garbe AI, Chakraborty T, Weiss S. Oral delivery of DNA vaccines using attenuated *Salmonella typhimurium* as carrier. FEMS Immunol Med Microbiol 2000; 27:341–349.
7. Shata MT, Stevceva L, Agwale S, Lewis GK, Hone DM. Recent advances with recombinant bacterial vaccine vectors. Mol Med Today 2000; 6:66–71.
8. Spreng S, Dietrich G, Niewiesk S, ter Meulen V, Gentschev I, Goebel W. Novel bacterial systems for the delivery of recombinant protein or DNA. FEMS Immunol Med Microbiol 2000; 27:299–304.
9. Levine MM. Typhoid fever vaccines. In: Plotkin SA, Orenstein WA, eds. Vaccines. 3rd ed. Philadelphia: WB Saunders, 1994:781–814.
10. Levine MM, Galen J, Barry E, Noriega F, Tacket C, Sztein M, Chatfield S, Dougan G, Losonsky G, Kotloff K. Attenuated *Salmonella typhi* and *Shigella* as live oral vaccines and as live vectors. Behring Inst Mitt 1997; 120–123.
11. Mascola JR, Stiegler G, VanCott TC, Katinger H, Carpenter CB, Hanson CE, Beary H, Hayes D, Frankel SS, Birx DL, Lewis MG. Protection of macaques against vaginal transmission of a pathogenic HIV-1/SIV chimeric virus by passive infusion of neutralizing antibodies. Nat Med 2000; 6: 207–210.
12. Baba TW, Liska V, Hofmann-Lehmann R, Vlasak J, Xu W, Ayehunie S, Cavacini LA, Posner MR, Katinger H, Stiegler G, Bernacky BJ, Rizvi TA, Schmidt R, Hill LR, Keeling ME, Lu Y, Wright JE, Chou TC, Ruprecht RM. Human neutralizing monoclonal antibodies of the IgG1 subtype protect against mucosal simian-human immunodeficiency virus infection. Nat Med 2000; 6:200–206.
13. Mascola JR, Lewis MG, Stiegler G, Harris D, VanCott TC, Hayes D, Louder MK, Brown CR, Sapan CV, Frankel SS, Lu Y, Robb ML, Katinger H, Birx DL. Protection of macaques against pathogenic simian/human immunodeficiency virus 89.6PD by passive transfer of neutralizing antibodies. J Virol 1999; 73:4009–4018.

14. Shibata R, Igarashi T, Haigwood N, Buckler-White A, Ogert R, Ross W, Willey R, Cho MW, Martin MA. Neutralizing antibody directed against the HIV-1 envelope glycoprotein can completely block HIV-1/SIV chimeric virus infections of macaque monkeys [comments]. Nat Med 1999; 5: 204–210.
15. Foresman L, Jia F, Li Z, Wang C, Stephens EB, Sahni M, Narayan O, Joag SV. Neutralizing antibodies administered before, but not after, virulent SHIV prevent infection in macaques. AIDS Res Hum Retroviruses 1998; 14:1035–1043.
16. Joag SV, Li Z, Wang C, Foresman L, Jia F, Stephens EB, Zhuge W, Narayan O. Passively administered neutralizing serum that protected macaques against infection with parenterally inoculated pathogenic simian-human immunodeficiency virus failed to protect against mucosally inoculated virus. AIDS Res Hum Retroviruses 1999; 15:391–394.
17. Van Rompay KK, Berardi CJ, Dillard-Telm S, Tarara RP, Canfield DR, Valverde CR, Montefiori DC, Cole KS, Montelaro RC, Miller CJ, Marthas ML. Passive immunization of newborn rhesus macaques prevents oral simian immunodeficiency virus infection. J Infect Dis 1998; 177:1247–1259.
18. Emini EA, Schleif WA, Nunberg JH, Conley AJ, Eda Y, Tokiyoshi S, Putney SD, Matsushita S, Cobb KE, Jett CM, et al. Prevention of HIV-1 infection in chimpanzees by gp120 V3 domain-specific monoclonal antibody. Nature 1992; 355:728–730.
19. Borrow P, Lewicki H, Hahn BH, Shaw GM, Oldstone MB. Virus-specific CD8+ cytotoxic T-lymphocyte activity associated with control of viremia in primary human immunodeficiency virus type 1 infection. J Virol 1994; 68:6103–6110.
20. Koup RA, Safrit JT, Cao Y, Andrews CA, McLeod G, Borkowsky W, Farthing C, Ho DD. Temporal association of cellular immune responses with the initial control of viremia in primary human immunodeficiency virus type 1 syndrome. J Virol 1994; 68:4650–4655.
21. Klein MR, van Baalen CA, Holwerda AM, Kerkhof Garde SR, Bende RJ, Keet IP, Eeftinck-Schattenkerk JK, Osterhaus AD, Schuitemaker H, Miedema F. Kinetics of Gag-specific cytotoxic T lymphocyte responses during the clinical course of HIV-1 infection: a longitudinal analysis of rapid progressors and long-term asymptomatics. J Exp Med 1995; 181:1365–1372.
22. Musey L, Hughes J, Schacker T, Shea T, Corey L, McElrath MJ. Cytotoxic-T-cell responses, viral load, and disease progression in early human immunodeficiency virus type 1 infection [comments]. N Engl J Med 1997; 337: 1267–1274.
23. Ogg GS, Jin X, Bonhoeffer S, Dunbar PR, Nowak MA, Monard S, Segal JP, Cao Y, Rowland-Jones SL, Cerundolo V, Hurley A, Markowitz M, Ho

DD, Nixon DF, McMichael AJ. Quantitation of HIV-1-specific cytotoxic T lymphocytes and plasma load of viral RNA. Science 1998; 279:2103–2106.

24. Rowland-Jones SL, Nixon DF, Aldhous MC, Gotch F, Ariyoshi K, Hallam N, Kroll JS, Froebel K, McMichael A. HIV-specific cytotoxic T-cell activity in an HIV-exposed but uninfected infant. Lancet 1993; 341:860–861.
25. De Maria A, Cirillo C, Moretta L. Occurrence of human immunodeficiency virus type 1 (HIV-1)-specific cytolytic T cell activity in apparently uninfected children born to HIV-1-infected mothers. J Infect Dis 1994; 170: 1296–1299.
26. Rowland-Jones S, Sutton J, Ariyoshi K, Dong T, Gotch F, McAdam S, Whitby D, Sabally S, Gallimore A, Corrah T, et al. HIV-specific cytotoxic T-cells in HIV-exposed but uninfected Gambian women. Nat Med 1995; 1(1):59–64. Erratum appears in Nat Med 1995; 1(6):598.
27. Pinto LA, Sullivan J, Berzofsky JA, Clerici M, Kessler HA, Landay AL, Shearer GM. ENV-specific cytotoxic T lymphocyte responses in HIV seronegative health care workers occupationally exposed to HIV-contaminated body fluids. J Clin Invest 1995; 96:867–876.
28. de Aizpurua HJ, Russell-Jones GJ. Oral vaccination. Identification of classes of proteins that provoke an immune response upon oral feeding. J Exp Med 1988; 167:440–451.
29. Herremans TM, Reimerink JH, Buisman AM, Kimman TG, Koopmans MP. Induction of mucosal immunity by inactivated poliovirus vaccine is dependent on previous mucosal contact with live virus. J Immunol 1999; 162: 5011–5018.
30. Hone DM, Shata MT, Pascual DW, Lewis GK. Mucosal vaccination with *Salmonella* vaccine vectors: past, present, and future. In: Patterson Y, ed. Intracellular Bacterial Vaccine Vectors: Immunology, Cell Biology, and Genetics. New York: Wiley and Sons, 1999:171–222.
31. Vazquez-Torres A, Fang FC. Cellular routes of invasion by enteropathogens. Curr Opin Microbiol 2000; 3:54–59.
32. Galan JE. Interaction of Salmonella with host cells through the centisome 63 type III secretion system. Curr Opin Microbiol 1999; 2:46–50.
33. Galan JE, Collmer A. Type III secretion machines: bacterial devices for protein delivery into host cells. Science 1999; 284:1322–1328.
34. Collazo CM, Galan JE. The invasion-associated type-III protein secretion system in *Salmonella*—a review. Gene 1997; 192:51–59.
35. Galan JE, Bliska JB. Cross-talk between bacterial pathogens and their host cells. Annu Rev Cell Dev Biol 1996; 12:221–255.
36. Galan JE. Molecular genetic bases of *Salmonella* entry into host cells. Mol Microbiol 1996; 20:263–271.

37. Collins LV, Attridge S, Hackett J. Mutations at rfc or pmi attenuate *Salmonella typhimurium* virulence for mice. Infect Immun 1991; 59:1079–1085.
38. Hone D, Morona R, Attridge S, Hackett J. Construction of defined galE mutants of *Salmonella* for use as vaccines. J Infect Dis 1987; 156:167–174.
39. Germanier R, Furer E. Immunity in experimental salmonellosis. II. Basis for the avirulence and protective capacity of gal E mutants of *Salmonella typhimurium*. Infect Immun 1971; 4:663–673.
40. Hoiseth SK, Stocker BA. Aromatic-dependent *Salmonella typhimurium* are non-virulent and effective as live vaccines. Nature 1981; 291:238–239.
41. Sigwart DF, Stocker BA, Clements JD. Effect of a purA mutation on efficacy of *Salmonella* live-vaccine vectors. Infect Immun 1989; 57:1858–1861.
42. McFarland WC, Stocker BA. Effect of different purine auxotrophic mutations on mouse-virulence of a Vi-positive strain of *Salmonella dublin* and of two strains of *Salmonella typhimurium*. Microb Pathog 1987; 3:129–141.
43. O'Callaghan D, Maskell D, Liew FY, Easmon CS, Dougan G. Characterization of aromatic- and purine-dependent *Salmonella typhimurium*: attention, persistence, and ability to induce protective immunity in BALB/c mice. Infect Immun 1988; 56:419–423.
44. Curtiss R 3rd, Kelly SM. *Salmonella typhimurium* deletion mutants lacking adenylate cyclase and cyclic AMP receptor protein are avirulent and immunogenic. Infect Immun 1987; 55:3035–3043. Live vaccines or as vectors for antigens of other pathogens.
45. Galan JE, Curtiss R 3rd. Cloning and molecular characterization of genes whose products allow *Salmonella typhimurium* to penetrate tissue culture cells. Proc Natl Acad Sci USA 1989; 86:6383–6387.
46. Miller SI, Kukral AM, Mekalanos JJ. A two-component regulatory system (phoP phoQ) controls *Salmonella typhimurium* virulence. Proc Natl Acad Sci USA 1989; 86:5054–5058.
47. Galan JE, Curtiss R 3rd. Virulence and vaccine potential of phoP mutants of *Salmonella typhimurium*. Microb Pathog 1989; 6:433–443.
48. Hone DM, Harris AM, Chatfield S, Dougan G, Levine MM. Construction of genetically defined double aro mutants of *Salmonella typhi*. Vaccine 1991; 9:810–816.
49. Servos S, Chatfield S, Hone D, Levine M, Dimitriadis G, Pickard D, Dougan G, Fairweather N, Charles I. Molecular cloning and characterization of the aroD gene encoding 3-dehydroquinase from *Salmonella typhi*. J Gen Microbiol 1991; 137:147–152.
50. Hone DM, Tacket CO, Harris AM, Kay B, Losonsky G, Levine MM. Evalu-

ation in volunteers of a candidate live oral attenuated *Salmonella typhi* vector vaccine. J Clin Invest 1992; 90:412–420.

51. Levine MM, Galen J, Barry E, Noriega F, Chatfield S, Sztein M, Dougan G, Tacket C. Attenuated *Salmonella* as live oral vaccines against typhoid fever and as live vectors. J Biotechnol 1996; 44:193–196.
52. Tacket CO, Sztein MB, Losonsky GA, Wasserman SS, Nataro JP, Edelman R, Pickard D, Dougan G, Chatfield SN, Levine MM. Safety of live oral *Salmonella typhi* vaccine strains with deletions in htrA and aroC aroD and immune response in humans. Infect Immun 1997; 65:452–456.
53. Tacket CO, Hone DM, Losonsky GA, Guers L, Edelman R, Levine MM. Clinical acceptability and immunogenicity of CVD 908 *Salmonella typhi* vaccine strain. Vaccine 1992; 10:443–446.
54. Tacket CO, Hone DM, Curtiss R 3rd, Kelly SM, Losonsky G, Guers L, Harris AM, Edelman R, Levine MM. Comparison of the safety and immunogenicity of delta aroC delta aroD and delta cya delta crp *Salmonella typhi* strains in adult volunteers. Infect Immun 1992; 60:536–541.
55. Tacket CO, Kelly SM, Schodel, F, Losonsky G, Nataro JP, Edelman R, Levine MM, Curtiss R 3rd. Safety and immunogenicity in humans of an attenuated *Salmonella typhi* vaccine vector strain expressing plasmid-encoded hepatitis B antigens stabilized by the Asd-balanced lethal vector system. Infect Immun 1997; 65(8):3381–3385. Erratum appears in Infect Immun 1997; 65(9):3981.
56. Noriega FR, Wang JY, Losonsky G, Maneval DR, Hone DM, Levine MM. Construction and characterization of attenuated delta aroA delta virG *Shigella flexneri* 2a strain CVD 1203, a prototype live oral vaccine. Infect Immun 1994; 62:5168–5172.
57. Johnson K, Charles, I, Dougan G, Pickard D, O'Gaora, P, Costa G, Ali T, Miller, I, Hormaeche C. The role of a stress-response protein in Salmonella typhimurium virulence. Mol Microbiol 1991; 5:401–407.
58. Strahan K, Chatfield SN, Tite J, Dougan G, Hormaeche CE. Impaired resistance to infection does not increase the virulence of *Salmonella* htrA live vaccines for mice. Microb Pathog 1992; 12:311–317.
59. Chatfield SN, Strahan K, Pickard D, Charles IG, Hormaeche CE, Dougan G. Evaluation of *Salmonella typhimurium* strains harbouring defined mutations in htrA and aroA in the murine salmonellosis model. Microb Pathog 1992; 12:145–151.
60. Tacket CO, Sztein MB, Wasserman SS, Losonsky G, Kotloff K, Wyant TL, Nataro JP, Edelmena R, Perry J, Bedford P, Brown D, Chatfield S, Dougan G, Levine MM. Phase 2 clinical trial of attenuated *Salmonella typhi* oral live vector vaccine CVD 908-*htrA* in U.S. volunteers. Infect Immun 2000; 68:1196–1201.

61. Jones BD, Falkow S. Salmonellosis: host immune responses and bacterial virulence determinants. Annu Rev Immunol 1996; 14:533–561.
62. Carter PB, Collins FM. The route of enteric infection in normal mice. J Exp Med 1974; 139:1189–1203.
63. Jones BD, Ghori N, Falkow S. *Salmonella typhimurium* initiates murine infection by penetrating and destroying the specialized epithelial M cells of the Peyer's patches [comments]. J Exp Med 1994; 180:15–23.
64. Jones B, Pascopella L, Falkow S. Entry of microbes into the host: using M cells to break the mucosal barrier. Curr Opin Immunol 1995; 7:474–478.
65. Kohbata S, Yokoyama H, Yabuuchi E. Cytopathogenic effect of *Salmonella typhi* GIFU 10007 on M cells of murine ileal Peyer's patches in ligated ileal loops: an ultrastructural study. Microbiol Immunol 1986; 30:1225–1237.
66. Clark MA, Jepson MA, Simmons NL, Hirst BH. Preferential interaction of *Salmonella typhimurium* with mouse Peyer's patch M cells. Res Microbiol 1994; 145:543–552.
67. Bockman DE, Cooper MD. Pinocytosis by epithelium associated with lymphoid follicles in the bursa of Fabricius, appendix, and Peyer's patches. An electron microscopic study. Am J Anat 1973; 136:455–477.
68. Owen RL, Jones AL. Epithelial cell specialization within human Peyer's patches: an ultrastructural study of intestinal lymphoid follicles. Gastroenterology 1974; 66:189–203.
69. Owen RL, Ermak TH. Structural specializations for antigen uptake and processing in the digestive tract. Springer Semin Immunopathol 1990; 12:139–152.
70. Neutra MR. Interactions of viruses and microparticles with apical plasma membranes of M cells: implications for human immunodeficiency virus transmission. J Infect Dis 1999; 179(suppl 3):S441–443.
71. Neutra MR. M cells in antigen sampling in mucosal tissues. Curr Top Microbiol Immunol 1999; 236:17–32.
72. Jones BD, Paterson HF, Hall A, Falkow S. *Salmonella typhimurium* induces membrane ruffling by a growth factor–receptor-independent mechanism. Proc Natl Acad Sci USA 1993; 90:10390–10394.
73. Hopkins SA, Kraehenbuhl JP. Dendritic cells of the murine Peyer's patches colocalize with *Salmonella typhimurium* avirulent mutants in the subepithelial dome. Adv Exp Med Biol 1997; 417:105–109.
74. Svensson M, Stockinger B, Wick MJ. Bone marrow–derived dendritic cells can process bacteria for MHC-I and MHC-II presentation to T cells. J Immunol 1997; 158:4229–4236.
75. Kraehenbuhl JP, Hopkins SA, Kerneis S, Pringault E. Antigen sampling

by epithelial tissues: implication for vaccine design. Behring Inst Mitt 1997; 98:24–32.
76. Marriott I, Hammond TG, Thomas EK, Bost KL. Salmonella efficiently enter and survive within cultured CD11c+ dendritic cells initiating cytokine expression. Eur J Immunol 1999; 29:1107–1115.
77. Takeuchi A. Electron microscope studies of experimental Salmonella infection. I. Penetration into the intestinal epithelium by *Salmonella typhimurium*. Am J Pathol 1967; 50:109–136.
78. Vazquez-Torres A, Jones-Carson J, Baumler AJ, Falkow S, Valdivia R, Brown W, Le M, Berggren R, Parks WT, Fang FC. Extraintestinal dissemination of Salmonella by CD18-expressing phagocytes. Nature 1999; 401: 804–808.
79. Mastroeni P, Villarreal-Ramos B, Hormaeche CE. Adoptive transfer of immunity to oral challenge with virulent salmonellae in innately susceptible BALB/c mice requires both immune serum and T cells. Infect Immun 1993; 61:3981–3984.
80. Gonzalez C, Hone D, Noriega FR, Tacket CO, Davis JR, Losonsky G, Nataro JP, Hoffman S, Malik A, Nardin E, et al. *Salmonella typhi* vaccine strain CVD 908 expressing the circumsporozoite protein of *Plasmodium falciparum*: strain construction and safety and immunogenicity in humans. J Infect Dis 1994; 169:927–931.
81. Wu S, Pascual DW, Lewis GK, Hone DM. Induction of mucosal and systemic responses against human immunodeficiency virus type 1 glycoprotein 120 in mice after oral immunization with a single dose of a Salmonella-HIV vector. AIDS Res Hum Retroviruses 1997; 13:1187–1194.
82. Steinman RM, Pack M, Inaba K. Dendritic cell development and maturation. Adv Exp Med Biol 1997; 417:1–6.
83. Yrlid BU, Wick MJ. Salmonella-induced apoptosis of infected macrophages results in presentation of a bacteria-encoded antigen after uptake by bystander dendritic cells. J Exp Med 2000; 191(4):613–624.
84. Powell RJ, Lewis GK, Hone DM, eds. Introduction of eukaryotic expression cassettes into animal cells using a bacterial delivery system. In: Brown F, Norrby E, Burton D, Mekalanos J, Burton D, eds. Vaccines '96: Molecular Approaches to Infectious Disease. Vol. 95. Cold Spring Harbor, NY: Cold Spring Harbor Press, 1996.
85. Sizemore DR, Branstrom AA, Sadoff JC. Attenuated *Shigella* as a DNA delivery vehicle for DNA-mediated immunization. Science 1995; 270:299–302.
86. Sizemore DR, Branstrom AA, Sadoff JC. Attenuated bacteria as a DNA delivery vehicle for DNA-mediated immunization. Vaccine 1997; 15:804–807.
87. Fouts TR, Lewis GK, Hone DM. Construction and characterization of a

Salmonella typhi-based human immunodeficiency virus type 1 vector vaccine. Vaccine 1995; 13:561–569.

88. Fouts TR, Tuskan RG, Chada S, Hone DM, Lewis GK. Construction and immunogenicity of *Salmonella typhimurium* vaccine vectors that express HIV-1 gp120. Vaccine 1995; 13:1697–1705.
89. Boyer JD, Cohen AD, Vogt S, Schumann K, Nath B, Ahn L, Lacy K, Bagarazzi ML, Higgins TJ, Baine Y, Ciccarelli RB, Ginsberg RS, MacGregor RR, Weiner DB. Vaccination of seronegative volunteers with a human immunodeficiency virus type 1 env/rev DNA vaccine induces antigen-specific proliferation and lymphocyte production of beta-chemokines. J Infect Dis 2000; 181:476–483.
90. Weiner DB, Kennedy RC. Genetic vaccines. Sci Am 1999; 281:50–57.
91. Haas J, Park EC, Seed B. Codon usage limitation in the expression of HIV-1 envelope glycoprotein. Curr Biol 1996; 6:315–324.
92. Andre S, Seed B, Eberle J, Schraut W, Bultmann A, Haas J. Increased immune response elicited by DNA vaccination with a synthetic gp120 sequence with optimized codon usage. J Virol 1998; 72:1497–1503.

10

Innate Immunity in HIV Infection

Thomas Lehner
Guy's, King's & St Thomas' School of Medicine
London, England

INTRODUCTION

Innate immunity is an ancient host defense system for the recognition of microorganisms (1). It is the first line of defense and functions during the early phase of infection, before the development of specific adaptive immune responses. The innate immune cells initially have effector functions, but act later as regulatory cells in adaptive immunity. Unlike the mechanisms of adaptive immunity, the innate immune cells do not use cell-surface immunoglobulins or T-cell receptors, they are not major histocompatibility complex (MHC) restricted and lack memory, which is essential in vaccination. An early, nonspecific protective response may limit microbial replication and dissemination, which allows adaptive immunity sufficient time to mount an effective protective response. The innate immune system can be characterized by a number of general features, which will be highlighted below (2,3). However, the role of innate immunity in controlling HIV infection has so far received only limited attention.

CELL-SURFACE RECEPTORS SUBVERTED BY HIV

HIV (or SIV) subverts a number of cell-surface receptors to gain entry into the host cells (Table 1). It is debatable whether all the receptors and molecules de-

Table 1 Cells, Receptors, and Soluble Mediators Involved in Innate Immunity of HIV Infection

Cells	Monocytes, macrophages, dendritic cells, NK cells, γδ T cells
Cell-surface receptors	
HIV binding	CD4 glycoprotein
	Chemokine receptors, CCR5, CXCR4
	DC-SIGN C-type lectin
	CR2 (CD21)
	Galactosyl ceramide
	Mannose receptors
	Heparin sulfate proteoglycan (HSPG)
Chemokine stimulation	CD80/86–CD28 interaction
	CD40–CD40L interaction
Th1-Th2	Th1: CCR5, CXCR3
	Th2: CCR3, CCR4, CCR8
Dendritic cells	Immature DC: CCR5, CCR2, CCR1
	Mature DC: CCR4, CXCR4, CCR7
Monocytes	CCR5, CXCR4, CCR2, CCR1
NK cells	KIR, ILT
	NKG2D
Soluble mediators	Th1 cytokines: IL-2, IL-12, IFN-γ
	Th2 cytokines: IL-4, IL-10
	Chemokines: RANTES, MIP-1α, MIP-1β, SDF1, MDC
	TNF-α, IL-1, IL-6
	Type 1 IFN
	Complement system

scribed below are part of the innate immune system. However, they constitute a noncognate mechanism that does not rely on prior sensitization by HIV, although immunological memory may greatly enhance some of the innate functions.

CD4 Glycoprotein

The 55 kDa CD4 glycoprotein is the principal receptor for HIV, and the targets for HIV appear to be CD4+ T cells, macrophages, and dendritic and Langerhans cells (4,5). The V1 domain of the CD4 glycoprotein binds the HIV gp120 envelope glycoprotein (6,7). The other three domains of CD4 may be involved in cell to cell fusion or syncytium formation (8,9). A crystal structure of gp120 complexed to two domains of CD4 and the Fab portion of a neutralizing monoclonal antibody (MAb) has revealed that the CD4 binding site is blocked by oligomeric

Table 2 Functions of Innate Immunity in HIV Infections

1. Rapid first-line defense
2. Chemoattraction of monocytes, dendritic, γδ T, NK, T, and B cells
3. Adjuvanticity by cytokines, chemokines, and C3d
4. Initiating and modulating adaptive immunity
5. Polarization of the immune response toward a Th1 or Th2 type of immunity

gp120 (10). This finding suggests that the critical epitope is protected from antibodies (11).

CCR5 and CXCR4 Coreceptors

A number of HIV or SIV coreceptors have been described belonging to the chemokine family. CCR5 appears to be the most important, as R5 (or M-tropic) HIV commonly initiates the infection (12–16). Later during HIV infection the X4 (T-tropic) HIV may take over, and this utilizes the CXCR4 coreceptor (17). Both CCR5 and CXCR4 molecules are expressed on CD4+ T cells, the former predominantly on Th1-type cells (18). CCR5 is a seven-transmembrane G-protein coupled molecule expressed on Th1 and Th0 cells (19), CD4+CD45 RO+ memory cells (20), macrophages, and immature dendritic cells (DC) (21,22). CCR5 regulates the traffic of mononuclear cells by binding CC chemokines and plays an essential role in inflammatory processes and autoimmunity. The receptor binds RANTES, MIP-1α, and MIP-1β. It now appears that HIV-1 tropism is generated largely by coreceptor selection, and HIV-1, HIV-2, and SIV strains can use coreceptors in the absence of CD4 for viral entry (23–26). Many primary SIV strains use CCR5 to infect simian cells in the absence of CD4, suggesting that CCR5 and not CD4 was the primordial SIV receptor.

DC-SIGN

DC-specific ICAM-3–grabbing nonintegrin (DC-SIGN) C-type lectin captures HIV at low titer, in the absence of CD4 or CCR5 and may harbor HIV for days without infecting the DC (27,28). These cells migrate to the regional lymph nodes where they transmit the virus to replication-permissive T cells.

CR2 (CD21) Receptors

CR2 (CD21) receptors are expressed on B cells that bind HIV-antibody-C3d immune complexes (29,30). As the immune complexes require antibodies to HIV, the B cell may be involved largely in disseminating HIV in seropositive subjects.

The CR2 molecule is a major recognition molecule of the innate immune system (3).

Galactosyl Ceramide

Galactosyl ceramide is found on rectal and vaginal epithelial cells. The possibility that Gal cerebroside may act as an epithelial receptor for HIV was first proposed some time ago (31,32). However, recently further in vitro evidence suggests that HIV transcytosis through epithelial cells is mediated by galactosyl ceramide (33), and this can be prevented by antibodies to HIV gp41 (34–37). Indeed, an epitope has been identified within gp41—peptide ELDKWA—and antibodies to HIV gp41 of the defined epitope may prevent HIV transcytosis in vitro (33) and to some extent in vivo (36,37).

Mannose Receptor

Mannose receptors have been identified on macrophages and immature DC (38). The receptors bind with great affinity mannose, *N*-acetyl glucosamine, fucose, and other sugars on glycosylated viral envelope proteins, such as HIV gp120 (39). Antigen is captured by the receptors and transported to the endosome-lysosomal compartment for degradation and to enter the HLA class I pathway. Mannose receptors on these cells play an important role in stimulating type I interferon (IFN) (40,41). The receptors are part of the innate immune system (2,3), and, although they can bind HIV gp120 glycoprotein, their role in HIV transmission has not been determined.

Heparin Sulfate Proteoglycan

Heparin sulfate proteoglycan (HSPG) expressed on the cell surface can bind oligomeric R4 type HIV-1 (42–44). Whereas epithelial and endothelial cells express high levels of HSPG, macrophages and primary CD4+ T cells have little HSPG (42–44). A potentially significant finding is that whereas X4-HIV attachment is greatly influenced by HSPG, this does not apply to R5 HIV (42–45).

PRINCIPAL INNATE IMMUNE CELLS INVOLVED IN HIV INFECTION

Macrophages

Macrophages, unlike monocytes, are readily infected by the R5 type of HIV, although it is not a replicating cell, by virtue of expressing CD4 and CCR5 receptors (46,47). Some cells may also express the DC-SIGN C-type lectin (27,28). HIV gp120 binds the CD4 glycoprotein and by conformational changes to the

CCR5 coreceptor produces a gp120–CD4–CCR5 complex, which initiates the fusion process of HIV to the host cell (10,48).

Dendritic Cells

Dendritic cells express not only CD4, CCR5, and CXCR4 receptors but also DC-SIGN, which enables the cells to bind HIV. DC-SIGN is a type II C-type lectin with a cytoplasmic tail and eight extracellular repetitive sequences with a C-type lectin domain. DC-SIGN is a receptor on DC that mediates binding to ICAM-3 on resting T cells and induces T-cell proliferation (27,28). ICAM-2 is also a ligand of DC-SIGN and it mediates DC trafficking (49). As a receptor for HIV-1 DC-SIGN does not mediate HIV entry, but captures HIV-gp120 with high affinity. DC-SIGN is found in DC of the lamina propria of the rectal and vaginal epithelium, but apparently not in Langerhans cells. Thus, the subepithelial dendritic cells encounter HIV directly after crossing the epithelial barrier and carry the virus to the regional lymph nodes (27,28). HIV-bound DC-SIGN transmits the virus to CD4+ T cells by a *trans* mechanism.

Natural Killer Cells

Natural killer (NK) cells function by integration of inhibitory and activating stimuli delivered by distinct receptors. The human inhibitory receptors KIR and ILT recognize MHC class I molecules (50, 51). These receptors inhibit NK cell cytotoxic responses, when target cells expressing normal levels of class I molecules are encountered. However, HIV-encoded nef protein interferes in the biosynthesis of HLA-A and -B but not HLA-C (52). By this strategy, HIV inhibits the cell-surface expression of HLA-A and -B, thereby preventing T-cell–mediated cytotoxicity. Furthermore, HIV allows cell-surface expression of HLA-C, the major ligand of KIR, thus inhibiting NK cell responses. As NK activity declines with the development of HIV-specific cytotoxic T lymphocytes (CTL), it has been suggested that NK cells might provide differentiation signals for CTL (53). The receptor NKG2D found on NK cells plays an essential role in triggering innate responses (54). NKG2D recognizes the two MHC class I–like molecules, MICA and MICB, which are weakly expressed in epithelial cells, fibroblasts, and possibly in endothelial cells (55,56). Heat shock or stress upregulates the level of expression of MIC, which prompts effector responses that are mediated by NKG2D-MIC interaction. NK cells are activated during viral infection by Type 1 IFN, IL-12, and other cytokines and they produce IFN-γ.

γδ T Cells

γδ T cells may play an important role in HIV infection, as they are involved in innate immunity (57) and mucosal protection (58), and they are upregulated in macaques protected from SIV infection (59). These cells produce Th1 or Th2 types of cytokines (60) and they lyse HIV- or SIV-infected target cells (61,62). $\gamma\delta$+ T cells also generate antiviral suppressor factors, RANTES, MIP-1α, and MIP-1β which can prevent SIV infection by binding to and downmodulating the CCR5 coreceptors (59). In HIV-infected humans, the Vγ1 subset of $\gamma\delta$+ T cells is upregulated, without or with upregulation of Vγ9, Vγ2-Vγ4 subsets (63–67). Recently, we have investigated the protective potential of $\gamma\delta$+ T cells in macaques, challenged rectally by SIV_{mac} 251 J5 molecular clone (59). This revealed a significant increase in $\gamma\delta$ T cells eluted from the rectal mucosa and the related iliac lymph nodes in protected as compared with infected macaques. As in NK cells, $\gamma\delta$ T cells express the inhibitory receptors KIR and ILT, which recognize MHC class I molecules, and these inhibit cytotoxic responses (50,51). The NKG2D receptor is also found on $\gamma\delta$ T cells (54) and recognizes MICA and MICB molecules. These are upregulated by stress, which elicits effector responses mediated by NKG2D-MIC interaction. However, the effect of HIV infection on the expression of MIC has not been studied.

M Cells

M cells are found among the epithelial cells covering Peyer's patches in the intestine (68). Lymphoid follicles with M cells have been reported in the rectal mucosa (69). Rodent M cells are capable of transmitting HIV to lymphoid cells (70).

SOLUBLE MEDIATORS INVOLVED IN INNATE IMMUNITY TO HIV INFECTION

Activation of the innate immune cells by LPS or HSP70 induces production of large number of chemokines and cytokines. Some of these will be discussed with particular reference to HIV infection (Table 1).

CC Chemokines

The CC chemokines RANTES, MIP-1α, and MIP-1β are produced by activation of macrophages, DC, T, NK, and $\gamma\delta$ T cells. The mechanism of upregulation of these chemokines is by ligation of either the B7 (CD80/86) molecule with CD28 (71,72) or CD40 with CD40 ligand (CD154) (73,74). It is of considerable significance that the two principal costimulatory molecules are involved which play an essential role as the second or noncognate signal in the cognate immune response; the first signal is the interaction between MHC-peptide and T-cell receptor. Indeed, the costimulatory molecules CD28-CD80/86 were considered part of innate immunity (2), and we suggest that this also applies to the CD40-CD40L molecules. The interactions of these two sets of costimulatory molecules and that of

MHC-peptide–T-cell receptor establishes an important bridge between innate and adaptive immunity.

There is a great deal of evidence that the three CC chemokines can block the CCR5 coreceptors and prevent HIV infection in vitro (75) or SIV infection in vivo (76). Indeed, the CC chemokines can be generated in vitro by activating CD8+ T cells nonspecifically by mitogens (PHA) or by cross-linking CD3. In vivo, the three chemokines were generated by immunization with SIV gp120 and p27 in alum, and the highest concentration of the chemokines was induced by targeting the iliac lymph nodes (76,77). Xenoimmunization in macaques (78) and alloimmunization in women (79) also greatly upregulated the concentrations of these CC chemokines. There is evidence both in vitro (80,81) and in vivo (79,82) that raised concentrations of CC chemokines downmodulate the cell-surface expression of CCR5. Whereas in vitro downmodulation of CCR5 treated with RANTES lasted about 20 minutes, alloimmunization of women upregulated the three CC chemokines and downmodulated the cell-surface expression of CCR5, the latter of which was evident up to 1 year (79). An inverse correlation was established between the concentration of the three CC chemokines and the proportion of cells expressing CCR5 in macaques immunized with SIV gp120 and p27 (82). This is the first in vivo evidence that the three CC chemokines may downmodulate cell-surface expression of CCR5. A novel and potent way of inducing upregulation of the three CC chemokines is by administration of HSP70 or HSP65 by the systemic or mucosal route (83). This finding will be further discussed in the context of adjuvanticity.

Stromal Derived Factor

Stromal derived factor (SDF-1) is the ligand of CXCR4 that is expressed on naive T cells (CD4 or CD8 CD45RA+) and monocytes (18). In vitro, SDF-1 binds and downmodulates CXCR4 (80). Unlike the CC chemokines, SDF-1 is produced by a large variety of cells, including T cells, monocytes, lung, brain, liver, heart, and kidney cells (84,85). There is no adequate explanation for the predominance of CCR5-dependent HIV infection at the mucosal surface. Indeed, even the transition over many years from the CCR5- to the CXCR4-dependent HIV (R5 to X4) takes place in a minority (about 20%) of clade C HIV and about half of clade B HIV infections (86,87). However, a recent finding of high concentrations of SDF-1 in the genital epithelial cells may account for the remarkable preference for the CCR5-dependent HIV (88).

Macrophage-Derived Chemokine

Macrophage-derived chemokine (MDC) inhibits a broad range of R5 and X4 HIV isolates (89,90). MDC binds CCR4, which does not seem to mediate HIV entry. MDC is highly expressed in lymphoid tissues (91–93). Langerhans cells migrating from epithelial site into lymph nodes upregulate MDC during a process of maturation (94). There has been some difficulty in determining the exact form of MDC that exerts the antiviral activity, as there is evidence that posttranslational processing may be required to generate HIV suppressor function (95).

Th1-Th2 Polarization and the Role of IL-12

Th1 and Th2 cytokines are generated by CD4 and CD8 T cells and have been implicated in the pathogenesis of AIDS. The evidence that Th1 cytokines are involved in protection against the development of AIDS (96), however, has not been demonstrated in protection against HIV infection. Th1 cytokines are required for the cellular functions, especially of CD8 cytotoxic cells and CD8+ suppressor factor against HIV (97). IL-12 may be particularly significant, as it stimulates maturation of Th1 cells (98,99) and promotes Th1 polarization with type 1 IFN (100). Expression of IL-12 receptor is necessary for maintenance of IL-12 responsiveness in Th1 polarization (101). However, the level of IL-12 production is controlled by the interaction between CD40 on DC and CD40L on T cells (102,103). A number of microbial agents stimulate the release of IL-12 mediated by CD40 (104,105), and this includes the terminal fragment of HSP70 (106). Leukocyte traffic is regulated by IL-12, which is critical in inducing selectins and the $\alpha 6\beta 1$ integrin to direct these cells to mucosal tissues (100). It is therefore significant that IL-12 production may be inhibited in HIV infection (107,108).

Since the primary function of chemokine receptors is in trafficking of leukocytes, it is noteworthy that Th1 cells express CCR5 and CXCR3, whereas Th2 cells express CCR3, CCR4, and CCR8 (19,109–111). Indeed, Th1 cell lines and clones synthesize the three CC chemokines (112). Furthermore, DNA-encoding RANTES and MCP-1 induces Th1, whereas MIP-1α favors Th2 polarization (113). These results suggest that chemokine-receptor mediated activation might affect Th1-Th2 polarization. Recent evidence indicates that MIP-1α, MIP-1β, and RANTES induce DC to produce IFN-γ and exert potent Th1 polarizing effect (114). Indeed, in vitro treatment of Th0 cells with MIP-1α induced Th1, whereas MCP-1 induced Th2 polarization (115), which is not consistent with the above DNA experiment (113).

Type 1 IFN

Type 1 IFN (α and β IFN) is produced in large amounts during the early innate phase of a viral infection by macrophages and DC. Type 1 IFN is released by the interaction between glycosylated envelope protein of the virus and mannose receptors on DC or macrophages (116). In addition to interfering with viral growth, type 1 IFN activates STAT 4 transcription factor to induce IFN and promote Th1 cell development, such as CD8+ CTL (117,118). IFN-α also prevents activated T cells from undergoing apoptosis, thereby keeping the T cells alive (119).

TNF-α

TNF-α is a homotrimer produced by Th1 and some Th2 cells' macrophages, and cytotoxic T cells, in soluble and membrane associated form. It is a proinflammatory cytokine that is increased both in plasma and tissues of patients with AIDS (120) or in vitro by macrophages infected with HIV or treated with HIV gp120 (121). TNF-α enhanced HIV replication in infected promonocytic and T-cell lines by activation of NF-κB, which stimulates the long terminal repeat of the provirus (122,123). However, TNF-α can induce cellular resistance to HIV transmission by selective inhibition of HIV entry into macrophages that is mediated by the 75 kDa TNF-R2 (124). CD40 ligation of macrophages by CD40L (125) or by the HSP70 fragment (106) induces secretion of TNF-α. TNF-α enables adhesion of phagocytes to endothelial cells, increases vascular permeability, and may induce apoptosis when interacting with TNF-R1. TNF-α with GM-CSF generates DC from human CD34+ cells and augments migration of Langerhans cells to the regional lymph nodes (126).

The Complement System

The complement system is an essential component of innate immunity (3), and activation of the classical complement or alternative pathway may be involved in the pathogenesis of HIV infection. Complement-dependent antibody-mediated enhancement of HIV infection has been demonstrated in vitro, but its relevance in vivo is not clear (127–129). High levels of circulating immune complexes are found in HIV-infected subjects (130,131), and these activate complement with raised concentrations of C3d, C4d, and Ba fragments (132). However, HIV has been known to be trapped as an immune complex with antibodies and complement in follicular dendritic cells (133,134). More recently HIV-antibody-complement (C3d) complexes were shown to bind B cells via the CD21 (CR2) complement receptors (29,30). These HIV virion–carrying B cells are not infected, but they can disseminate the virus to HIV-permissive CD4+ T cells in blood and lymphoid tissues. CR2 (CR1 and CR3) are major recognition molecules of the innate immune system (3).

ADJUVANT COMPONENTS IN VACCINES TRIGGER THE INNATE IMMUNE RESPONSE ESSENTIAL FOR INITIATING AND MODULATING ADAPTIVE IMMUNITY

Most vaccines, with the exception of replicating viruses, require an adjuvant to initiate adaptive immunity. The mechanism of adjuvanticity is complex and outside the remit of this review, but a number of reviews have been published (135,136). An attractive concept has been proposed that adjuvants induce the innate system to activate adaptive immunity by virtue of pathogen-associated molecular pattern (PAMP), found in adjuvants (2). These will induce costimulatory signals that activate lymphocytes and generate cytokines. We have recently demonstrated that the adjuvanticity of HSP70 and HSP65, both systemic and mucosal, is dependent on stimulation of the production of CC chemokines (83). These attract monocytes, immature DC, T cells, and B cells, which are the principal cells involved in generating an immune response (137–139). The innate or CC chemokine–generating component of HSP70 is linked with a specific peptide that resides in the pocket of HSP70. Specific immunity to the peptide is greatly enhanced by the HSP70-chaperoned peptide being taken up and presented by the accumulation of antigen processing and presenting cells to T and B cells. As HSP70 binds CD40 in stimulating macrophages or DC to generate CC chemokines (140), the target appears to be another costimulatory molecule, which may function in concert with B7-CD28 and play a part in adjuvanticity (2).

Another function of HSP70 is that it favors Th1 polarization by virtue of stimulating the production of IL-12 when administered in the truncated form (106). This function, linked with that of HSP70 translocating molecules from outside the cell into the HLA class I pathway, enables HSP70 to elicit CTL as well as IgG2a antibody responses. HSP70 is a major inhibitor of apoptosis, downstream of caspase-3 protease activity, thereby keeping the cells alive (141). Furthermore, mucosal administration of HSP70 linked to SIV antigens in macaques functions as an effective adjuvant and elicits sIgA and IgG antibodies (83). The innate immune function elicited by HSP70 is greatly enhanced in HSP70-primed macaques, the CD8 cells of which yield significantly higher concentrations of RANTES, MIP-1α, and MIP-1β than those from unimmunized animals.

MUCOSAL INNATE IMMUNITY AS THE FIRST LINE OF DEFENSE IN HIV INFECTION

As HIV infection is transmitted by the vaginal or rectal mucosa or foreskin in about 80% of cases, mucosal innate immunity is of considerable significance and has received little attention.

Cellular Components

Noncognate immune responses may play a role in protection of HIV infection, with Langerhans cells in vaginal and foreskin epithelia (142) and γδ+ T cells in rectal and vaginal epithelia. Furthermore, macrophages and DC are present in the subepithelial tissues. Cell-surface CCR5 is expressed by Langerhans cells (143) and the other cells, so blocking and downmodulating these receptors with the CC chemokines may inhibit HIV transmission. Indeed, resting or activated

CD8-enriched cells eluted from normal rectal mucosa generated a large number of RANTES- and MIP-1β–secreting cells (83). This might be due to stimulation by the large number of gram-negative and gram-positive bacteria residing in the rectum, as these contain heat-shock protein (HSP) and lipopolysaccharide (LPS), both of which induce CC chemokines that immobilize T and B cells, DC, and macrophages in the rectal mucosa. Consistent with these findings is the larger number of RANTES- and MIP-1β–secreting cells in the iliac compared with the axillary lymph nodes (83), as the former drain the rectal mucosa, with its indigenous microbial population, unlike the axillary lymph nodes, which drain the relatively aseptic skin.

γδ T cells are an important innate component of mucosal tissues, and they home preferentially from the internal iliac lymph node (LN) to the genital and rectal mucosa after targeted iliac lymph node (TILN) immunization, and this is consistent with localization of protective immunity in the mucosal-regional LN complex (76). It is also noteworthy that after TILN immunization, higher proportions of PKH-26–labeled γδ+ T cells are found in the rectal and vaginal mucosa and inferior mesenteric LN, but not the superior mesenteric or submaxillary LN (59). This is consistent with preferential homing of mononuclear cells from the iliac LN to the rectal and vaginal mucosa but not to the unrelated LN (144).

Microbial Heat-Shock Protein

HSP in microorganisms may function as a natural adjuvant generating CC chemokines, somewhat akin to microbial agents stimulating the complement pathway to generate C3d, which has potent adjuvant activity (145). This concept is also consistent with the "danger hypothesis" of infection (146), with HSP alerting the innate system to secrete CC chemokines and to mobilize the immune repertoire of cells and generate specific immune responses against the invading organism. The presence of HSP in most gut microorganisms (147,148) may also be responsible for upregulation of γδ T cells in the intestinal epithelium. Activation of CD8+ T cells with HSP (59), a proportion of which are γδ cells, generates the three CC chemokines. γδ T cells, with their CC chemokine–generating potential, localize the innate immune mechanism at the mucosal barrier, between the gut microbial flora and the lamina propria of the intestine. Indeed, a large number of RANTES- and MIP-1β–secreting cells are found in the rectal epithelium (59), which may attract the cellular repertoire responsible for adaptive cellular and humoral immunity against the invading microorganisms. Innate immunity-initiating and -modulating adaptive immunity at the mucosal barrier (2,3) is a potent protective mechanism against microbial infection. Moreover, in SIV or HIV infection there is an additional factor, in that the CC chemokines and antiviral factors generated by macrophages, DC, NK, and γδ T cells may prevent the viral infection mediated by the CCR5 coreceptors.

Soluble Mediators

Complement proteins, especially C3, have been found in low concentrations in secretions, but it is doubtful if these are fully functional. Chemokines have been demonstrated in cervico-vaginal washings from HIV-infected women (149). The concentration and frequency of these chemokines were found in the following descending order: IL-8, RANTES, and MIP-1α. It is of interest that the concentration of IL-8 levels correlated significantly with those of IL-1β and IgG, whereas RANTES correlated with those of C1q, C3, and C4 (149). These data suggest that RANTES and MIP-1α might be protective at the surface of the cervico-vaginal mucosa.

SDF-1 was not assayed in genital fluids. However, high concentrations of SDF-1 are expressed constitutively by human cervico-vaginal and rectal epithelial cells, and this was correlated with low cell-surface expression of CXCR4 (88). Since CXCR4 mRNA was readily detectable in these epithelial cells by RT-PCR, this is consistent with SDF-1 downmodulating CXCR4 in vivo. Surprisingly, human intestinal intraepithelial lymphocytes expressed high levels of CCR5 but low levels of CXCR4 on flow cytometry (88). This is consistent with the quantitative RT-PCR studies showing that CCR5 is expressed 10 times more frequently than CXCR4 in cervical biopsies of women with and without sexually transmitted diseases (150). An important factor is the level of progesterone, which increased CCR5 and CXCR4 expression in lymphocytes and or macrophages of PBMC treated in vitro (151). However, in vivo progesterone inhibited IL-2–induced upregulation of CCR5 and CXCR4 and reduced HIV infectivity in vitro (151).

The remarkable preference for R5-dependent (M-tropic) HIV transmission through the mucosal epithelia is difficult to explain. However, at least three innate mucosal factors may account for this selectivity:

1. High concentrations of SDF-1 found in genital epithelial cells may block and downmodulate CXCR4, thus preventing X4-dependent HIV transmission (88).
2. HSPG expressed by epithelial cells bind predominantly X4-HIV, which is therefore prevented from infecting permissive cells, unlike R5-HIV, which can pass through the epithelial cells and infect permissive CD4+CCR5+ cells (45).
3. Cervico-vaginal intraepithelial Langerhans cells do not express DC-SIGN (28) but do express CD4 and CCR5 (143), which enables selective transmission of R5-HIV. However, subepithelial DC-SIGN+ cells in genital or rectal mucosa do not differentiate between R5- and X4-dependent HIV (28).

REFERENCES

1. Hoffmann JA, Kafatos FC, Janeway CA Jr, Ezekowitz RAB. Phylogenetic perspectives in innate immunity. Science 1999; 284:1313–1318.

2. Medzhitov RM, Janeway CA Jr. Innate immunity: impact in immunology on the adaptive immune response. Curr Opin Immunol 1997; 9:4–9.
3. Fearon DT, Locksley RM. The instructive role of innate immunity in the acquired immune response. Science 1996; 272:50–53.
4. Dalgleish AG, Berverley PC, Clapham PR, Crawford DH, Greaves MF, Weiss RA. The CD4 (T4) antigen is an essential component of the receptor for the AIDS retrovirus. Nature 1984; 312:763-767.
5. Klatzmann D, Champagne E, Chamaret S, Gruest J, Guetard D, Hercend T, Glukman JC, Montagnier L. T-lymphocyte T4 molecule behaves as the receptor for human retrovirus LAV. Nature 1984; 767–768.
6. Maddon P, Molineaux SM, Maddon DE, Zimmerman KA, Godfrey M, Alt FW, Chess L, Axel R. Structure and expression of the human and mouse T4 genes. Proc Natl Acad Sci USA 1987; 84:9155–9159.
7. Arthos J, Deen K, Chaikin M, Fornwald J, Sathe G, Sattentau Q, Clpham P, Weiss R, McDougal J, Pietropaolo C, Axel R, Truneh A, Maddon P, Sweet R. Identification of the residues in human CD4 critical for the binding of HIV. Cell 1989; 57:469–481.
8. Camerini D, Seed B. A CD4 domain important for HIV-mediated syncytium formation lies outside the virus binding site. Cell 1990; 60:747–754.
9. Healey D, Didanda L, Moore JP, McDougal JS, Moore MJ, Estess P, Buck D, Kwong PD, Beverly PCL, Sattentau QJ. Novel anti-CD4 monoclonal antibodies separate human immunodeficiency virus infection and fusion of CD4+ cells from virus binding. J Exp Med 1990; 172:1233–1242.
10. Kwong PD, Wyatt R, Robinson J, Sweet RW, Sodroski J, Hendrikson WA. Structure of an HIV gp120 envelope glycoprotein in complex with the CD4 receptor and a neutralizing human antibody. Nature 1998; 393: 648–659.
11. Moore JP, Binley J. Envelopes letters boxed into shape. Nature 1998; 393: 630–631.
12. Deng H, Liu R, Ellmeier W, Choe S, Unutmaz D, Burkhart M, Marzio PD, Marmon S, Sutton RE, Hill CM, Davis CB, Peiper SC, Schall TJ, Littman DR, Landau NR. Identification of a major co-receptor for primary isolates of HIV-1. Nature 1996; 381:661–666.
13. Dragic T, Litwin V, Allaway GP, Martin SR, Huang Y, Nagashima KA, Cayanan C, Maddon PJ, Koup RA, Moore JP, Paxton WA. HIV-1 entry into CD4+ cells is mediated by the chemokine receptor CC-CKR-5. Nature 1996; 381:667–673.
14. Chen Z, Zhou P, Ho DD, Landau NR, Marx PA. Genetically divergent strains of simian immunodeficiency virus use CCR5 as a coreceptor for entry. J Virol 1997; 71:2705–2714.
15. Edinger AL, Adaemee A, Miller K, Doranz BJ, Endress M, Sharron M, Samson M, Lu Z-H, Clements JE, Murphey-Corb M, Peiper SC, Parmentier M, Broder CC, Doms RW. Differential utilization of CCR5 by macro-

phage and T cell tropic simian immunodeficiency virus strains. Proc Natl Acad Sci USA 1997; 94: 4005–4010.

16. Hill CM, Deng HK, Unutmaz D, Kewalramani VN, Bastiani L, Gorny MK, Zolla-Pazner S, Littman DR. Envelope glycoproteins from HIV-1, HIV-2 and SIV can use human CCR5 as coreceptor for viral entry and make direct CD4-dependent interactions with this chemokine receptor. J Virol 1997; 71:6296–6304.
17. Feng Y, Broder CC, Kennedy PE, Berger EA. HIV-1 entry cofactor: functional cDNA cloning of a seven transmembrane, G protein-coupled receptor. Science 1996; 272:872–877.
18. Berger EA, Murphy PM, Farber JM. Chemokine receptors as HIV-1 coreceptors: toles in viral entry, tropism and disease. Annu Rev Immunol 1999; 17:657–700.
19. Sallusto F, Lenig D, Mackay CR, Lanzavecchia A. Flexible programs of chemokine receptor expression on human polarized T helper 1 and 2 lymphocytes. J Exp Med 1998; 187:875–883.
20. Ostrowski MA, Justement SJ, Catanzaro A, Hallahan CA, Ehler LA, Mizell SB, Kumar PN, Mican JA, Chun T-W, Fauci AS. Expression of chemokine receptors CXCR4 and CCR5 in HIV-1-infected and uninfected individuals. J Immunol 1998; 161:3195–3201.
21. Sallusto F, Schaerli P, Loetscher P, Schaniel C, Lenig D, Mackay CR, Qin S, Lanzavecchia A. Rapid and coordinated switch in chemokine receptor expression during dendritic cell maturation. Eur J Immunol 1998; 28: 2760–2769.
22. Sallusto F, Lanzavecchia A, Mackay CR. Chemokines and chemokine receptors in T-cell priming and Th1/Th2-mediated responses. Immunol Today 1998; 19:568–574.
23. Edinger AL, Mankowski JL, Doranz BJ, Marguilies BJ, Lee B, Rucker J, Sharron M, Hoffman TL, Berson JF, Zink MC. CD4-independent CCR5-dependent infection brain capillary endothelial cells by a neurovirulent simian immunodeficiency virus strain. Proc Natl Acad Sci USA 1997; 94: 14742–14747.
24. Endreas MJ, Clapham PR, Marsh M, Ahuja M, Turner JD, McKnight A, Thomas JF, Stoebenau-Haggarty B, Choe S, Vance PJ, Wells TN, Power CA, Sutterwala SS, Doms RW, Landau NR, Hoxie JA. CD4-independent infection by HIV-2 is mediated by fusin/CXCR4. Cell 1996; 87:745–756.
25. Reeves JD, McKnight A, Potempa S, Simmons G, Gray PW, Power CA, Wells T, Weiss RA, Talbot SJ. CD4-independent infection by HIV-2 (ROD/B): use of the 7-transmembrane receptors CXCR4, CCR3 and V28 for entry. Virology 1997; 231:130–134.
26. Hoffman T L, LaBranche CC, Zhang W, Gabriella C, Robinson J, Chaiken

I, Hoxie JA, Doms RW. Stable exposure of the coreceptor-binding site in a CD4-independent HIV-1 envelope protein. Proc Natl Acad Sci USA 1999; 96:6359–6364.

27. Geijtenbeek TBH, Torensma R, van Vilet SJ, van Duijnhoven GCF, Adema GJ, van Kooyk Y, Figdor CG. Identification of DC-SIGN, a novel dendritic cell-specific ICAM-3 receptor that supports primary immune responses. Cell 2000; 100:575–585.
28. Geijtenbeek TBH, Kwon DS, Torensma R, van Viliet SJ, van Duijnhoven GCF, Middel J, Cornelissen ILMHA, Nottet HSLM, KewalRamani VN, Littman DR, Figdor CG, van Kooyk Y. DC-SIGN, a dendritic cell-specific HIV-1 binding protein that enhances trans-infection of T cells. Cell 100: 587–597.
29. Moir S, Malaspina A, Li Y, Chun T-W, Lowe T, Adelsberger J, Baseler M, Ehler LA, Liu S, Davey RT, Mican JAM, Fauci AS. B cells of HIV-1-infected patients bind virions through CD21-complement interactions and transmit infectious virus to activated T cells. J Exp Med 2000; 192: 637–643.
30. Jakubik JJ, Saifuddin M, Takefman DM, Spear GT. Immune complexes containing human immunodeficiency virus type 1 primary isolates bind to lymphoid tissue B lymphocytes and are infectious for T lymphocytes. J Virol 2000; 74:552–555.
31. Yahi N, Baghdiguian S, Moreau H, Fantini J. Galatosyl ceramide (or a closely related molecule) is the receptor for human immunodeficiency virus type 1 on human colon epithelial HT29 cells. J Virol 1992; 66:4848–4854.
32. Furata Y et al. Infection of vaginal and colonic epithelial cells by the human immunodeficiency virus type 1 is neutralised by antibodies raised against conserved epitopes in the envelope glycoprotein gp120. Proc Natl Acad Sci USA. 1994; 91:12559–12563.
33. Bomsel M. Transcytosis of infectious human immunodeficiency virus across a tight human epithelial cell line barrier. Nat Med 1997; 3:42–47.
34. Muster T, Steindl F, Purtscher M, Trkola A, Kilma A, Himmler G, Ruker F, Katinger H. A conserved neutralizing epitope on gp41 of human immunodeficiency virus type 1. J Virol 1993 67:6642–6647.
35. Trkola A, Pomales AB, Yuan H, Korber B, Maddon PJ, Allaway GP, Katinger H, Barbas CF, Burton DR, Ho DD, Moore Jp. Cross-clade neutralisation of primary isolates of human immunodeficiency virus type 1 by human monoclonal antibodies and tetrameric CD4-IgG. J Virol 1995; 69:6009–6617.
36. Mascola JR, Steigler G, Vancott TC, Katinger H, Carpenter CB, Hanson CE, Beary H, Hayes D, Frankel SS, Birx DL, Lewis MG. Protection of macaques against vaginal transmission of a pathogenic HIV-1/SIV chime-

ric virus by passive infusion of neutralizing antibodies. Nat Med 2000; 6: 207–210.
37. Baba TW, Liska V, Hoffmann-Lehmann R, Vlasak J, Xu W, Ayehunie S, Cavacini LA, Posner MR, Katinger H, Steigler G, Bernacky BJ, Rizvi TA, Schmidt R, Hill LR, Keeling ME, Lu Y, Wright JE, Chou T-C, Ruprecht RM. Human neutralizing monoclonal antibodies of the IgG1 subtype protect against mucosal simian-human immunodeficiency virus infection. Nat Med 2000; 6:200–206.
38. Pontow SE, Kery V, Stahl PD. Mannose Receptor. Int Rev Cytol B 1992; 137:221–244.
39. Milone MC, Fitzgerald-Bocarsly P. The mannose receptor mediates induction of IFN-I in peripheral blood dendritic cells by enveloped RNA and DNA viruses. J Immunol 1998; 161:2391–2399.
40. Capobianchi M, Ansel H, Amelglio F, Paganelli P, Pizzoli P, Dianzani F. Recombinant glycoprotein 120 of human immunodeficiency virus is a potent interferon inducer. AIDS Res Hum Retroviruses 1992; 8:575–579.
41. Francis ML, Meltzer MS. Induction of IFN-α by HIV-1 in monocyte enriched PBMC requires gp120-CD4 interaction but not virus replication. J Immunol 1993; 151:2208–2216.
42. Roderiquez G, Oravecz T, Yanagishita M, Bou-Habib DC, Mostowski H, Norcross MA. Mediation of human immunodeficiency virus type 1 binding by interaction of cell surface heparan sulfate proteoglycans with the V3 region of envelope gp120-gp41. J Virol 1995; 69:2233–2239.
43. Patel M, Yanagishita M, Roderiquez G, Bou-Habib DC, Oravecz T, Hascall VC, Norcross MA. Cell-surface heparin sulfate proteoglycan mediates HIV-1 infection of T-cell lines. AIDS Res Hum Retroviruses 1993; 9: 167–174.
44. Ohshiro Y, Murakami T, Matsudo K, Nishioka K, Yoshida K, Yamamoto N. Role of cell surface glycosaminoglycans of human T cells in human immunodeficiency virus type-1 (HIV-1) infection. Microbiol Immunol 1996; 40:827–835.
45. Ugolini S, Mondor I, Sattentau QJ. HIV-1 attachment: another look. Trends Microbiol 1999; 7:144–149.
46. Di Marzio P, Tse J, Landau NR. Chemokine receptor regulation and HIV type 1 tropism in monocyte-macrophages. AIDS Res Human Retroviruses 1998; 14:129–138.
47. Wang J, Roderiquez G, Oravecz T, Norcross MA. Cytokine regulation of human immunodeficiency virus type 1 entry and replication in human monocytes/macrophages through modulation of CCR5 expression. J Virol 1998; 72:7642–7647.
48. Wyatt R, Sodroski J. The HIV-1 envelope glycoproteins: fusogens, antigens and immunogens. Science 1998; 280:1884–1888.

49. Geijtenbeek TBH, Kroopshoop DJEB, Bleijs DA, van Vliet SJ, van Duijnhoven GCF, Grabovsky V, Alon R, Figdor CG, van Kooyk Y. DC-SIGN-ICAM-2 interaction mediates dendritic cell trafficking. Nat Immunol 2000; 1:353–357.
50. Campbell KS, Dessing M, Lopez-Botet M, Cella M, Colonna M. Tyrosine phosphorylation of a human killer inhibitory receptors recruits protein tyrosine phosphatase 1C. J Exp Med 1996; 184:93–100.
51. Colonna M, Navarro F, Bellon T, Llano M, Garcia P, Samaridis J, Angman L, Cella M, Lopez-Botet M. A common inhibitory receptor for MHC class I molecules on human lymphoid and myelomonocytic cells. J Exp Med 1997; 186:1809–1818.
52. Cohen GB, Gandhi RT, Davis DM, Mandelboim O, Chen BK, Strominger JL, Baltimore D. The selective downregulation of class I major histocompatibility complex proteins by HIV-1 protects HIV-infected cells from NK cells. Immunity 1999; 10:661–671.
53. Giavendoni LD, Velasquillo MC, Parodi LM, Hubbard GB, Hodara VL. Cytokine expression, natural killer cell activation, and phenotypic changes in lymphoid cells from rhesus macaques during acute infection with pathogenic simian immunodeficiency virus. J Virol 2000; 74:1648–1657.
54. Moretta L, Biassoni R, Bottino C, Mingari MC, Moretta A. Human NK-cell receptors. Immunol Today 2000; 21:420–422.
55. Bauer S, Groh V, Wu J, Stenle A, Phillips JH, Lainer LL, Spies T. Activation of NK cells and T cells by NKG2D, a receptor for stress-inducible MICA. Science 1999; 285:727–729.
56. Colonna M, Samaridis J, Cella M, Angman L, Allen R, O'Callaghan C, Dunbar R, Ogg G, Cerundolo V, Rolink A. Human myelomonocytic cells express an inhibitory receptor for classical and non-classical MHC class I molecules. J Immunol 1998; 160:3096–3100.
57. Boismenu R, Havran WL. An innate view of γδ T cells. Curr Opin Immunol 1997; 9:57–63.
58. Carding SR, Allan W, Kyes S, Hayday A, Bottomly K, Doherty PC. Late dominance of the inflammatory process in murine influenza by γδ+ T cells. J Exp Med 1990; 172:1225–1231.
59. Lehner T, Mitchell E, Bergmeier L, Singh M, Spallek R, Cranage M, Hall G, Dennis M, Villinger F, Wang Y. The role of γδ T cells in generating antiviral factors and β-chemokines in protection against mucosal simian immunodeficiency virus infection. Eur J Immunol 2000; 30:2245–2256.
60. Ferrick DA, Schrenzel MD, Mulvania T, Hsieh B, Ferlin WA, Lepper H. Differential production of IFN-γ and IL-4 in response to Th1- and Th2-stimulating pathogens by γδ T cells in vivo. Nature 1995; 373:255–257.
61. Malkovsky M. The function and specificity of γδ T cells. Vaccine Res 1992; 1:183–191.

62. Wallace M, Bartz SR, Chang W-L, MacKenzie D, Pauza CD, Malkovsky M. γδ T lymphocyte responses to human immuno-deficiency virus. Clin Exp Immunol 1996; 103:177–184.
63. Autran B, Triebel F, Katlama C, Rozenbaum W, Hercend T, Debre P. T-cell receptor $\gamma\delta^+$ lymphocyte subsets during HIV infection. Clin Exp Immunol 1989; 75:206–210.
64. De Paoli P, Gennari D, Martelli P, Basaglia G, Crovatto M, Battistin S. A subset of lymphocytes is increased during HIV-1 infection. Clin Exp Immunol 1991; 83:187–191.
65. De Maria A, Ferrazin A, Ferrini S, Ciconne E, Terragna A, Moretta L. Selective increase of a subset of T cell receptor of γδ T lymphocytes in the peripheral blood of patients with HIV-1 infection. J InfectDis 1992. 165:917–919.
66. Hinz T, Wesch D, Friese K, Reckziegel A, Arden B, Kabelitz D. T cell γδ repertoire in HIV-1 infected individuals. Eur J Immunol 1994; 24: 3044–3049.
67. Boullier S, Cochet M, Poccia F, Gougeon M-L. CDR3-independent γδ $V\delta1^+$ T cell expansion in the peripheral blood of HIV-infected persons. J Immunol 1995; 154:1418–1431.
68. Owen RL, Nemanic P. Antigen processing structures of the mammalian intestinal tract: an SEM study of lymphoepithelial organs. Scanning Electron Microsc 1978; 2:367–378.
69. O'Leary AD, Sweeney EC. Lymphoglandular complexes of the colon: structure and distribution. Histopathology 1986; 10:267–283.
70. Amerongen HM, Weltzin R, Farnet CM, Michetti P, Haseltine WA, Neutra MR. Transepithelial transport of HIV-1 by intestinal M cells: a mechanism for transmission of AIDS. J AIDS 1991; 4:760–765.
71. Herold KC, Lu J, Rulifson I, Vezys V, Taub D, Grusby MJ, Bluestone JA. Regulation of C-C chemokine production by murine T cells by CD28/B7 costimulation. J Immunol 1997; 159:4150–4153.
72. Riley JL, Carroll RG, Levine BL, Bernstein W, St Louis DC, Weislow OS, June CH. Intrinsic resistance to T cell infection with HIV type 1 induced by CD28 costimulation. J Immunol 1997; 158:5545–5553.
73. Kornbluth RS, Kee K, Richman DD. CD40 ligand (CD154) stimulation of macrophages to produce HIV-1 suppressive β-chemokines. Proc Natl Acad Sci USA 1998; 95:5205–5210.
74. McDyer JF, Dybul M, Goletz TJ, Kinter AL, Thomas EK, Berzofsky JA, Fauci AS, Seder RA. Differential effects of CD40 ligand/trimer stimulation on the ability of dendritic cells to replicate and transmit HIV infection: evidence for CC-chemokine-dependent and independent mechanisms. J Immunol 1999; 162:3711–3717.

75. Cocchi F, DeVico AL, Garzino-Demo A, Arya SK, Gallo RC, Lusso P. Identification of RANTES, MIP-1α and MIP-1β as the major HIV- suppressive factors produced by CD8$^+$ T cells. Science 1995; 270:1811–1815.
76. Lehner T, Wang Y, Cranage M, Bergmeier LA, Mitchell E, Tao L, Hall G, Dennis M, Cook N, Brookes R, Klavinskis L, Jones I, Doyle C, Ward R. Protective mucosal immunity elicited by targeted iliac lymph node immunisation with a subunit SIV envelope and core vaccine in macaques. Nat Med 1996; 2:767–775.
77. Aubertin A-M, Wang Y, Le Grand R, Beyer C, Tao L, Neildez O, Barre-Sinoussi F, Hurtel B, Moog C, Lehner T, Girard M. Generation of CD8-suppressor factor and β-chemokines by targeted iliac lymph node immunization in monkeys challenged with SHIV by the rectal route. AIDS Res Hum Retroviruses 2000; 16:381–392.
78. Wang Y, Tao L, Mitchell E, Bogers WMJM, Doyle C, Bravery CA, Bergmeier LA, Kelly CG, Heeney JL, Lehner T. Generation of CD8 suppressor factor and β chemokines, induced by xenogeneic immunization, in the prevention of simian immunodeficiency virus infection in macaques. Proc Natl Acad Sci USA 1998; 95:5223–5228.
79. Wang Y, Tao L, Mitchell E, Bravery C, Berlingieri P, Armstrong P, Vaughan R, Underwood J, Lehner T. Allo-immunization elicits CD8+ T cell-derived chemokines, HIV suppressor factors and resistance to HIV infection in women. Nat Med 1999; 5:1004–1009.
80. Amara A, Gall SL, Schwartz O, Salamero J, Montes M, Loetscher P, Baggiolini M, Virelizier JL, Arenzana-Seisdedos F. HIV coreceptor downregulation as antiviral principle: SDF-1 alpha-dependent internalization of the chemokine receptor CXCR4 contributes to inhibition of HIV replication. J Exp Med 1997; 186:139–146.
81. Mack M, Lucklow B, Nelson PJ, Cihak J, Simmons G, Clapham PR, Signoret N, Marsh M, Stangassinger M, Borlat F, Wells TN, Schondorff D, Proudfoot AE. Aminooxypentane-RANTES induced CCR5 internalization but inhibits recycling: a novel inhibitory mechanism of HIV infectivity. J Exp Med 1998; 187:1215–1224.
82. Lehner T, Wang Y, Cranage M, Tao L, Mitchell E, Bravery C, Doyle C, Pratt K, Hall G, Dennis M, Villinger FL, Bergmeier L. Upregulation of β-chemokines and downmodulation of CCR5 co-receptors inhibit simian immunodeficiency virus transmission in non-human primates. Immunology 2000; 99:569-577.
83. Lehner T, Bergmeier LA, Tao L, Singh M, Spallek R, van der Zee R. Heat shock proteins generate β-chemokines which function as innate adjuvants enhancing adaptive immunity. Eur J Immunol 2000; 30:594–603.

84. Bleul CC, Farzan M, Choe H, Parolin C, Clark-Lewis I, Sodroski J, Springer TA. The lymphocyte chemoattractant SDF-1 is a ligand for LESTR/fusin and blocks HIV-1 entry. Nature 1996; 382:829–833.
85. Oberlin E, Amara A, Bachelerie F, Bessia C, Virelizier JL, Arenzana-Seisdedos F, Schwartz O, Heard JM, Clark-Lewis I, Legler DF, Loetscher M, Baggiolini M, Moser B. The CXC chemokine SDF-1 is the ligand for LESTR/fusin and prevents infection by T-cell-line adapted HIV-1. Nature 1996; 382:833–835.
86. DeRoda Husman AM, van Rij RP, Blaak H, Broersen S, Schuitemaker H. Adaptation to promiscuous usage of chemokine receptors is not a prerequisite for human immunodeficiency virus type 1 disease progression. J Infect Dis 1999; 180:1106–1115.
87. Peeters M, Vincent R, Perret JL, Lasky M, Patrel D, Liegeois F, Courgnard V, Seng R, Matton T, Molinger S, Delaporte E. Evidence of differences in MT2 cell tropism according to genetic subtypes of HIV-1: syncytium-inducing variants seem rare among subtype C HIV-1 viruses. J AIDS Hum Retrovirol 1999; 20:115–121.
88. Agace WW, Amara A, Roberts AI, Pablos JL, Theien S, Uguccioni MG, Li XY, Marsal J, Arenzana-Seisdedos F, Delaunauy T, Ebert EC, Moser B, Parker CM. Constitutive expression of stromal derived factor-1 by mucosal epithelia and its role in HIV transmission and propagation. Curr Biol 2000 10:325–328.
89. Pal R, Garzino-Demo A, Markham PD, Burns J, Brown M, Gallo RC, DeVico AL. Inhibition of HIV-1 infection by the J chemokine MDC. Science 1997; 278:695–698.
90. Godiska R, Chantry D, Raport CJ, Sozzani S, Allavena P, Leviten D, Mantovani A, Gray PW. Human macrophage-derived chemokine (MDC), a novel chemoattractant for monocytes, monocyte-derived dendritic cells and natural killer cells. J Exp Med 1997; 185:1595–1604.
91. Andrew DP, Chang MS, McNinch J, Wathen ST, Rihanek M, Tseng J, Spellberg JP, Elias CG. STCP-1 (MDC) CC chemokine acts specifically on chronically activated Th2 lymphocytes and is produced by monocytes on stimulation with Th2 cytokines IL-4 and IL-13. J Immunol 1998; 161: 5027.
92. Chang MS, McNinch J, Elias C III, Manthey CL, Grosshans D, Meng T, Boone T, Andrew DP. Molecular cloning and functional characterization of a novel CC chemokine, stimulated T cell chemotactic protein (STCP-1) that specifically acts on activated T lymphocytes. J Biol Chem 1997; 272: 25229–25237.
93. Schaniel C, Pardali E, Sallusto F, Speletas M, Ruedl C, Shimizu T, Seidl T, Andersson J, Melchers F, Rolink AG, Sideras P. Activated murine B

lymphocytes and dendritic cells produce a novel CC chemokine which acts selectively on activated T cells. J Exp Med 1998; 188:451–463.
94. Tang HL, Cyster JG. Chemokine up-regulation and activated T cell attraction by maturing dendritic cells. Science 1999; 284:819–822.
95. Garzino-Demo A, DeVico AL, Cocchi F, Gallo RC. β-chemokine and protection from HIV type 1 disease. AIDS Res Hum Retroviruses 1998; 14:177–184.
96. Clerici M, Shearer GM. A Th1-Th2 switch is a critical step in the etiology of HIV infection. Immunol Today 1993; 14:107–111.
97. Barker E, Mackewicz CE, Levy J. Effects of TH1 and TH2 cytokines on $CD8^+$ cell response against human immunodeficiency virus: Implications for long-term survival. Proc Natl Acad Sci USA 1995; 92:11135–11139.
98. Hsieh CS, Macatonia SE, Tripp CS, Wolf SF, O'Garra A, Murphey KM. Development of Th1 CD4+ T cells through IL-12 produced by listeria-induced macrophages. Science 1993; 260:547–549.
99. Afonso LCC, Sharton M, Vieira LQ, Wysocka M, Trinchieri G, Scott P. The adjuvant effect of interleukin-12 in a vaccine against Leishmania major. Science 1994; 263:235.
100. Sinigaglia F, D'Ambrosia D, Panina-Bordignon P, Rogge L. Regulation of the IL-12/IL-12R axis: a critical step in T-helper cell differentiation and effector function. Immunol Rev 1999; 170:65–72.
101. Szabo SJ, Dighe AS, Gubler U, Murphy KM. Regulation of the interleukin (IL)-12R β2 subunit expression in developing T helper 1 (Th1) and Th2 cells. J Exp Med 1997; 185:817–824.
102. Verhagen CE, de Boer T, Smits HH, Verreck FAW, Wierenga EA, Kurimoto M, Lammas DA, Kumararatne DS, Sanal O, Kroon FP, van Dissel JT, Sinigaglia F, Ottenhoff THM. Residual type 1 immunity in patients genetically deficient for interleukin 12 receptor β1 (IL-12Rβ1): Evidence for an IL-12Rβ1-independent pathway of IL-12 responsiveness in human T cells. J Exp Med 2000 192:517–528.
103. Cella M, Scheidegger D, Palmerlehmann K, Lane P, Lanzavecchia A, Alber G. Ligation of CD40 on dendritic cells triggers production of high levels of interleukin-12 and enhances T cell stimulatory capacity: T-T help via APC activation. J Exp Med 1996; 184:747–752.
104. Gately MK, Renzetti LM, Magram J, Stern AS, Adorini L, Gabler U, Presky DH. The interleukin-12/interleukin-12-receptor system: role in normal and pathologic immune responses. Annu Rev Immunol 1998; 16: 495–521.
105. Reis e Sousa C, Hieny S, Scharton-Kersten T, Charest H, Jankovic D, Germain RN, Sher A. In vivo microbial stimulation induces rapid CD40L-

independent production of IL-12 by dendritic cells and their re-distribution to T cell areas. J Exp Med 1997; 186:1819–1829.

106. Wang Y, Kelly CG, Singh M, Phipps P, Lehner T. The effect of truncation of the peptide binding fragment of HSP70 on stimulation of CC chemokines and cytokines. In preparation.
107. Chougnet C, Wynn TA, Clerici M, Landay AL, Kessler HA, Rusnak J, Melcher GP, Sher A, Shearer GM. Molecular analysis of decreased interleukin-12 production in persons infected with human immunodeficiency virus. J Inf Dis 1996; 174:46–53.
108. Chehimi J, Starr SE, Frank I, D'Andrea A, Ma X, MacGregor RR, Sennelier J, Trinchieri G. Impaired interleukin 12 production in human immunodeficiency virus-infected patients. J Exp Med 1994; 179:1361–1366.
109. Sallusto F, Mackay CR, Lanzavecchia A. Selective expression of the eotaxin receptor CCR3 by human T helper 2 cells. Science 1997; 277:2005–2007.
110. Bonecchi R, Bianchi G, Bordignon PP, D'Ambrosio D, Lang R, Borsatti A, Sozzani S, Allavena P, Gray PA, Mantovani A, Sinigaglia F. Differential expression of chemokine receptors and chemotactic responsiveness of type 1 T helper cells (Th1s) and Th2s. Differential expression of chemokine receptors and chemotactic responsiveness of type 1 T helper cells (Th1s) and Th2s). J Exp Med 1998; 187:129–134.
111. Zingoni A, Soto H, Dedrick JA, Stopacciaro A, Storiazzi CT, Sinigaglia F, D'Ambrosio D, O'Garra A, Robinson D, Rocchi M, Santoni A, Zlotnik A, Napolitano M. The chemokine receptor CCR8 is preferentially expressed in Th2 but not in Th1 cells. J Immunol 1998; 161:547–551.
112. Schrum S, Probst P, Fleischer B, Zipfel PF. Synthesis of the CC-chemokine MIP-1 alpha, MIP-1 beta and RANTES is associated with a type 1 immune response. J Immunol 1996; 15:3598–3604.
113. Kim JJ, Nottingham LK, Sin JI, Tsai A, Morrison L, Oh J, Dang K, Hu Y, Kazahaya K, Bennett M, Dentchev T, Wilson DM, Chalain AA, Boyer JD, Agadjanyan MG, Weiner DB. CD8 positive T cells influence antigen-specific immune response through the expression of chemokines. J Clin Invest 1998; 102:1112–1124.
114. Zou W, Borvak J, Marches F, Wei S, Galanaud P, Emilie D, Curiel TJ. Macrophage-derived dendritic cells have strong Th1-polarizing potential mediated by β-chemokines rather than IL-12. J Immunol 2000; 165:4388–4396.
115. Karpus WJ, Kennedy KJ. MIP-1 alpha and MCP-1 differentially regulate acute and relapsing autoimmune encephalomyelitis as well as Th1/Th2 lymphocyte differentiation. J Leukocyte Biol 1997; 62:681–687.
116. Milone MC, Fitzgerald-Bocarsly P. The mannose receptor mediates induc-

tion of IFN-alpha in peripheral blood dendritic cells by enveloped RNA and DNA viruses. J Immunol 1998; 161:2391–2399.
117. Rogge L, D'Ambrosio D, Biffi M, Penna G, Minetti LJ, Presky DH, Adorini L, Sinigaglia F. The role of STAT4 in species-specific regulation of Th cell development by type 1 IFNs. J Immunol 1998; 161:6567–6574.
118. Cho SS, Bacon CM, Sudarshan C, Rees RC, Finbloom D, Pine R, O'Shea JJ. Activation of STAT4 by IL-12 and IFN-α. Evidence for the involvement of ligand-induced tyrosine and serine phosphorylation. J Immunol 1996; 157:4781–4789.
119. Marrack P, Kappler J, Mitchell T. Type 1 interferons keep activated T cells alive. J Exp Med 1999; 189:521–530.
120. Fauci AS. Multifactorial nature of human immunodeficiency virus disease: implications for therapy. Science 1993; 262:1011–1018.
121. Merrill JE, Koyanagi Y, Chen ISY. Interleukin-1 and tumor necrosis factor alpha can be induced from mononuclear phagocytes by human immunodeficiency virus type 1 binding to the CD4 receptor. J Virol 1989; 63:4404–4408.
122. Duh EJ, Maury WJ, Folks TM, Fauci AS, Rabson AB. Tumor necrosis factor activates human immunodeficiency virus type 1 through induction of nuclear factor binding to the NF-κB sites in the long terminal repeat. Proc Natl Acad Sci USA 1989; 86:5974–5978.
123. Osborn L, Kunkel S, Nabel GJ. Tumor necrosis factor I and interleukin-1 stimulate the human immunodeficiency virus enhancer by activation of the nuclear factor κB. Proc Natl Acad Sci USA 1989; 86:2336–2340.
124. Herbein G, Montaner LJ, Gordon S. Tumor necrosis factor alpha inhibits entry of human immunodeficiency virus type 1 into primary human macrophages: a selective role for the 75-kilodalton receptor. J Virol 1996; 70: 7388–7397.
125. Kiener PA, Moran-Davis P, Rankin BM, Wahl AF, Aruffo A, Hollengaugh D. Stimulation of CD40 with purified soluble gp39 induces proinflammatory responses in human monocytes. J Immunol 1995; 155:4917–4925.
126. Banchereau J, Steinman RM. Dendritic cells and the control of immunity. Nature 1998; 392:245–252.
127. Szabo J, Prohaszka Z, Toth FD, Gyuris A, Segesdi J, Banhegyi D, Ujhelyi E, Minarovits J, Fust G. Strong correlation between the complement-mediated antibody-dependent enhancement of HIV-1 infection and plasma viral load. AIDS 1999; 13:1841–1849.
128. Montefiori DC, Lefkowitz LB, Keller RE, Holmberg V, Sandstrom E, Phair JP. Absence of a clinical correlation for complement-mediated, infection-enhancing antibodies in plasma or sera from HIV-1 infected in-

dividuals. Multicenter AIDS Cohort Study Group. AIDS 1991; 5:513–517.
129. Robinson WE, Montefiori DC Jr, Mitchell WM. Antibody-dependent enhancement of human immunodeficiency virus type 1 infection. Lancet 1988; 1:790–794.
130. McDougal JS, Hubbard M, Nicholson JK, Jones BM, Holman RC, Roberts J, Fishbein DB, Jaffe HW, Kaplan JE, Spira TJ. Immune complexes in the acquired immunodeficiency syndrome (AIDS): relationship to disease manifestation, risk group and immunologic defect. J Clin Immunol 1985; 5:130–138.
131. McHugh TM, Stites DP, Busch MP, Krowka JF, Stricker RB, Hollander H. Relation of circulating levels of human immunodeficiency virus (HIV) antigen, antibody to p24, and HIV-containing immune complexes in HIV-infected patients. J Infect Dis 1988; 158:1088–1091.
132. Senaldi G, Peakman M, McManus T, Davies ET, Tee DEH, Vergani D. Activation of the complement system in human immunodeficiency virus infection: relevance of the classical pathway to pathogenesis and disease severity. J Infect Dis 1990; 162:1227–1232.
133. Heath SL, Tew JG, Edgar LC, Whelan G, Rook AH, Fauci AS. Abnormalities of B-cell activation and immunoregulation in patients with the acquired immunodeficiency syndrome. N Engl J Med 1983; 309:453–458.
134. Tenner-Racz K, Racz P, Nofill M, Schulz-Meyer A, Dietrich M, Kern P, Weber J, Pinching AJ, Veronese-Dimarzo F, Popovic M. HTLV-III/LAV viral antigens in lymph nodes of homosexual men with persistent generalized lymphadenopathy and AIDS. Am J Pathol 1986; 123:9–15.
135. Vogel FR, Powell MF. A compendium of vaccine adjuvants and excipients. In: Powell MF, Newman M, eds. Vaccine Design. The Subunit and Adjuvant Approach. New York: Plenum Press, 1995:141–228.
136. Cox JC, Coulter AR. Adjuvants: a classification and review of their modes of action. Vaccine 1997; 15:248–256.
137. Kim JJ, Nottingham LK, Sin JI, Tsai A, Morrison L, Oh J, Dang K, Hu Y, Kazahaya K, Bennett M, Dentchev T, Wilson DM, Chalian AA, Boyer JD, Agadjanyan MG, Weiner DB. CD8 positive T cells influence antigen-specific immune responses through the expression of chemokines. J Clin Invest 1998; 102:1112–1124.
138. Sallusto F, Mackay CR, Lanzavecchia A. The role of chemokine receptors in primary, effector and memory immune responses. Annu Rev Immunol 2000; 18:593–620.
139. Lusso P. Chemokines and Viruses: The Dearest Enemies. Virol 2000; 273: 228–240.
140. Wang Y, Kelly CG, Karttunen JT, Whittall T, Lehner PJ, Duncan L, Younson JS, Singh M, Cheng G, Bergmeier L, Lehner T. CD40 functions as a

cellular receptor for heat shock protein 70 stimulation of CC-chemokines. Immunity. In press.

141. Jaattela M, Wissing D, Kokholm K, Kallunki T, Egeblad M. Hsp70 exerts its anti-apoptotic function downstream of caspase-3-like proteases. EMBO J 1998; 17:6124–6134.

142. Hussain L, Lehner T. Comparative investigation of Langerhans cells and potential receptors for HIV in oral, genitourinary and rectal epithelia. Immunology 1995; 85:475–484.

143. Zaitseva M, Blauvelt A, Lee S, Lapham CK, Klaus-Kovtun V, Mostowski H, Manischewitz J, Golding H. Expression and function of CCR5 and CXCR4 on human Langerhans cells and macrophages: implications for HIV primary infection. Nat Med 1997; 3:1369–1375.

144. Mitchell EA, Bergmeier LA, Doyle C, Brookes R, Hussain LA, Wang Y, Lehner T. Homing of mononuclear cells from iliac lymph nodes to the genital and rectal mucosa in non-human primates. Eur J Immunol 1998; 28:3066–3074.

145. Dempsey PW, Allison MED, Akkaraju S, Goodnow CC, Fearon DT, C3d of complement as a molecular adjuvant: bridging innate and acquired immunity. Science 1996; 271:348–350.

146. Matzinger P. Tolerance, danger and the extended family. Annu Rev Immunol 1994; 12:991–1045.

147. Thole JER, van Schooten WCA, Keulen WJ, Hermans PWM, Janson AM, de Vries RRP, Kolk AJH, van Embden JDA. Use of recombinant antigens expressed in *Escherichia coli* K-12 to map B-cell and T-cell epitopes on the immunodominant 65-kilodalton protein of *Mycobacterium bovis* BCG. Infect Immun 1988; 56:1633–1640.

148. Ivanyi J, Sharp K, Jackett P, Bottomley G. Immunological study of defined constituents of mycobacteria. Springer Semin Immunopathol 1988; 10: 279–300.

149. Spear GT, Sha BE, Saarloos MN, Benson CA, Rydman R, Massad LS, Gilmore R, Landay AL. Chemokines are present in the genital tract of HIV-seropositive and HIV-seronegative women. J AIDS Hum Retrovir 1998; 18:454–459.

150. Patterson BK, Landay A, Andersson J, Brown C, Behbahani H, Jiyamapa D, Burki Z, Stanislawski D, Czerniewski MA, Garcia P. Repertoire of chemokine receptor expression in the female genital tract. Am J Pathol 1998; 153:481–490.

151. Vassiliadou N, Tucker L, Anderson DJ. Progesterone-induced inhibition of chemokine receptor expression on peripheral blood mononuclear cells correlates with reduced HIV-1 infectability in vitro. J Immunol 1999; 162: 7510–7518.

11

The Role for Nonhuman Primate Models in the Development and Testing of AIDS Vaccines

C. David Pauza
University of Maryland Biotechnology Institute
Baltimore, Maryland

Marianne Wallace
University of Wisconsin
Madison, Wisconsin

INTRODUCTION

Lentiviruses related to human immunodeficiency virus type 1 (HIV-1) but not identical, can establish productive infection and cause disease in nonhuman primates. At the molecular level, the simian immunodeficiency viruses (SIV) and related HIV-2 strains have similar genome organization to HIV-1 but are distinct from HIV-1 in many ways (1,2). The TAR regions mediating responses to Tat protein are different in SIV/HIV-2 viruses (3), even though HIV-1 TAR decoys inhibit both SIV and HIV-1 Tat transactivation (4), and there are several differences in the family of accessory genes found roughly in the middle of the virus genome (2). The SU envelope glycoprotein of SIV/HIV-2 lacks a clearly defined V3 loop, and cell tropism determinants are scattered throughout this envelope gene sequence (5,6), while cell tropism determinants are mainly, but not exclusively, found in the V3 loop of HIV-1 (7–9). The idea has been advanced that SIV/HIV-2 and HIV-1 viruses evolved from a single precursor and that HIV-1 is most closely related to SIVcpz isolated from chimpanzees (10) and may have entered human populations by zoonotic transmission in the course of close contact with nonhuman primate species. The HIV-1 and the SIV/HIV-2 virus families have many similarities, but the viruses are clearly distinct at the sequence level, and the virus families have different genetic maps.

Differences between human and nonhuman primate infections are also apparent in the pathogenic outcomes. A disease course measured in decades for human beings may be measured in days to months for nonhuman primates. Such a difference may be due partly to the effects of virus dose during inoculation. The effects of inoculum size and virus variation on HIV-1 transmission are not well known, and animal doses are adjusted to produce a high frequency of infection in order to maximize the efficient use of limited animal resources. As a result, animal models of AIDS use virus inoculation doses that are likely to be higher than the amounts required for epidemic HIV-1 transmission, thus making experimental virus challenges more stringent than might be encountered during an average natural exposure to HIV-1 (11,12). As a result of selecting virulent virus isolates through interspecies transmission and then choosing the most susceptible nonhuman primate species, disease progression rates in animals are much more rapid than in humans. It is common to observe full disease progression and death in SIV-infected macaques within 6 months to 1 year after intravenous inoculation (13–16), with the notable exception of SIVpbj infection in *Macaca nemestrina*, where the acutely fatal disease course may be completed within 2 weeks (17). It is important to note that death after experimental infection mostly occurs via euthanasia that is ordered to curtail undue suffering. Thus, the time to death reflects the best judgment of attending veterinarians and not the time necessary to expire as a result of terminal disease progression.

The spectrum of disease outcomes is also different compared to HIV-1 infection in humans. SIV-infected macaque cohorts produce approximately 30% of animals that are virus positive, seronegative, and have rapidly progressing disease (14,16), a frequency much higher than observed for seronegative, rapid progressors after HIV-1 infection in humans (18). Although not as well studied, it is likely that the frequency of long-term nonprogressors in SIV or SHIV models is also higher than for HIV-1 infection. Thus, SIV or SHIV infection in macaques tends to flatten the curve that represents disease outcomes (in terms of survival), and this exaggerates the proportion of animals with extremely short or extremely long survival times. We should also note that macaques live in highly controlled environments that do not adequately mimic the exposure to intercurrent infections that is so problematic in AIDS. All of these concerns must be added to the fact that current vaccine research utilizes at least five different nonhuman primate species and at least five types of challenge viruses, not including a wide variety of molecularly cloned viruses and independent passages of common virus stocks. Considering these issues and restrictions on nonhuman primate studies imposed by the need for special facilities, one can understand the difficult problems confronting the application of this animal model to the development of HIV vaccines.

Despite the many problems associated with nonhuman primate models for AIDS, there are few options for early-stage vaccine development and testing. Hence, researchers struggle to find solutions when possible and to make accommodations when necessary. This brief discussion of the role for animal models in HIV vaccine research does not provide a comprehensive listing of current vaccine studies, as this has been done recently by others (19). Rather, our goal is to highlight key problems with using nonhuman primate models for HIV-1 vaccine development and to show how these problems are confronted by workers in the field. Finally, we will propose a scheme for integrating data from nonhuman primate vaccine research that seeks to derive the greatest value from existing and proposed studies. We tried to approach the issue of ''perspective,'' as mandated by the title of this volume, by evaluating nonhuman primate studies in the larger context of the urgent need to produce effective HIV-1 vaccines. However, we must face the reality that animal models involve a great number of choices about individual species, desired rates of infection, types of disease, and types of viruses, along with the practical problems of animal availability, housing space, and the need for substantial expertise in the laboratory staff. A great deal of *perspective* is necessary to comprehend the progress in nonhuman primate AIDS vaccine research, and *perspective* is also needed to plan the next stages of research that will (hopefully) inform about appropriate vaccine candidates for clinical evaluation.

VIRUSES, HOST SPECIES, AND FACTORS AFFECTING DISEASE PROGRESSION IN NONHUMAN PRIMATE MODELS FOR AIDS

Early reports of AIDS-like diseases in macaques occurred in the early 1980s. Laboratories at Harvard and the New England Regional Primate Research Center reported the isolation and serological characterization of retroviruses related to HTLV-III (as HIV-1 was then known) from unhealthy macaques (20–22). Early virus isolates were obtained from serial transmission studies where the aim was to identify infectious, lymphomagenic agents. Instead of lymphoma, critical evaluation of the unusual disease in exposed animals suggested a unique pathology and eventually led researchers to the SIVmac251 biological isolate that has been a foundation for much subsequent research in this field (14). However, the issue was not so clear at the time of these discoveries, because a group from the California Regional Primate Research Center was reporting a different AIDS-inducing virus from macaques. The California group uncovered a Type D retrovirus from

Macaca nigra that induced clinical signs similar to HIV in humans or to the recently described SIV when it was used in susceptible macaque species. The Type D virus had a unique manifestation because it also induced retroperitoneal fibromatosis (23) and is among the small group of directly transforming, nondefective retroviruses. Excitement grew around the California Primate Center discovery, with a report of preventive immunization using a simple, formalin-inactivated particle vaccine (24) and publication of the nucleotide sequence for simian retrovirus type 1 (SRV-1) (25).

Controversy was apparent in the first reports on nonhuman primate models for AIDS, with papers supporting the use of two different viruses. Both viruses induced wasting disease and immune system debilitation in susceptible macaque species, both were retroviruses, and by 1988 both viruses had been captured as pathogenic, infectious molecular clones (26,27). Inspection of viral sequences and genome organization quickly showed that SIV was more similar to HIV-1 than was the SRV-1 isolate, and it evolved subsequently as the main choice in nonhuman primate models for AIDS. This choice was fortunate in using a virus with a genomic organization similar to HIV-1, but it was unfortunate in that SRV-1 infection had already been prevented by a simple inactivated virus vaccine (24), and this model could have provided a platform for developing conventional inactivated particle or split vaccines. By choosing SIV as the model for HIV-1 infection, researchers were influenced by considerations about molecular structure and some aspects of disease progression that seemed more similar to human AIDS. At some future time we will be able to evaluate the wisdom of choosing SIV as the virus for modeling AIDS in nonhuman primates, and we will be able to assess the costs of this decision in terms of whether it accelerated or delayed progress toward a practical HIV-1 vaccine.

The key to developing animal models for AIDS has been inter-species transmission of retroviruses. The SIV_{mac} family of viruses descends mostly from original isolates at Harvard and the New England Primate Center (20,21) and is related to viruses found in sooty mangabeys (28). Endogenous and often indolent SIV have been observed in a wide range of nonhuman primate species (Table 1). For example, studies performed in African green monkeys showed that persistent infection with SIVagm did not lead to immune system dysfunction or apparent disease (29–31). Broader surveillance studies have discovered a great variety of SIV strains (for examples, see Ref. 32), including the SIV_{cpz} that has been advanced as the missing link between nonhuman primate and human AIDS viruses (10). The absence of obvious disease is the rule rather than the exception for SIV in their natural hosts (33,34), and the appearance of HIV-1 and AIDS in humans is thought to be a zoonosis for this promiscuous virus family. Interspecies transmission from a natural (coevolved) host to a new species often results in increased viral virulence. This observation emphasizes the fact that virulence is never a property of one virus type or one species alone but always represents the profile

Table 1 Animal Species and Their Endemic Viruses

Nonhuman primate species	Common name	SIV
Cercocebus torquatus atys	Sooty mangabey	SIV_{sm}/SIV_{smm}
Macaca mulatta	Rhesus macaque	SIV_{mac}
Macaca arctoides	Stumptail macaque	SIV_{stm}
Macaca nemestrina	Pigtailed macaque	SIV_{mne}
Macaca fascicularis	Cynomologus	SIV_{cyn}
Cercopithecus aethiops super species	African green monkeys	SIV_{agm}
Cercopithecus aethiops	Grivet monkey	SIV_{agmgri}
Cercopithecus pygerythrus	Vervet monkey	SIV_{agmver}
Cercopithecus sabaeus	Sabaeus monkey	SIV_{agmsab}
Cercopithecus tantalus	Tantalus monkey	SIV_{agmtan}
Pan troglodytes troglodytes	Chimpanzee	SIV_{cpz}

Source: Adapted from Ref. 32.

of disease in one combination of virus and species. The Asian subspecies of rhesus macaques (*Macaca mulatta*) has emerged as one of the major species for nonhuman primate AIDS research. Rhesus macaques develop progressing disease after infection with SIV_{mac} family of viruses and are also susceptible to several simian/human immunodeficiency (SHIV) variants. By the extensive use of rhesus macaques and SIV_{mac} viruses, we have emphasized efficient virus transmission and virulent outcomes as the key features of our model. For perspective, it is important to remember that we are modeling natural HIV-1 infection that has inefficient transmission, moderate to low virulence, and a disease course measured in decades for most human populations.

In addition to the rhesus macaque, several other species have also been used, including the pigtailed macaque (*Macaca nemestrina*), the cynomolgus macaque (*Macaca fasicularis*), members of the genus *Cercopithecus*, including grivet and vervet monkeys (African green monkeys, and the stump-tailed macaque (*Macaca arctoides*) (29–31,35,36). The virulence in each model depends on the combination of virus and host species. For example, high-level virus replication has been noted in African green monkeys infected with SIV_{agm}, yet there are no apparent signs of clinical disease (33), even in newborn animals (37). Similar observations have been made for sooty mangabeys infected with their cognate SIV_{smm} (38), yet these viruses can cause acutely fatal disease in rhesus or cynomolgus macaques (39). The panel of choices for virus–species combinations provides a great variety of options from essentially avirulent infections all the way to acutely lethal viral diseases (Table 2). When evaluating the outcomes of infection in terms of whether they represent the events in human disease, the impact of these many choices must be considered.

Table 2 The Most Common Virus–Host Combinations in Nonhuman Primate Models for AIDS in Order of Increasing Virulence (top to bottom)

	Months[a]	Model	Comments	Ref.
No disease	—	SIV_{mac251} IV/rhesus (molecular clone)		81
	—	SHIVhxbc2 IV/rhesus		31
	—	SIV_{agm}/vervets		37
Slow	60	SIV_{delta} nef IV/rhesus	Pathogenic in young macaques	54
	48	SHIV89.6P IV/cynomolgus	Projected from unpublished data	71
	36	SIV_{mac251} IR/rhesus		16
	24	SIV_{mne} IV/pigtailed macaques		30
	18	SIV_{mac239} IV/rhesus (molecular clone)		96
Moderate	12	SHIVku IV/pigtailed macaques	Adapted pathogenic isolate	47
	12	SIV_{mac251} IV/rhesus		14
	12	SHIV89.6PD IR/rhesus	Adapted pathogenic isolate	50
Rapid	6	SHIV89.6PD IV/rhesus	Adapted pathogenic isolate	48
	1	SIV_{pbj14} IV/pigtailed macaques	Some animals resist acute disease and become moderate progressors	97

Survival times are approximate and provide only a general comparison among models. Accurate survival times are often not reported, partly due to the expense of maintaining animals for the full duration of disease. In some cases, survival data are not yet available, as for SHIV89.6P in cynomolgus macaques. Comments indicate some of the problems involved in these types of generalizations, especially in the SIV_{pbj14} infections, with which some animals die from acute disease while others have a more moderate disease.

[a] Approximate time for 50% mortality.

IV = Intravenous inoculation; IR = intrarectal inoculation.

A new type of interspecies infection was created when researchers developed chimeric viruses containing portions of both the SIV and HIV-1 genomes and now relied on the HIV-1 envelope glycoprotein to mediate infection in nonhuman primates. Recombinant viruses were constructed that contained SIV long terminal repeat regions and the 5′ portion of SIV coupled to the envelope, Tat and Rev regions of HIV. These viruses were infectious for macaque cells in vitro (40) and established persistent infections in macaques (41–43) or baboons (44). Despite persisting infection, these early SHIV constructs did not cause a typical disease in nonhuman primates, but could induce a protective immune response that blocked a subsequent challenge with pathogenic SIV (45). When nonpathogenic SHIV were passaged repeatedly in naïve animals, fast replicating, pathogenic variants emerged and caused rapid CD4+ T-cell depletion and accelerated disease progression (46,47). The pathogenic SHIV were highly infectious by intravenous and intramucosal routes (48,49). In approximately half of each animal cohort infected with one pathogenic SHIV isolate, the CD4+ T-cell and CD20+ B-cell populations were depleted rapidly, and animals progressed to death within 6 months to one year after intrarectal inoculation (50). Because of the sequences shared with HIV-1, their efficient intramucosal transmission, and pathogenic potential, SHIV has many advantages as a vaccine challenge virus in macaques (51). The SHIV infection offers both advantages and disadvantages that must be weighed when selecting an appropriate model for a particular vaccine experiment. The presence of HIV-1 sequences facilitates tests on vaccines directed at envelope or regulatory gene regions however, nonpathogenic SHIV already protects against SIV infection (45), suggesting that responses to virus genes other than envelope (52) were also important for protection against the heterologous challenge stock. The rapid disease progression after SHIV infection helps to provide data on vaccine efficacy within a short period after challenge, but also brings the risk that the model virus is far more aggressive than HIV-1 in humans. Whether the particular vaccine studies utilize SIV or SHIV challenge models, it is important to appreciate how each model is likely to influence the potential for achieving protective immunization.

Selection of appropriate nonhuman primate models for AIDS demands critical choices about the virus isolate, the animal species, the age of test animals, virus preparation, virus delivery, and endpoint criteria for evaluating outcomes. With so many choices it is not surprising that a wide variety of results have been reported, ranging from barely detectable disease to fulminant infection with acute disease and death. The four factors most important for virulence in nonhuman primates are virus type, animal species, route, and dose for inoculation. We discussed above the types of choices for animal species and virus isolates. We will now review the influence of virus dose and route for inoculation, beginning with a few comments about the methods for establishing the standard dose for inoculation and virus challenge.

The minimum infectious dose for a specific virus isolate and a selected macaque species is determined by an *in vivo* titration of the virus inoculum. The doses can be represented by the designation AID (animal infectious dose) followed by the route of inoculation, e.g., AIDiv for intravenous administration. To perform the titration, 10-fold dilutions of virus are inoculated into macaques. Intramucosal routes include oral exposure (po), intrarectal (ir) inoculation (generally delivered to the distal colon), and intravaginal (ivag), including virus doses placed on the vaginal wall or applied to the ectocervix. These three routes are listed in the approximate order of susceptibility, meaning that oral inoculation requires lower doses than either intrarectal or intravaginal routes. Titration experiments have shown that the minimum dose required for a given virus isolate to establish productive infection with progressing disease, depends on both the virus dose and route for inoculation. In a case where one AIDiv of SIVmac251 is required for productive infection and disease in rhesus monkeys, approximately 1000 AIDiv were necessary to achieve infection of ≥90% of age-matched animals when the virus isolate was applied to the rectal mucosa (16). For complex biological isolates such as the SIVmac251, the AIDiv is approximately equivalent to the tissue culture infectious dose (TCID), and for a first approximation, infection via intrarectal inoculation requires around 1000 TCID in order to obtain a high frequency of persistently infected animals. For a high frequency of infection after a single intravaginal exposure, the required doses may be up to 10 times higher than for intrarectal inoculation (49,53). For oral inoculation, the intrarectal doses are generally sufficient if not slightly higher than necessary, depending very much on the age of selected animals, with lower doses required in infant macaques (54). One can represent these data as: 10,000 AIDiv ≈ 10 AIDir or AIDpo ≈ 1 AIDivag. Of course, this is a very crude approximation and can vary depending on the method for inoculation and unique properties of individual virus isolates.

Rhesus macaques that were exposed intrarectally to 10, 1, or 0.1 AIDiv of the SIVmac251 biological isolate were virus isolation negative and had undetectable antibodies to SIV. We described these animals as transiently infected due to the presence of viral DNA–positive lymphocytes in blood and a brief interval of very low level plasma antigenemia, despite the lack of overt signs of infection (16,55,56). Transiently infected macaques failed to develop clinical signs of SIV disease and resisted a high-dose intrarectal challenge with the homologous SIV isolate (55). However, animals with transient viremia after low-dose intrarectal inoculation were not protected against a subsequent intravenous virus challenge, suggesting specificity in the types of immune responses. These experiments are the precursors to later studies with attenuated viruses, where it was shown that inoculation with low replicating strains provided immune protection against subsequent challenge (57). Our studies also showed that local immunity to virus was possible and could be durable. However, we note that virus reemerged at 3.5

years after infection in one of seven transiently infected animals from a single study (55). The animal had been housed alone and had no physical contact with other macaques. Moreover, this animal had been negative for virus isolation from PBMC or lymph node biopsy materials throughout the 3.5 years. Despite this apparently negative condition, the virus that reemerged was clearly derived from the original SIVmac251 stock, but sequence variation in the envelope gene region implied that replication had continued throughout this time (55). In addition, the reemerged virus caused a rapid decline in CD4 counts with rapidly progressing disease, showing that the host was not protected against disease despite the long period of exposure.

Infection studies with long-term follow-up showed that disease progression rates were slower after intrarectal inoculation compared to intravenous infection. In general, one can expect disease progression to be around 50% as rapid for intrarectal inoculation compared to intravenous routes (11). There are a number of possible explanations for slower disease progression after mucosal exposure. The host may gain valuable time to develop and recruit early mechanisms of immune defense at or near the mucosal surface that are simply not possible after the immediate intravenous introduction of virus and rapid seeding to secondary lymphoid tissues. Sequence analysis of SIV present in the transiently infected macaques showed that a limited subset of virus present in the complex SIVmac251 biological isolate was able to cross the mucosal surface when the virus inoculum was limiting (56). Thus, mucosal exposure acts as a bottleneck that reduces the complexity of virus populations that are established during the acute infection interval. The genetic bottleneck may be due either to selection for particular virus strains that transit more efficiently across the mucosal barrier as proposed for HIV-1 (58,59) or to the fact that mucosal inoculations may be nearer to the true minimal dose, and we observe the results of something approaching a limiting dilution. Large-scale sequencing studies with SIVmac251 and intrarectal transmission (55,56) failed to adequately resolve these issues. For experimental infection or vaccine challenge studies in macaque species, choices about the virus dose and route for inoculation are critically important for influencing disease outcomes. The age of the animal is another factor that can influence outcome. For example, viruses lacking the *nef* gene and other portions were highly attenuated in adult rhesus macaques exposed by intravenous infection, and this type of virus was proposed as a candidate attenuated viral vaccine (57). When the route was changed to oral inoculation and infant macaques were used in place of adult animals, there was a substantial increase in virulence, with most animals progressing to AIDS and death (60). The viruses were identical in both cases, but other choices about the model had drastic impacts on the outcome.

Within a model that uses a single virus isolate, a single route for inoculation, and a single species, there is still substantial variation in terms of disease progression (see Refs. 50 and 61). Each infected cohort usually includes rapid, intermediate, and slow progressor groups in the approximate proportions of 1:1:1, and there are reproducible differences among these groups. A rapid course of SIV-infection is characterized by persistent, high level viremia, weak or undetectable SIV specific antibody responses, and a rapid loss of circulating CD4+ T cells that is often accompanied by losses of circulating CD8+ T cells and B cells as well (32,61). Rapid progressors are often euthanized between 4 and 6 months after infection due to opportunistic infections, wasting, and other complications of AIDS. Macaques with an intermediate level of disease progression may not develop AIDS until about 1 year after intravenous SIV infection, and these animals manifest plasma viral antigenemia during acute infection and then again during late stage disease. They often develop strong antibodies to SIV that decline later in disease, and they experience a moderately rapid loss of CD4+ T cells. Slow progressors may experience an early antigenemia and develop strong and durable SIV-specific antibody responses. T-cell subset losses are minimal during the prolonged period; they remain free of clinical infection signs and may remain healthy for up to 5 years. Studies have shown that the quantity of plasma viral RNA stabilizes rapidly after the first few months of acute SIV infection and is predictive for the rate of disease progression (62,63) as it is in humans infected with HIV-1 (64). There are several good correlates of disease progression and time to death, including peak plasma antigenemia, rate of CD4+ or CD20+ lymphocyte losses (50,61), plasma interferon-α levels (65), efficiency of virus isolation (66), and viral RNA at set-point (62,63). These factors (Table 3) can be used to evaluate challenge studies within 8–13 weeks after inoculation and obviate the need to wait for the full disease course before concluding about vaccine efficacy

Table 3 Correlation of Laboratory Markers and Survival After Immunodeficiency Virus Infection of Rhesus Macaques

	p-value[a]	
	SIV_{mac251}[b]	SHIV89.6PD[c]
Virus-binding antibody	<0.005	0.005
Neutralizing antibody	<0.05 (7 weeks)	0.005
Plasma antigenemia	<0.05	<0.005
CD4 T-cell count	Not significant	<0.02
CD20 B-cell count	<0.05	<0.02

[a] Correlation between assay values and survival times.
[b] SIV_{mac251} data are 13 weeks after intravenous inoculation except where noted (61).
[c] SHIV89.6PD data are 2 weeks after intrarectal inoculation (50).

(50,61). However, it is important to remember that high viral loads alone do not always lead to disease as evidenced by African green monkeys infected with SIV_{agm} and sooty mangabeys infected with SIV_{sm} in nature, as described above. The relationship between these hosts and their viruses may have changed from pathogenic into nonpathogenic infections as the virus and host coevolved (33).

Recent progress in the quantitative analysis of immunodeficiency virus infection in the rhesus monkey model has facilitated our ability to assess disease outcome and inform future attempts of vaccination and therapy. Methods to detect viral RNA and viral DNA have increased sensitivity over the early assays. Virus isolation techniques have become more rigorous with the routine assessment of several millions of lymphocytes in coculture with cell lines exhibiting strong cytopathic effect upon virus infection. In parallel, means to measure specific immune responses toward viral infection and aspects of innate immunity have become more sophisticated as researchers understand more about the rhesus macaque immune system and have developed tools to better investigate it. The analysis of macaque T-cell repertoires, estimates of cytotoxic T lymphocyte (CTL) frequencies using tetramer binding assays, the assessment of cytokine and chemokine production at the single cell level and by ELISA are among some of the newer assays now routinely employed in many macaque studies and vaccine trials.

Recent research in HIV-1 infection and in nonhuman primates infected with SIV or SHIV emphasizes the critical importance of events during acute infection and how they dictate subsequent disease progression rates. In our laboratory we view the acute infection interval as a competition between virus dissemination and the host's ability to evolve antiviral immune responses. We believe that the virus set-point which has been so useful for disease prognosis (62,63) is actually a consequence of the ''host set-point,'' which describes the level of immunity that survives acute infection, and here we are emphasizing the MHC class II–restricted, T-helper repertoire that will be needed to sustain cellular and humoral effector mechanisms (67). Therefore, to design novel vaccines, we need to understand acute infection and how this dictates subsequent disease progression rates. Qualitative and quantitative differences in lymphocyte activation, apoptosis rates, and virus replication in the first few weeks after infection are correlated with rates of disease progression, even though the full disease course may stretch to years. For these studies, we used SHIV89.6PD in rhesus macaques. In order to slow disease progression to rates that are more suitable for experimental analysis, we elected to use intrarectal inoculation instead of intravenous virus challenge. The resulting model creates highly pathogenic infections where high viral loads peak at around 2 weeks after intrarectal infection and 90% or more of circulating CD4+ T cells may be lost within 4–6 weeks (49,50). Peak viremia is reached within about 1 week after intravenous inoculation, and all other rates are also about twice as rapid as for intrarectal infection examples (49). High levels of

CD4+ T-cell activation and an inability of T cells to respond in vitro to mitogenic stimuli (because of activation-induced cell death during the interval of acute infection) predicted a rapid disease course in intrarectally infected macaques (67) and were coincident with extinguishing preexisting lymphoproliferative responses to viral proteins (68,69). These studies were designed to emphasize acutely virulent infections, which might allow better observation of lymphocyte activation events related to disease progression. Careful evaluation of acute infection lymphocyte activation pathways at both the molecular and cellular levels is already providing new information about the essential elements of virulence in AIDS, and these findings may elucidate novel vaccine targets and new measurement approaches for vaccine evaluation.

SCHEMES FOR USING NONHUMAN PRIMATE MODELS IN VACCINE DEVELOPMENT AND TESTING PROGRAMS

How then can we best apply nonhuman primate studies to the practical problem of developing efficacious vaccines against HIV-1 in humans? Experimental vaccination and challenge studies in macaques are most useful for evaluating new types of immunization schemes or for comparing vaccine products. In general, vaccine studies in nonhuman primates fall into two broad categories. Early-stage studies with new immunization schemes can be described as *concept evaluation* efforts that seek to establish a need for additional research on a particularly novel approach. Once the activity of a novel vaccine has been documented at some reasonable level, the next stage is to conduct *comparative testing* studies that validate the relative efficacy of a new vaccine in relation to distinct products (in order to prioritize multiple vaccines) or in relation to modifications in adjuvant, dose, or immunization protocol (to optimize a single vaccine). Mixed prime boost studies, where multiple vaccine products are combined, also fall into the concept testing or comparative evaluation categories, depending on the experimental plan. The distinction between types of vaccine studies is critical for our ability to assess the results and their implications for vaccines against HIV-1 in humans.

Until now there have been at least six types of AIDS vaccine *concept testing* studies in nonhuman primate models. They include conventional inactivated or split vaccines, subunit vaccines, low replicating (attenuated) viruses, chimeric viral vectors, recombinant bacterial or mycobacterial vectors, and naked DNA vaccines. A detailed list of vaccine and challenge studies, including challenge doses and outcomes, has been compiled by Warren and Levinson (19). To avoid a nearly endless complexity, we are not mentioning the number of different adjuvants and immunization protocols that have been employed. Concept testing studies have reported three general types of results including full protection against virus challenge (sterilizing immunity), disease attenuation, and no effect of immunization (see Ref. 19 for details).

Concept testing studies generally aim to provide preliminary evidence that an immunization method has value as a protective or therapeutic vaccine. Concept testing studies often use small numbers of animals with a consequent lack of statistical validity. Smaller animal groups may be necessary because these studies occur early in the development of a new approach and may not yet have earned sufficient resources to support larger, statistically valid experiments. Concept testing has a high risk/reward ratio but is still an essential part of the HIV vaccine program because it is the source of new methods that might include the crucial discovery for success. Unfortunately, the lack of statistical validation often produces results that are best characterized as being ''consistent with protection,'' ''supporting further investigation,'' or similar syllogisms representing the investigator's best conclusion in the absence of rigorous testing. Careful and conservative interpretation of these data, and a subsequent retesting using larger animal groups, is the best method for realizing value from concept testing projects. New vaccines that prove their potential in follow-up studies are excellent candidates for comparative evaluation studies.

The *comparative evaluation* study tests distinct types of vaccines or modifications of a single vaccine product in parallel. This type of study uses a single macaque species and a single virus isolate (preferably the same production lot of virus), along with standardized assay protocols. The comparative evaluation study depends ultimately on statistical testing to distinguish among various groups, and it is essential to include enough animals in each control or immunized group. It is often difficult to conduct all arms of a comparative study contemporaneously, but the best experiments will work toward this goal. In our own experience and in consultation with biostatisticians, animal groups of eight or more macaques are generally needed to ensure statistical significance for the results (70). However, if the experiments are performed with animals of a single haplotype or are subjected to other rigorous selection criteria, it is not always possible to have groups of eight or more macaques. In these cases, we should expect to lose the potential for statistical validation, and the studies will tend to resemble concept testing experiments.

Formally, comparative evaluation studies seek to prioritize individual candidate vaccines, and they require an ability to distinguish efficacy using statistically valid criteria. Endpoint criteria may include sterilizing immunity, although comparative evaluations based on viral burden, blood CD4 counts, duration of survival, or other surrogate markers may be equally valid. Note that comparative evaluation studies need not make assumptions about whether the vaccine candidate induces sterilizing immunity, is specific only to a single virus type, or other considerations even if they are ultimately important for promoting a vaccine candidate to human clinical trials. In this phase of research, the principal goal is to prioritize among a group of candidates. It is likely that subsequent rounds of comparative testing, involving head-to-head comparisons of the best candidates from many independent comparative studies, will be needed to reduce the number of candidates proposed for clinical testing. Thus, a logical progression from concept testing to comparative evaluation promotes the best selection of promising candidate vaccines and makes the best use of nonhuman primate data. It is unwise to presume that the effects of a vaccine in one particular model are directly relevant to a similar vaccine that will be tested against HIV-1 in humans. The strategy of evolving from concept testing to comparative evaluation ultimately relies on the ability to generate any acceptable and statistically valid evidence that one vaccine candidate is superior to others.

We can see the potential for applying this strategy in the recent studies on vaccines directed at the HIV-1 Tat protein. For example, a new candidate vaccine might elicit protective immunity during a concept testing study that used a low-virulence model. The recent report that Tat vaccine protected cynomolgus macaques from SHIV89.6P infection (71) is an example of using a low-virulence model to emphasize the protective activities of vaccination, because this virus is weakly pathogenic in cynomolgus macaques. Peak virus titers in the cynomolgus model reached only around 10^6 viral RNA copies per mL in plasma, and most control animals were orders of magnitude lower (71). In a larger concept-testing study, this same type of vaccine might not provide the same degree of protection when using a higher virulence model. As an example, our laboratory selected a high virulence model for studying the effects of vaccinating rhesus macaques with chemically inactivated Tat toxoid, followed by intrarectal challenge with the SHIV89.6PD (nearly identical to SHIV89.6P). In contrast to the study mentioned above, our control animals showed peak levels in the range of 10^9 viral RNA per mL of plasma, with obvious signs of clinical disease progression. We showed that Tat toxoid vaccination provided a statistically valid attenuation of disease progression but was on its own not protective (65,70). Both of these experiments support further development of preventive or therapeutic vaccines that include Tat protein, but expectations about the performance of this vaccine are greatly influenced by model choices. The ability to induce protective immunity in the low-virulence infection (71) was as much a product of the model as a consequence of immunization, and predictions that a Tat vaccine would be equally protective in human beings were not supported by the data. Comparative evaluation studies in macaques will help to select the best Tat vaccine candidate among several products. However, we must recognize that vaccine efficacy in humans may be greater, similar, or less than comparable products tested in nonhuman primate models. The efficacy of Tat vaccines in humans will only be learned through Tat vaccination studies in humans.

IMMUNE RESPONSES IN NONHUMAN PRIMATE MODELS

Finally, what type of immune responses can we expect in animal model studies, and how are these responses related to protection? The subject of immune correlates of protection is a difficult and confusing area for AIDS vaccine research. Opinions drift with the times and with changing technology. Very early studies suggested that the best correlate of protection was the lymphoproliferative response (72,73) until better assays revealed a stringent relation between virus-binding serum antibody levels and disease progression (14,50,61). With the development of cytotoxic T-lymphocyte assays (74,75) facilitated by the availability of MHC class I tetramer reagents that label epitope-specific cells (76), attention turned to CTL as the hope for vaccine protection. In our experience, CTL activities and virus-binding serum antibody levels are usually related in SIV- or SHIV-infected macaques. That is to say, rapid progressors demonstrate very low responses in both the cellular and humoral arms of immunity, while slow progressors have high responses in both categories. This observation would tend to promote the view that both strong CTL and antibody responses will be required for protection, and this will necessarily involve vaccines that can also elicit sufficient T-helper responses to maintain effector immunity through the difficult interval of acute infection.

However, HIV-1 and SIV have many negative effects on lymphocytes, including the action of directly toxic proteins encoded by the viruses. Inappropriate T-cell activation leading to activation-induced cell death (67,77) and apoptosis (78) is a danger during acute infection, and this must be avoided in vaccine protocols and products. There are many reports of the proapoptotic effects of envelope glycoprotein (e.g., Ref. 79), and this was the original justification for developing the therapeutic vaccine product Remune, which is depleted of gp120 (80). The suspected cellular toxicities of nef protein made it a target for deletion in attenuated virus strains (81). The many toxic effects of Tat protein, including promoting apoptosis (82–85) suggest that this might be a important target for vaccination. These and other components of the SIV and HIV-1 viruses may be directly toxic as native proteins and are thus unsuitable vaccines. An example of how to approach this problem is provided by our recent studies on chemically inactivated Tat toxoid vaccines.

The Tat protein of HIV-1 is secreted by infected cells and has multiple effects on uninfected cells (reviewed in Ref. 86), which promote virus replication and T-cell destruction. In our view the actions of extracellular Tat are an essential element of infection that distinguishes HIV-1 from simpler retroviruses and makes this agent such a devastating killer and so hard to prevent by vaccination. As Tat promotes activation (87) and apoptosis of uninfected T helper cells, the subpopulation that is responding to virus antigen in support of effector responses is at great risk of elimination. This mechanism will undoubtedly work against most vaccine effects, as Tat works to degrade the immunity built so carefully during prolonged immunization. Tat also acts to increase virus dissemination, principally by upregulating vital chemokine receptors that are required for virus entry (88,89) and possibly through direct transactivation of proviral LTR to increase virus production (90). In studies from our laboratory (70) and others (71), immunization with Tat or a safer inactivated version designated Tat toxoid (91–94) attenuated disease in macaques challenged with SHIV. We believe that Tat toxoid is an important and necessary component in any HIV-1 vaccine and will produce the crucial distinction between vaccines that barely fail and those that succeed in providing protection. Administration of Tat toxoid is also envisioned as an important approach for therapeutic vaccination and is intended to preserve vital T-cell immunity that withstands virus recrudescence after cessation of anti-retroviral therapy.

SUMMARY

Nonhuman primate models for AIDS have contributed enormously to the understanding of viral pathogenesis in AIDS. There has also been substantial progress in vaccine research and development, although the complexities of model choices may have obscured these contributions from uninitiated eyes. The nonhuman primate models have a defined role in the future process of vaccine development and testing but should not be overinterpreted or assumed to provide direct prognostications for vaccine mechanisms or efficacy in humans. Nonhuman primate models will continue to be required for the evolution and rapid evaluation of new vaccine concepts but should not be advanced to the role of gatekeeper that might prevent clinical evaluation of potential vaccine products.

REFERENCES

1. Colombini S, Arya S, Reitz M, Jagodzinski L, Beaver B, Wong-Staal F. Structure of simian immunodeficiency virus regulatory genes. Proc Natl Acad Sci 1989; 86:4813–4817.
2. Franchini G, Gurgo C, Guo HG, et al. Sequence of simian immunodeficiency virus and its relationship to the human immunodeficiency viruses. Nature 1987; 328:539–542.
3. Berkhout B. Structural features in TAR RNA of human and simian immunodeficiency viruses: a phylogenetic analysis. Nucleic Acids Res 1992; 20: 27–31.
4. Lisziewicz J, Sun D, Smythe J, et al. Inhibition of human immunodeficiency virus type 1 replication by regulated expression of a polymeric Tat activation response RNA decoy as a strategy for gene therapy in AIDS. Proc Natl Acad Sci USA 1993; 90:8000–8004.
5. Kodama T, Mori K, Kawahara T, Ringler DJ, Desrosiers RC. Analysis of simian immunodeficiency virus sequence variation in tissues of rhesus macaques with simian AIDS. J Virol 1993; 67:6522–6534.
6. Mori K, Ringler DJ, Kodama T, Desrosiers RC. Complex determinants of macrophage tropism in env of simian immnuodeficiency virus. J Virol 1992; 66:2067–2075.

7. Harrowe G, Cheng-Mayer C. Amino acid substitutions in the V3 loop are responsible for adaptation to growth in transformed T-cell lines of a primary human immunodeficiency virus type 1. Virology 1995; 210:490–494.
8. Trujillo JR, Wang W-K, Lee T-H, Essex M. Identification of the envelope V3 loop as a determinant of a CD4-negative neuronal cell tropism for HIV-1. Virology 1996; 217:613–617.
9. Kim FM, Kolson DL, Balliet JW, Srinivasan A, Collman RG. V3-independent determinants of macrophage tropism in a primary human immunodeficiency virus type 1 isolate. J Virol 1995; 69:1755–1761.
10. Gao F, Bailes E, Robertson DL, et al. Origin of HIV-1 in the chimpanzee *Pan troglodytes troglodytes*. Nature 1999; 397:436–441.
11. Pauza CD, Horejsh D, Wallace M. Mucosal transmission of virulent and avirulent lentiviruses in macaques. AIDS Res Hum Retrovir 1998; 14:S83–87.
12. Pauza CD, Malkovsky M, Salvato MS. SIV transmission across the mucosal barrier. AIDS Res Hum Retrovir 1994; 10:7–10.
13. Letvin NL, Daniel MD, Sehgal PK, et al. Induction of AIDS-like disease in macaque monkeys with T-cell tropic retrovirus STLV-III. Science 1985; 230:71–73.
14. Daniel MD, Letvin NL, Sehgal PK, et al. Long-term persistent infection of macaque monkeys with the simian immunodeficiency virus. J Gen Virol 1987; 68:3183–3189.
15. Pauza CD, Emau P, Salvato S, et al. Transmission of SIV by intrarectal inoculation in rhesus monkeys. Colloque des ''Cent Gardes'', 7th, Marnes-la-Coquette, Paris, France, Oct 22–24, 1992. Proceedings: Retroviruses of Human AIDS and Related Animal Diseases. Girard M, Vallette L, eds. Lyon: Foundation Marcel Merieux, 1993:151–156.
16. Pauza CD, Emau P, Salvato MS, et al. Pathogenesis of SIVmac251 after atraumatic inoculation of the rectal mucosa in rhesus monkeys. J Med Primatol 1993; 22:154–161.
17. Fultz PN, Stricker RB, McClure HM, Anderson DC, Switzer WM, Horaist C. Humoral response to SIV/SMM infection in macaque and mangabey monkeys. J AIDS 1990; 3:319–329.
18. Michael NL, Brown AE, Voigt RF, et al. Rapid disease progression without seroconversion following primary human immunodeficiency virus type 1 infection: evidence for highly susceptible human hosts. J Infect Dis 1997; 175:1352–1359.
19. Warren JT, Levinson MA. AIDS preclinical vaccine development: biennial survey of HIV, SIV, and SHIV challenge studies in vaccinated nonhuman primates. J Med Primatol 1999; 28:249–273.
20. Daniel MD, Letvin NL, King NW, et al. Isolation of T-cell tropic HTLV-III-like retrovirus from macaques. Science 1985; 228:1201–1204.

21. Kanki PJ, McLane MF, King NW, et al. Serologic identification and characterization of a macaque T-lymphotropic retrovirus closely related to HTLV-III. Science 1985; 228:1199–1201.
22. Kannagi M, Kiyotaki M, Desrosiers RC, et al. Humoral immune responses to t cell tropic retrovirus simian T Lymphotropic virus type III in monkeys with experimentally induced acquired immune deficiency-like syndrome. J Clin Invest 1986; 78:1229–1236.
23. Marx P, Bryant M, Osborn K, et al. Isolation of a new serotype of simian acquired immune deficiency syndrome type D retrovirus from Celebes black macaques (*Macaca nigra*) with immune deficiency retroperitoneal fibromatosis. J Virol 1986; 56:571–578.
24. Marx P, Pedersen N, Lerche N, et al. Prevention of simian acquired immune deficiency syndrome with a formalin-inactivated type D retrovirus vaccine. J Virol 1986; 60:431–435.
25. Power M, Marx P, Bryant M, Gardner M, Barr P, Luciw P. Nucleotide sequence of SRV-1, a type D acquired immune deficiency syndrome retrovirus. Science 1986; 231:1567–1572.
26. Naidu Y, Kestler H, Li C, et al. Characterization of infectious molecular clones of simian immunodeficiency virus (SIV_{mac}) and human immunodeficiency virus type 2: persistent infection of rhesus monkeys with molecularly cloned SIV mac. J Virol 1988; 62:4691–4696.
27. Heidecker G, Lerche N, Lowenstine L, et al. Induction of simian AIDS (SAIDS) with a molecular clone of a type D SAIDS retrovirus. J Virol 1987; 61:3066–3071.
28. Hirsch VM, Olmstead RA, Murphy-Corb M, Purcell RH, Johnson PR. SIV from sooty mangabeys: an African non-human primate lentivirus closely related to HIV-2. Nature 1989; 339:389–392.
29. Baier M, Garber C, Müller C, Cichutek K, Kurth R. Complete nucleotide sequence of a simian immunodeficiency virus from African green monkeys: a novel type of intragroup divergence. Virology 1990; 176:216–221.
30. Benveniste RE, Raben D, Hill RW, et al. Molecular characterization and comparison of simian immunodeficiency virus isolates from macaques, mangabeys, and African green monkeys. J Med Primatol 1989; 18:287–303.
31. Li Y, Naidu Y, Daniel M, Desrosiers R. Extensive genetic variability of simian immunodeficiency virus from African green monkeys. J Virol 1989; 63:1800–1802.
32. Hirsch VM, Johnson PR. Pathogenic diversity of simian immunodeficiency viruses. Virus Res 1994; 32:183–203.
33. Hartung S, Boller K, Cichutek K, Norley ST, Kurth R. Quantitation of a lentivirus in its natural host: simian immunodeficiency virus in African green monkeys. J Virol 1992; 66:2143–2149.

34. Norley SG, Kraus G, J, Bonilla J, König H, Kurth R. Immunological studies of the basis for the apathogenicity of simian immunodeficiency virus from African green monkeys. Proc Natl Acad Sci USA 1990; 87:9067–9071.
35. Novembre FJ, Hirsch VM, McClure HM, Fultz PN, Johnson PR. SIV from stump-tailed macaques: molecular characterization of a highly transmissible primate lentivirus. Virology 1992; 186:783–787.
36. Hirsch VM, Dapolito G, Johnson PR, et al. Induction of AIDS by simian immunodeficiency virus from an African green monkey: species-specific variation in pathogenicity correlates with the extent of in vivo replication. J Virol 1995; 69:955–967.
37. Beer B, Denner J, Brown CR, et al. Simian immunodeficiency virus of African green monkeys is apathogenic in the newborn natural host. J AIDS 1998; 18:210–220.
38. Rey-Cuille MA, Berthier JL, Bomsel-Demontoy MC, et al. Simian immunodeficiency virus replicates to high levels in sooty mangabeys without inducing disease. J Virol 1998; 72:3872–3886.
39. Lewis MG, Zack PM, Elkins WR, Jahrling PB. Infection of rhesus and cynomolgus macaques with a rapidly fatal SIV (SIVSMM/PB_j) isolate from sooty mangabeys. AIDS Res Hum Retroviruses 1992; 8:1631–1639.
40. Shibata R, Kawamura M, Sakai H, Hayami M, Ishimoto A, Adachi A. Generation of a chimeric human and simian immunodeficiency virus infectious to monkey peripheral blood mononuclear cells. J Virol 1991; 65:3514–3520.
41. Li J, Lord C, Haseltine W, Letvin N, Sodroski J. Infection of cynomolgus monkeys with a chimeric HIV-1/SIV that expresses the HIV-1 envelope glycoproteins. J AIDS 1992; 5:639–646.
42. Sakuragi S, Shibata R, Mukai R, et al. Infection of macaque monkey with a chimeric human and simian immunodeficiency virus. J Gen Virol 1992; 73:2983–2987.
43. Li JT, Halloran M, Lord CI, et al. Persistent infection of macaques with simian-human immunodeficiency viruses. J Virol 1995; 69:7061–7071.
44. Allan JS, Ray P, Broussard S, et al. Infection of baboons with simian/human immunodeficiency viruses. J AIDS Hum Retrovirol 1995; 9:429–441.
45. Letvin NL, Li J, Halloran M, Cranage MP, Rud EW, Sodroski J. Prior infection with a nonpathogenic chimeric simian immunodeficiency virus does not efficiently protect macaques against challenge with simian immunodeficiency virus. J Virol 1995; 69:4569–4571.
46. Reimann KA, Li JT, Veazy R, et al. A chimeric simian/human immunodeficiency virus expressing a primary patient human immunodeficiency virus type 1 isolate env causes an AIDS-like disease after in vivo passage in rhesus monkeys. J Virol 1996; 70:6922–6928.

47. Joag SV, Li Z, Foresman L, et al. Chimeric simian/human immunodeficiency virus that causes progressive loss of CD4+ T cells and AIDS in pig-tailed macaques. J Virol 1996; 70:3189–3197.
48. Lu Y, Brosio P, Lafaile M, et al. Vaginal transmission of chimeric simian/ human immunodeficiency viruses in rhesus macaques. J Virol 1996; 70: 3045–3050.
49. Lu YC, Pauza CD, Lu XS, Montefiori DC, Miller CJ. Rhesus macaques that become systemically infected with pathogenic SHIV89.6-PD after intravenous, rectal, or vaginal inoculation and fail to make an antiviral antibody response rapidly develop AIDS. J AIDS Hum Retrovirol 1998; 19: 6–18.
50. Steger KK, Dykhuizen M, Mitchen J, et al. CD4+ T cell and CD20+ B cell changes that predict rapid disease progression after SHIV89.6PD inoculation of rhesus macaques. J Virol 1998; 72:1600–1605.
51. Lu Y, Salvato MS, Pauza CD, et al. Utility of SHIV for testing HIV-1 vaccine candidates in macaques. J AIDS Hum Retrovirol 1996; 12:99–106.
52. Voss G, Li J, Manson K, Wyand M, Sodroski J, Letvin NL. Human immunodeficiency virus type 1 envelope glycoprotein-specific cytotoxic T lymphocytes in simian-human immunodefiency virus-infected rhesus monkeys. Virology 1995; 208:770–775.
53. Miller C, Alexander N, Sutjipto S, et al. Genital mucosal transmission of simian immunodeficiency virus: animal model for heterosexual transmission of human immunodeficiency virus. J Virol 1989; 63:4277–4284.
54. Baba TW, Trichel AM, An L, et al. Infection and AIDS in adult macaques after nontraumatic oral exposure to cell-free SIV. Science 1996; 272:1486–1489.
55. Trivedi P, Horejsh D, Hinds SB, et al. Intrarectal transmission of simian immunodeficiency virus in rhesus macaques: selective amplification and host responses to transient or persistent viremia. J Virol 1996; 70:6876–6883.
56. Trivedi P, Meyer KK, Streblow DN, Preuninger BL, Schultz KT, Pauza CD. Selective amplification of simian immunodeficiency virus genotypes after intrarectal inoculation of rhesus monkeys. J Virol 1994; 68:7649–7653.
57. Daniel MD, Kirchhoff F, Czajak SC, Sehgal PK, Desrosiers RC. Protective effects of a live attenuated SIV vaccine with a deletion in the nef gene. Science 1992; 258:1938–1941.
58. Zhu T, Wang N, Carr A, et al. Genetic characterization of human immunodeficiency virus type 1 in blood and genital secretions: evidence for viral compartmentalization and selection during sexual transmission. J Virol 1996; 70:3098–3107.
59. Zhu T, Mo H, Wang N, et al. Genotypic and phenotypic characterization of HIV-1 patients with primary infection. Science 1993; 261:1179–1181.

60. Baba TW, Liska V, Khimani AH, et al. Live, attenuated, multiply deleted simian immunodeficiency virus causes AIDS in infant and adult macaques. Nature Med 1999; 5:194–203.
61. Dykhuizen M, Mitchen J, Montefiori DC, et al. Determinants of disease in the SIV-infected rhesus macaque: characterizing animals with low antibody responses and rapid progression. J Gen Virol 1998; 79:2461–2467.
62. Nowak MA, Lloyd AL, Vasquez GM, et al. Viral dynamics of primary viremia and antiretroviral therapy in simian immunodeficiency virus infection. J Virol 1997; 71:7518–7525.
63. Watson A, Ranchalis J, Travis B, et al. Plasma viremia in macaques infected with simian immunodeficiency virus: plasma viral load early in infection predicts survival. J Virol 1997; 71:284–290.
64. Mellors JW, Kingsley LA, Rinaldo CR Jr., et al. Quantitation of HIV-1 RNA in plasma predicts outcome after seroconversion. Ann Intern Med 1995; 122:573–579.
65. Pauza CD, Trivedi P, Wallace M, et al. Vaccination with Tat toxoid attenuates disease in simian/human immunodeficiency virus-challenged macaques. Proc Natl Acad Sci USA 2000; 97:3515–3519.
66. Joag SV, Stephens EB, Adams RJ, Foresman L, Narayan O. Pathogenesis of SIVmac infection in Chinese and Indian rhesus macaques: effects of splenectomy on virus burden. Virology 1994; 200:436–446.
67. Wallace M, Waterman PM, Mitchen J, et al. Lymphocyte activation during acute SHIV89.6PD infection in macaques. J Virol 1999; 73:10236–10244.
68. Steger KK, Pauza CD. Immunization of Macaca mulatta with aroA-attenuated *Salmonella typhimurium* expressing SIV p27 antigen. J Med Primatol 1997; 26:44–50.
69. Steger KK, Valentine P, Heffron F, So M, Pauza CD. Recombinant, attenuated *Salmonella typhimurium* stimulate cell-mediated immune responses to SIV capsid antigen in rhesus macaques. Vaccine 1999; 17:923–932.
70. Pauza CD, Trivedi P, Wallace M, et al. Immunization with Tat toxoid attenuates SHIV89.6PD infection in rhesus macaques. In: Girard M, Dodet B, eds. Colloque des "Cent Gardes," 12th, Marnes-la-Coquette, Paris, France, 25–27 October 1999, Proceedings: Retroviruses of Human AIDS and Related Animal Diseases. Lyon: Foundation Marcel Merieux, 2000:83–86.
71. Cafaro A, Caputo C, Fracasso C, et al. Control of SHIV-89.6P-infection of cynomolgus monkeys by HIV-1 tat protein vaccine. Nat Med 1999; 5: 643–650.
72. McGraw TP, Vowels BR, Gardner MB, Ahmed-Ansari A, Gershwin ME. Simian immunodeficiency virus-specific T-cell-mediated proliferative response of infected rhesus macaques. AIDS 1990; 4:191–198.
73. Salvato MS, Emau P, Malkovsky M, Schultz KT, Johnson E, Pauza CD. Cellular immune responses in rhesus macaques infected rectally with low dose simian immunodeficiency virus. J Med Primatol 1994; 23:125–130.

74. Miller MD, Lord CI, Stallard V, Mazzara GP, Letvin NL. Gag-specific cytotoxic T lymphocytes in rhesus monkeys infected with the simian immunodeficiency virus of macaques. J Immunol 1990; 144:122.
75. Yamamoto H, Miller MD, Tsubota H, et al. Studies of cloned simian immunodeficiency virus-specific T lymphocytes: gag-specific cytotoxic T lymphocytes exhibit a restricted epitope specificity. J Immunol 1990; 144: 3385–3391.
76. Egan M, Kuroda M, Voss G, et al. Use of major histocompatibilty complex class I/peptide/b2M tetramers to quantitate CD8+ cytotoxic T lymphocytes specific for dominant and nondominant viral epitopes in simian-human immunodeficiency virus-infeted rhesus monkeys. J Virol 1999; 73:5466–5472.
77. Steger KK, Waterman PM, Pauza CD. Acute effects of pathogenic SHIV challenge on vaccine-induced cellular and humoral responses to Gag in rhesus macaques. J Virol 1999; 73:1853–1859.
78. Muro-Cacho CA, Pantaleo G, Fauci AS. Analysis of apoptosis in lymph nodes of HIV-infected persons: Intensity of apoptosis correlates with the general state of activation of the lymphoid tissue and not with stage of disease or viral burden. J Immunol 1995; 154:5555–5566.
79. Banda NK, Bernier J, Kurahara DK, et al. Crosslinking CD4 by human immunodeficiency virus gp120 primes T cells for activation-induced apoptosis. J Exp Med 1992; 176:1099–1106.
80. Salk J, Bretscher PA, Salk PL, Clerici M, Shearer GM. A strategy for prophylactic vaccination against HIV. Science 1993; 260:1270–1272.
81. Kestler H, Ringler D, Mori K, et al. Importance of the nef gene for maintainence of high virus loads and for development of AIDS. J Virol 1991; 65:651–662.
82. Katsikis PD, Garcia-Ojeda ME, Torres-Roca JF, Greenwald DR, Herzenberg LA. HIV type 1 Tat protein enhances activation-but not Fas (CD95)-induced peripheral blood T cell apoptosis in healthy individuals. Int Immunol 1997; 9:835–841.
83. Kruman, II, Nath A, Mattson MP. HIV-1 protein Tat induces apoptosis of hippocampal neurons by a mechanism involving caspase activation, calcium overload, and oxidative stress. Exp Neurol 1998; 154:276–288.
84. Li CJ, Friedman DJ, Wang C, Metelev V, Pardee AB. Induction of apoptosis in uninfected lymphocytes by HIV-1 Tat protein. Science 1995; 268:429–431.
85. Westendorp MO, Frank R, Ochsenbauer C, et al. Sensitization of T cells to CD95-mediated apoptosis by HIV-1 Tat and gp120. Nature 1995; 375: 497–500.
86. Gallo RC. Tat as one key to HIV-induced immune pathogenesis and Tat (correction of Pat) toxoid as an important component of a vaccine. Proc Natl Acad Sci USA 1999; 96:8324–8326.

87. Li CJ, Ueda Y, Shi B, et al. Tat protein induces self-perpetuating permissivity for productive HIV-1 infection. Proc Natl Acad Sci USA 1997; 94: 8116–8120.
88. Secchiero P, Zella D, Capitani S, Gallo R, Zauli G. Extracellular HIV-1 Tat protein up-regulates the expression of surface of CXC-chemokine receptor 4 in resting CD4 T cells. J Immunol 1999; 162:2427–2431.
89. Huang L, Bosch I, Hofmann W, Sodroski J, Pardee AB. Tat protein induces human immunodeficiency virus type 1 (HIV-1) coreceptors and promotes infection with both macrophage-tropic and T-lymphotropic HIV-1 strains. J Virol 1998; 72:8952–8960.
90. Frankel AD, Pabo CO. Cellular uptake of the tat protein from human immunodeficiency virus. Cell 1988; 55:1189–1193.
91. Gringeri A, Santagostino E, Muca-Perja M, et al. Safety and immunogenicity of HIV-1 Tat toxoid in immunocompromised HIV-1-infected patients. J Hum Virol 1998; 1:293–298.
92. Zagury JFea. Antibodies to the HIV-1 Tat protein correlated with nonprogression to AIDS: a rational for the use of Tat toxoid as an HIV-1 vaccine. J Hum Virol 1998; 1:282–292.
93. Le Buanec H, Lachgar A, Bizzini B, et al. A prophylactic and therapeutic AIDS vaccine containing as a component the innocuous Tat toxoid. Biomed Pharmacother 1998; 52:431–435.
94. Gringeri A, Santagostino E, Muca-Perja M, et al. Tat toxoid as a component of a preventive vaccine in seronegative subjects. J AIDS 1999; 20:371–375.
95. Kestler HWd, Naidu YN, Kodama T, et al. Use of infectious molecular clones of simian immunodeficiency virus for pathogenesis studies. J Med Primatol 1989; 18:305–309.
96. Kestler H, Kodama T, Ringler D, et al. Induction of AIDS in rhesus monkeys by molecularly cloned simian immunodeficiency virus. Science 1990; 248:1109–1112.
97. Dewhurst S, Embretson J, Anderson D, Mullins J, Fultz P. Sequence analysis and acute pathogenicity of molecularly cloned $SIV_{SMM\text{-}PBj14}$. Nature 1990; 345:636–640.

12

International Perspectives on HIV Vaccine Development

Seth Berkley
The International AIDS Vaccine Initiative
New York, New York

INTRODUCTION

Despite almost 20 years of global effort to control the HIV epidemic, the virus continues to spread. More than 60 million people have been infected; more than 15,000 new infections occur daily. Although the epidemic was initially recognized in industrialized countries, it is spreading most rapidly in the developing world. Today more than 95% of new infections occur in less developed countries (LDCs); the epidemic is growing fastest in sub-Saharan Africa, South Asia, and the former socialist republics. Many of these countries are doubly cursed by inadequate resources: they can neither effectively implement prevention programs across populations at risk nor cope with the financial burden of treatment and of the epidemic's social consequences.

As the rest of this book has described, there is great promise in the field of HIV vaccinology. But significant scientific challenges remain. If these challenges are to be overcome, a substantial effort will be required. Until recently, however, HIV vaccine research and development (R&D) received relatively low priority compared with other areas of HIV research, particularly therapeutics R&D. The creation of candidate vaccines specifically targeted towards developing countries has been virtually nonexistent. A vaccine is an international public good. Its effects will go well beyond those who invest in the vaccine, or even those who take it. New efforts to accelerate vaccine development—particularly those targeted at the parts of the world where it is needed most—are urgently necessary. Furthermore, full involvement of developing country scientists—as full partners in the effort—will help to minimize problems in creating and using these products.

Since 95% of new infections occur in the developing world, it is critical that any successful HIV vaccine products be appropriate for use in those environments. Given the magnitude and global nature of the HIV pandemic, it is appropriate that we use all of the expertise—in science, manufacturing, testing, and distribution—the world has to offer in accelerating the effort. But all of the effort will be for naught if the resulting products are not made available where they are needed most. The current paradigm of vaccine development is not encouraging. Public sector research institutions generally conduct basic research on topics related to vaccines, leaving industry to do the actual vaccine development. Currently, for-profit vaccine manufacturers develop vaccines for the industrialized world market and sell it at a high profit margin during the initial period, while they are the sole supplier, to rapidly recoup R&D costs. Vaccines only trickle down to developing countries 10–15 years later, when prices drop as patents expire and competition enters the marketplace. Such a paradigm should be unacceptable for any vaccine but is especially alarming for a vaccine against HIV. A new strategy is necessary to assure that any vaccine be made available simultaneously in both developed and developing countries and to all those who need it.

THE ROLE OF HIV VACCINATION

Vaccines are the traditional way to control viral infections. Through vaccination the world has been able to control polio, eradicate smallpox, and, more recently, begin to dramatically reduce measles. Historically, vaccination is one of the most cost effective interventions to control disease. For example, it is estimated that for every dollar invested in immunization in the United States, between $2 and $29 in medical costs are saved (1). With new vaccines, however, costs are higher, and it is not clear that they will always be cost effective. For example, the new conjugated vaccine against the *Pneumococcus* bacteria is priced at $232 for a four-dose series, more expensive then all other childhood immunizations combined. The calculated cost-effectiveness is $80,000 per life saved. This cost is so high that it became the first vaccine in U.S. history that fails to produce a clearly acceptable cost savings to society. As a result, the U.S. government advisory panel voted to consider its use only in those 24–59 months old, with priority for higher-risk black and Native American children (2,14). In developing countries, interventions are usually considered cost effective if they cost less than $100 per disability adjusted life-year (DALY) saved (3). Calculations for the current EPI vaccines are very favorable; less than $10 per DALY gained for measles immunization and less than $25 for a combination of polio plus DPT (3). Thus, cost-effectiveness criteria is a value easy for the traditional vaccines to meet but perhaps more difficult for novel and more complicated vaccines. However, given the enormous cost of HIV in the developing world and the lack of cost-effective therapeutic options, it is likely that all but the most expensive and complicated HIV vaccines are likely to be cost-effective.

Moreover, new vaccines targeted primarily at developing countries may not be developed because private companies are unable to foresee a good return on their investment. For example, no vaccine has been successfully developed to control an endemic infection in developing countries since the development of yellow fever vaccine by the Rockefeller Foundation more than 50 years ago. All of the new currently available vaccines were developed for industrialized countries and have been priced as described above. It is often 15–25 years after introduction before the product reaches maturity and is made widely available in developing countries. For example, even though the burden of hepatitis cases and resultant liver cancer (1 million deaths annually) is enormous in developing countries and an effective hepatitis B vaccine has been available for 19 years, it is still not widely used in most of the world's immunization programs. This is despite an almost 40-fold reduction from its initial offering price to $1.50, which is still, however, about 1½ times the cost of a full course of all of the currently used childhood immunizations (BCG, OPV, DPT, measles) in developing countries. Another example is the *Haemophilus influenzae* type b vaccine. Although it has virtually eliminated this infection as a major cause of ill health in children in industrialized countries, this vaccine has not been put routinely into immunization programs in developing countries. Lest one think that this is only seen in the fairly limited vaccine market, this similar challenge of huge need and market failure applies to drugs: of 1223 drugs developed between 1975 and 1997, only 13 were for tropical conditions. Even of these, only four were the result of efforts by pharmaceutical companies to create human products. The other nine came from military or veterinary efforts.

Given the complexity and cost of HIV vaccine development and the capital costs of vaccine plant production, it is likely any HIV vaccine will initially be priced quite high unless there is a significant public sector intervention. This intervention—to resolve pricing and availability issues—must be done well before the vaccine is finalized, produced, and released.

TECHNICAL CHARACTERISTICS OF A GLOBAL VACCINE

An ideal preventive HIV vaccine intended for global use would have all the technical characteristics listed in Table 1. It is unlikely that the first successful vaccine will have all these characteristics. However, some of these factors are more critical in developing countries (such as simplicity in delivery, temperature stability, and cost) than they would be in industrialized countries. In fact, a low-cost, single-dose vaccine may be more useful in some settings even if it is of slightly lower efficacy than a comparable vaccine that is costly and requires many inoculations.

Although complete safety is the ideal, the tolerable risk-to-benefit ratio varies by population. In some populations, particularly those without access to other interventions, the very high risk of infection may justify use of a vaccine that has side effects that would make it unattractive in lower HIV risk situations. One example of this changing risk/benefit ratio is oral polio vaccine (OPV), the standard vaccine for more than two decades in the United States. Now, with the recent elimination of naturally occurring polio, the small but consistent risk of vaccine-induced paralysis has led the United States to recommend switching to enhanced inactivated polio vaccine for the first two doses. OPV, however, remains the standard in most other populations of the world, where the threat of contracting polio still vastly outweighs the risk associated with vaccination. This example demonstrates why local decision making about the acceptable risk asso-

Table 1 Ideal Characterisitics of an HIV Vaccine

Protection: Able to stimulate the production of durable, functional protective immune responses against most, if not all, subtypes of HIV to which an individual is likely to be exposed and from all potential routes of exposure.

Safety: Safe in both the short and long term. The vaccine should also be safe to deliver without prior screening for HIV infection (i.e., the vaccine should not induce any adverse reactions when given to HIV-infected individuals).

Delivery: Provide long-lasting protection with a minimum number of doses (preferably one), have a long shelf life, be heat stable, and be simple to administer (preferably oral).

Unambiguous marker for seroconversion: Provide health care professionals with a marker that enables seroconversion due to vaccination and seroconversion due to infection to be distinguished rapidly, easily, and inexpensively.

Cost: Final price of the vaccine should be such that it will be affordable for wide-scale distribution to all at risk of infection throughout the world.

Manufacturing: Vaccine should be able to be manufactured in large volume, packaged simply, and ideally able to be transferred to selected developing country sites or manufactured locally.

ciated with bringing specific vaccines to trial will be critical. Until recently, however, this has not been the norm (see the ethical discussion below).

THE CURRENT ENVIRONMENT FOR VACCINE DEVELOPMENT AND PRODUCTION

Although much of the basic science underlying vaccine development comes from national research agencies of industrialized countries, commercial industry conducts most of the world's new vaccine product research and development.

It is important to note that the world's vaccine market is rather small (approximately \$3 billion) as compared to the global sales of medical drugs (\$300 billion) (4,5). Unlike most drugs, however, vaccines are an essential part of public health programs, and at least some are recommended as public policy by virtually all countries. There are over 170 vaccine producers, the vast majority of which are under the direct control of governments and produce one or more of the basic six Expanded Programme on Immunization (EPI) vaccines. Bulk purchase and sales to multinational organizations account for more than 60% of the world's commercially produced doses but a very small percentage of the profit. For example, purchases by UNICEF account for approximately 23% of the volume of vaccines sold globally, but because of the low public sector price and profit margin, they account for only 6% of the global revenues (6). However, because vaccine manufacturing is a fixed-cost businss (approximately 85% of the costs are fixed), the marginal cost of vaccine production for this large number of doses is quite small. With large-scale production, efficiency usually also increases and therefore when the costs are spread over a larger number of doses, profits per dose for the primary (and most profitable) market also increase. This can occur because price "tiering" (vaccines offered at different prices in different markets) for the EPI vaccines has been quite steep. The vaccine pricing spans a very broad range with an average price differential of 70 times between the poorest and wealthiest markets (7). As a result, overall only 14% of the total vaccine dosage volume is sold in standard commercial markets, but this small percentage accounts for 75–80% of the market value (8). Currently, six leading companies control about 70% of the commercial market, and most of their profit is generated by a few new vaccines (priced substantially higher than older ones) sold in the OECD countries as described above. These large multinational companies are the largest investors in research and development and in production facilities and would logically be the organizations to invest heavily in HIV vaccine development.

There are barriers to their involvement, however. Vaccine development is expensive and is becoming moreso. On average it takes 10–12 years to develop a new product and bring it to market. Development costs are reported to be in excess of \$250 million, although this includes the losses of abandoned and unsuccessful products, opportunity costs, and industrial and marketing overhead and does not include tax credits. A more realistic sum may be around $57 million as an average R&D cost after taxes, which still accounts for the cost of unsuccessful projects (8). Furthermore, vaccine development is commercially very risky: only about 22% of vaccines that leave the pre-clinical stage end up entering the market (9).

Over the past few decades, the vaccine industry has consolidated and vaccine companies have become subsidiaries of the broader pharmaceutical industry. This pharmaceutical industry is highly profitable. For example, in 1996, the average profit margin of the 10 largest drug firms was 30% (5). As a result of the way these new companies are structured, the vaccine components are often held to this standard. This is particularly challenging: the life of a patent is only 20 years, and experience has shown that it often takes more than a decade just to recoup the R&D costs for a new vaccine.

THE NEED FOR PUBLIC–PRIVATE COLLABORATION

Industrial investment in HIV vaccines R&D is seen as particularly high risk and specific investment in HIV vaccines for developing countries commercially non-justifiable. There are several reasons for this:

1. The science is difficult and there are controversies within the scientific community as to what approaches might work.
2. The HIV activist community, in its attempts to be heard, has created discomfort within some leaders of industry.
3. Infection with HIV is still stigmatized.
4. The market for an HIV vaccine is largest in some of the poorest developing countries.
5. There are inherent opportunity costs for working in this area.

As a result, what started out as a broad-based effort by the pharmaceutical industry in the mid-1980s has contracted considerably. As a recent industry publication noted, "the pharmaceutical industry has virtually turned its back on HIV-vaccine research, leaving the biotechnology industry as the gate-keepers of hope for a preventive vaccine, yet the number of biotechnology companies in the field is small and getting smaller" (10).

Given that an HIV vaccine is an international public good, there is a critical global need to assure it is made as soon as possible. The commercial sector will not do this because there is a "market failure." It is, therefore, the responsibility of the public sector to step in. To get industry to invest heavily in HIV vaccine development, either research costs must be supplemented and/or the vaccine market will need to be made more attractive. If specific vaccines for developing countries are needed, given the low price that the market will bear, the barriers will be even higher. If vaccines that will serve *only* those living in the poorest developing countries are needed, then a new mechanism will be required.

IAVI AS A MODEL

The International AIDS Vaccine Initiative (IAVI) was established in 1996, when the global effort to create and AIDS vaccine reached its nadir. Its mission is to ensure the development of safe, effective, accessible, preventive HIV vaccines for use throughout the world. IAVI works as a global scientific organization using public-private partnerships to implement its activities. In many ways it operates like a virtual vaccine company. It has four strategies that are still relevant today as approaches for accelerating the effort.

GLOBAL DEMAND

A critical first need was to create demand—from all sectors—for HIV vaccines. Because the AIDS activist community was made up mostly of HIV-infected persons, its primary concern was treatment. The voice advocating for AIDS vaccines within that community was limited. More interesting was the lack of interest from either the public health community or developing country leadership. Successful vaccine research, development, and deployment will require the participation of scientists, industrial vaccine developers, community groups, educators, funders, journalists, ethicists, policy makers, etc. As a result, broad-based education and involvement of these communities in developed and developing countries are necessary. In fact, lessons from the Thailand and Ugandan trials suggest that, despite the best intentions of scientists, public concerns and questions will be raised once the decision has been made to proceed with trials. Excellent communication efforts are critical to minimize misunderstanding.

Fortunately, after years of hard work, increasing attention is being paid to HIV vaccines. There is now a growing chorus of leaders who understand the importance of AIDS vaccine development. A group of eight leaders of the largest economies (G-8) have referred to the need for an AIDS vaccine in their last three annual sessions; President Clinton (United States) and Prime Minister Vajpayee (India) declared it a national goal; and President Mandela (South Africa) and Prime Minister Blair (United Kingdom) also spoke publicly about the need. There has been a flurry of interest in AIDS vaccines from the press, with articles on the importance and the state of the effort in papers around the world. Finally, scientists have begun to take this critical need more seriously—at the 2000 International AIDS Conference in Durban, there were approximately 10 times as many sessions on HIV vaccines as were held at the previous international conference 2 years earlier.

Creating constituencies for an HIV vaccine will be critical to this effort. Although it is important to keep the "HIV community" up to date and involved, they are not the only constituency necessary. Potential additional advocates for HIV vaccines include mothers, the development community, health advocates, children's advocates, etc. We must create an environment in which attention to the tough issues of garnering resources for vaccine development, overcoming ethical challenges, and planning for eventual delivery will be taken seriously.

APPLIED SCIENCE

A strong foundation of basic science is critical in moving vaccines forward. After almost two decades of HIV research, there have been many useful discoveries that may contribute to vaccine R&D. However, without perfect animal models or known correlates of protection, we cannot avoid testing vaccines in humans in order to determine efficacy. Complicating the science is the variability of the virus. Although the immunotypes of HIV are not yet known (we have not yet determined what immune response is necessary for protection), we do know that the virus undergoes enormous genetic variation. Current circulating strains have been divided into many subgroups, or clades, based on the genetic makeup of their envelopes. Although the significance of these subgroups remains unknown, a recent scientific review of the data suggested that until there is more data on the practical importance of genetic variation, the vaccine strain should be as closely matched to the local circulating strain as practically possible (UNAIDS Advisory Committee Meeting, April 2000).

Despite the global need, the pipeline for AIDS vaccines has been woefully inadequate. Although there have been more than 25 candidate vaccines tested in humans for safety and immunogenicity, these represent only a few different vaccine approaches, and most are made from the strains of the virus circulating in developed countries. Almost 17 years into the vaccine effort, only one product has entered efficacy testing, and a second new one is in phase II testing. Table 2 lists all of the vaccines that have been tested in developing countries since the beginning of the epidemic. Clearly more products, a range of different approaches, made from different strains and tested in different locations, is necessary if we are to find a viable vaccine in the foreseeable future. Using the best science available to create a vaccine candidate, testing that candidate, and then using the results from the study to improve the candidate, has been the time-tested process for vaccine development.

However, the process of vaccine development is very different from that of academic research. Product development is an applied science that requires a team of people with skills in design, manufacturing, project management, process engineering, regulatory and clinical trial expertise, etc. Critical to this process is industrial product management expertise, which assures an efficient, milestone-driven product development effort. Although these skills are fully present in most large companies, small companies and academic institutions may be lacking in

Table 2 Candidate HIV Vaccines Evaluated in Developing Countries

Product	Strain	Company	Trial site	Begun	Status
Phases 1–2					
V3-MAPS	B	UBI	China	1994	Completed; inactive
V3-MAPS	B	UBI	Thailand	1994	Completed; inactive
V3-MAPS	B	UBI	Brazil	1994	Completed; inactive
rgp120	B	Chiron	Thailand	1995	Completed; in bivalent B+E
rgp120	B	VaxGen	Thailand	1995	Completed; in bivalent B+E
V3 peptides	Multi B	CIGB	Cuba	1996	Ongoing w/new adjuvant
rgp120	B+E	VaxGen	Thailand	1998	Completed; expanded to phase 3
Canarypox	B	PMC	Uganda	1998	Recently completed
rgp120	E	Chiron	Thailand	1998	Ongoing
rgp120	B+E	Chiron	Thailand	1998	Ongoing
Canarypox	B	PMC	Thailand	1999	Ongoing
Canarypox	E	PMC	Thailand	2000	Ongoing
rgp140	E	PMC	Thailand	2000	Ongoing
DNA multiepitope	A	Oxford/IAVI	Kenya	2000	Completed
MVA multiepitope	A	Oxford/IAVI	Kenya	2002	To start
Canarypox	A env	PMC	Uganda	2002	Planned
Phase 3					
rgp120	B+E	VaxGen	Thailand	1999	Ongoing

some or all of this expertise. As a result, IAVI has created a cadre of staff and consultants who can work with companies and academic institutions to move candidates forward rapidly and assist in the broad range of development activities.

IAVI believes that it is critical to involve all partners at the beginning of the project. Its model is vaccine development partnerships, which bring together a working team of vaccine designers, manufacturers and developing country clinical trial expertise to be responsible for design, manufacturer and testing of the vaccine in as rapid a time period as possible. Vaccines are constructed from viral isolates circulating in the area in which the vaccine will be tested. To date, IAVI has launched four partnerships based on live viral vectors: a DNA/modified vaccinia Ankara approach made from clade A, which will be tested in the United Kingdom and Kenya; a clade C–based Venezuelan equine encephalitis replicon, which will be tested in South Africa and the United States; and a adeno-associated virus vectored approach made from Clades A&D, which will also be tested in East Africa; and an attenuated *Salmonella* vector, which can be taken orally and which is being made from clade A and will be tested in East Africa. All show excellent immunogenicity in various animal models, and most promise in the macaque SIV challenge model. Critical to the success of this vaccine development program will be minimizing the time it takes for these vaccines to arrive in the clinic. Through active project management, each of these is expected to go from research bench to clinical testing in 18–24 months.

To assure that the results of these partnerships would be made available if they were successful, IAVI developed the concept of ''social venture capitalism.'' If a traditional venture capitalist invested in a small biotechnology company, he would accumulate substantial equity as a result of that investment. IAVI permits the company to keep its equity and intellectual property (IP). In return for IAVI's investment, the company must commit that, if the vaccine is successful, it must make it available at cost plus a reasonable profit (defined) for the public sector of the developing world. If it does not, IAVI has the rights to transfer the IP to another manufacturer. The company can price its product at whatever the market will bear in their other (public and private industrialized as well as private developing country) markets. Through such an arrangement, IAVI uses the tools and incentives of the private capital markets combined with public investment to maximally accelerate vaccine development. IAVI also works with these companies to maximize their success, assisting them with searches for staff talent, with the regulatory process, with process engineering issues, with clinical trials, with contract manufacturing, project management, and in engaging the assistance of other companies if appropriate.

In certain large countries or those with substantial scientific and manufacturing capabilities, IAVI has worked with local governments and institutions to create national vaccine programs. Their purpose is to create comprehensive programs to cover all aspects of preventive HIV vaccine development, from creating demand, through applied science, to creating an enabling environment for industrial production if appropriate. As a result of these interventions, there are now growing national programs in China, India, and South Africa. In each, vaccine programs are moving forward with substantial political leadership.

To assure global distribution and appropriate tiered pricing, there may be a key role for vaccine manufacturing in selected developing countries. If this is to occur, it will be important to assure that there are appropriate national control authorities in place and that the facility has established the requisite scientific and quality-control procedures. Although there are a few hundred developing country vaccine manufacturers, most produce only one or two of the EPI vaccines and many are not of adequate quality. There is also no assurance that production of vaccines in developing countries will be cheaper than production in a large-scale facility in a large vaccine company in the industrialized world. It is important, however, to prepare for both scenarios. IAVI visited to numerous facilities in developing countries and is doing Good Manufacturing Practice (GMP) audits before considering technology transfers. IAVI is working closely with the WHO to assure vaccine quality globally.

ENABLING ENVIRONMENT

Where market failures prevent development of a vital public good, public policies must be adopted to correct or diminish these market disincentives. Given the necessary role that industry plays in HIV vaccine development and taking into account the enormous direct and opportunity costs for them to be involved, it is critical to provide appropriate incentives to overcome the serious barriers to their entry. These can be done through a combination of push-and-pull initiatives to encourage greater industrial participation (Table 3). Furthermore, because the current low level of private industry involvement in the HIV vaccine field stems from multiple market disincentives, encouraging greater private sector participation will require pursuit of multiple public policy approaches. Public policies must differentiate between the smaller biotech companies that are vital to early HIV vaccine R&D and the larger private entities that will be required to support production scale-up and ultimate marketing and distribution. For small, minimally capitalized biotechnology companies, the most important need is current finance to move forward their intellectual property. Furthermore, smaller biotechnology companies may not have the substantial tax liabilities that will allow them to benefit from tax credits—unless they are permitted to pass the credits on to their investors. Larger companies that are substantially capitalized need incentives that will shift internal decision-making towards using scarce human, infrastructure, and capital resources on HIV vaccine development—particularly for developing countries. In this case, ensuring adequate markets, distribution systems, regulatory simplicity, mechanisms to minimize the risk of legal liability, etc. may be as important, or even more important, than financing up-front R&D.

Another important area for action is to simplify the morass of country-by-country rules governing approval and licensure of vaccines, which discourages investment in vaccines for developing countries. International mechanisms to harmonize and expedite procedures for licensure and approval, such as the Euro-

Table 3 Public Policy Mechanisms to Encourage AIDS Vaccine Research

Push mechanisms to lower costs and risk of R&D or remove barriers	Pull mechanisms to provide incentives for industrial investment
Fund basic research	Create a market in developing countries (vaccine purchase funds)
Fund applied R&D	Tax credits for sales
Tax credits for R&D	Political support for tiered pricing
Assistance with phase III trials	Purchase and use of existing underutilized vaccines
Regulatory harmonization	Legislate product liability reform

pean Commission are attempting, may be very important in assuring rapid dissemination of new vaccine technologies. In devising policies to encourage vaccine development, it is critical that policymakers remind themselves that the ultimate goal is not merely to develop a vaccine, but to ensure that it is actually used by people in developing countries. Attention to distribution issues on the front end is critical; distribution costs for currently available vaccines represent over 90% of their cost, as discussed above.

Particularly attractive is the growing movement by industrialized nations and multilateral institutions to work together to guarantee a market for HIV vaccines prospectively (before the vaccine is developed and licensed). One mechanism under active consideration by the World Bank and others is the development of a global fund for the purchase of HIV vaccines for developing countries. Although no HIV vaccine is currently available to be purchased, funds should be obligated in advance—through contingent pledges or yearly contributions by OECD countries—in order to convince private companies to make the investments required to support expensive clinical testing, production scale-up, and preparations for marketing and distribution (13).

Another important mechanism for assuring accessibility is to attempt to tier the pricing. Companies should be allowed to charge higher prices for HIV vaccines in industrialized countries than in developing countries, where annual per capita health expenditures are sometimes less than $10. As with the vaccine purchase fund concept, tiered pricing will allow OECD countries to cross-subsidize vaccine purchases in developing countries. One way to approach this is to amortize R&D and other development expenses in the OECD market, which is where they normally would amortize the costs anyway (as the developing country markets would not be initially served). This would allow sales in poor countries to take place at the marginal cost of production plus a reasonable profit.

Finally, as a strategy for building confidence in the world's commitment to ensure a market for HIV vaccines in developing countries, international efforts should be made to stimulate the market in such countries for existing non-HIV vaccines. As mentioned above, a number of cost-effective vaccines are licensed and being used in developed countries that are not being used in developing countries. This leaves industry with the conviction that the public sector may not be able to deliver on its promises to make cost effective newer vaccines available. The newly created Global Alliance for Vaccines and Immunization (GAVI) is working with all of its partners to solve this problem. Initiatives would include improving vaccine distribution infrastructure in developing countries and increasing funding for international vaccine purchase mechanisms.

ACCESSIBILITY

A number of characteristics of HIV—and of a preventive vaccine against it—will make accessibility particularly challenging (Table 4). However, it should be

Table 4 Special Access Issues for an HIV/AIDS Vaccine

Initially, the vaccine will need to be delivered to high risk groups:
Migrants, commercial sex workers, intravenous drug users
Adolescents, both attending and not attending schools
Vaccine will need to be given along with other prevention methods, including barrier methods, behavior change education, testing and counseling, etc.
Those seeking vaccine may be stigmatized because of their self-identified risk behavior
Depending on the vaccine, those immunized may test falsely positive on HIV screening tests, which may lead to stigmatization
Vaccine may be considered controversial and be opposed by those who are prejudiced against those at risk
The international public good aspect of an HIV vaccine may mean that the public health authorities may want persons to be vaccinated even if not personally perceived to be at highest risk.

noted that all vaccines have important access and distribution issues in developing countries. Historically, from 1974 to 1990 a global effort was able to increase worldwide immunization of children from 5% to close to 80%. This effort, driven by a global coalition of United Nations, governmental, and private agencies, can be counted as one of the last century's greatest accomplishments. To do this, not only was it critical to have adequate supplies of heat-stable, inexpensive vaccines, but also to create a quality-controlled chain of management and delivery systems. As described above, these systems currently account for more than 90% of the cost of delivering these vaccines and are complicated to establish and maintain. For example, it has been calculated that if one could reduce the current five contacts to fully immunize children in the EPI program to one encounter, the costs of the program could be reduced by as much as 70% (3). Given that the HIV vaccine is unlikely to be as inexpensive as these older vaccines and that a delivery system does not exist, it is likely that accessibility will be one of the formidable challenges to success using an HIV vaccine.

Although an ideal vaccine should be one that is given orally, once, at birth, and provides lifetime protection, this ideal is unlikely to be met in the first or second generation of vaccines. Even if we were successful in initially creating such a vaccine, to have any vaccine impact the epidemic today, it would need to be delivered to those currently at high risk of infection—such as commercial sex workers, migrants, soldiers, drug users, and adolescents. There are no specific mechanisms in place to reach any of these groups in developing countries. Furthermore, simple mechanisms such as school delivery are unlikely to cover the highest risk persons in that cohort; those out of school in most developing countries are at higher risk than those attending school. Other challenges include the possibility that those seeking vaccination will be stigmatized for declaring themselves at risk (drug users, commercial sex workers, men who have sex with men) or that those immunized will test false positive on simple screening assays for HIV. Finally, even if a vaccine was 100% effective, unlike other vaccines, the delivery of an HIV vaccine will require simultaneous provision of other preventive strategies,—including counseling and testing, behavior change education, the provision of barrier methods to prevent other reproductive tract infections or unwanted pregnancies, etc.

For some vaccines, such as tetanus, the effect on the disease is only at the level of the individual (or a mother plus her unborn infant). In this case, provision of a vaccine has no effect on the overall ecology of the disease. For other infections which are transmissible and for which humans serve as the reservoir, immunization of members of the population results in a "herd immunity," which ultimately reduces the risk of infection for others even if they are not immunized. HIV is likely to fall into the latter category and as a result may be indicated as a mandatory vaccine in high-risk areas as a public health measure. This, however, may clash with those who stigmatize HIV or who believe that a preventive vaccine will lead to irresponsible sexual behavior. Telling examples include recent attempts to stop routine use of hepatitis B vaccine for infants by some groups in the United States because they believe that vaccination encourages children to use intravenous drugs or pursue a "homosexual lifestyle."

ETHICAL ISSUES

The overarching ethical question regarding HIV vaccines is why there has not been more of a global effort to create one given the catastrophic nature of the pandemic? That being said, there are specific ethical challenges to be addressed. All vaccine testing requires the establishment of local ethical review bodies as well as an educating of the local population so that they can be good consumers of the information provided. From this author's perspective, ethical principles are global; however, acceptable risk-benefit ratios change based on the local severity of the epidemic and on the availability of other interventions. As a result, it is critical to empower local decision on the testing of vaccines.

Historical abuses of developing country subjects in biomedical research have led to codes of ethics that are—perhaps—too paternalistic. For example, the International Ethical Guidelines for Biomedical Research Involving Human Subjects published by the Council for International Organizations of Medical Science (CIOMS) stated that "phase I and II vaccine studies should be conducted only in developed communities of the country of the sponsor" (11). This meant that industrialized country (where most of the vaccine R&D is undertaken) policymakers and ethicists were able to control access of other countries to potential benefits of science. For example, if a vaccine was developed by scientists in an industrialized country and there was no interest in testing that vaccine locally (because it is made from developing country strains, the IP position is not adequate to justify significant investment or the risk-benefit ratio is too high for local use), it could not, under these guidelines, be made available to scientists in developing countries for testing. These guidelines, however, are seen by developing countries to be ''paternalistic or imperialistic and to pre-empt the sovereign rights of developing countries to make decisions that profoundly affect the health of their people''(12).

UNAIDS recently released ethical guidelines that put forward a set of recommendations for the clinical testing of HIV vaccines, which takes into account the needs and rights of developing countries (www.UNAIDS.org). Unfortunately, these remain controversial.

Better access to ethics training for developing country scientists and policymakers would help. Although many developing countries have rich traditions of ethical dialogue on their terms, academic ethicists in the west often do not take these spokespersons seriously. Providing them with dual training to articulate local values as well as assist the Western ethicists in understanding local decision making would be a useful addition to the cause. The role of UNAIDS in bridging the local and global ethical debates cannot be overestimated. Having a neutral globally mandated agency that can reassure the global community that local decision making has done ''due diligence'' is critical if we are to empower countries to share technology and move forward as rapidly as possible.

FUTURE STRATEGIES AND SUMMARY

Although HIV has become a truly global pandemic, developing countries are now bearing the full brunt of the crisis. A vaccine represents our best hope to end it. However, vaccine development efforts have been a poor stepchild to other research efforts, particularly those vaccines directed at developing countries. Many of the issues related to vaccine development may be different for developing countries and therefore demand attention. Furthermore, creating a policy environment that will assure that when appropriate products are developed, they will be produced and distributed, is not a simple challenge. It must be addressed now. If we do, we cannot only speed the development of an AIDS vaccine but also maximize its impact on the global epidemic. In no previous vaccine development effort was a vaccine delivered simultaneously in the north and south—with HIV we have the opportunity to create a new paradigm that will make it possible to end this scourge and the ones that follow it.

REFERENCES

1. Bloom BR, Widdus R. Vaccine visions and their global impact. Nat Med 1998; 4:480–484.
2. Lieu TA. Projected cost-effectiveness of pneumococcal vaccination of healthy infants and young children. JAMA 2000; 283:1460–1468.

3. World Bank. World Development Report 1993: Investing in Health. New York: Oxford University Press, 1993.
4. Report on the United States Vaccine Industry. New York: Report to the U.S. Department of Health and Human Services by Mercer Management Consulting, 1995.
5. The pharmaceutical industry: the alchemists. The Economist Insert, Feb 21, 1998.
6. A commercial perspective of vaccine supply. New York: Report to UNICEF by Mercer Management Consulting, 1994.
7. Batson A. Win-win interactions between the public and private sectors. Nat Med Vaccine Suppl 1998; 4: 487–491.
8. Gregersen J-P. Vaccine development: the long road from initial idea to product licensure. In: Levine MM, Woodrow, GC, Kaper JB, eds. New Generation Vaccines. 2d ed. New York: Marcel Dekker, 1997:1165–1177.
9. Struck MM. Vaccine R&D success rates and development times. Nat Biotechnol 1996; 14:591–593.
10. Glaser V. Number of biotechnology companies pursuing HIV vaccines begins to dwindle. Genetic Eng News Jan. 1, 1997, pp 14, 44.
11. The International Ethical Guidelines for Biomedical Research Involving Human Subjects. Geneva: CIOMS, 1993.
12. Bloom BR. The highest attainable standard: ethical issues in AIDS vaccines. Science 1998; 279:186–188.
13. Barton JH. Financing of vaccines. Lancet 2000; 355:1269–1270.
14. Preventing pneumococcal disease among infants and young children: recommendations of the Advisory Committee on Immunization Practices (ACIP). MMWR 2000; 49(RR-9):1–35.

Index

About the Editors

Flossie Wong-Staal is Florence Riford Chair in AIDS Research and Professor of Biology and Medicine, University of California, San Diego. A world-renowned authority in molecular virology and recognized internationally as a pioneer in AIDS research for cloning, sequencing, and characterizing novel pathogenic human retroviruses, including HIV, Dr. Wong-Staal serves on the editorial board of numerous journals and many national and international scientific committees and advisory panels. She received the B.A. degree (1968) in bacteriology and the Ph.D. degree (1972) in molecular biology from the University of California, Los Angeles.

Robert C. Gallo is Director of the Institute of Human Virology and Professor of Medicine, Microbiology, and Immunology, University of Maryland, Baltimore. Universally recognized for his achievements in pioneering the field of human retrovirology, he has lectured worldwide and is the author of more than 1000 scientific publications. A member of numerous professional and honorary societies, he is the recipient of numerous awards and received the B.A. degree (1959) in biology from Providence College, Rhode Island, and the M.D. degree (1963) from Jefferson Medical College, Philadelphia, Pennsylvania.

ISBN 0-8247-0645-5

90000

9 780824 706456